New PET Radiotracers

Guest Editor

ROBERT H. MACH, PhD

PET CLINICS

www.pet.theclinics.com

Consulting Editor
ABASS ALAVI, MD,
MD (Hon), PhD (Hon), DSc (Hon)

January 2009 • Volume 4 • Number 1

SAUNDERS an imprint of ELSEVIER, Inc.

W.B. SAUNDERS COMPANY
A Division of Elsevier Inc.

1600 John F. Kennedy Boulevard • Suite 1800 • Philadelphia, Pennsylvania 19103-2899

http://www.theclinics.com

PET CLINICS Volume 4, Number 1
January 2009 ISSN 1556-8598, ISBN 10: 1-4377-0524-3, ISBN-13: 978-1-4377-0524-9

Editor: Barton Dudlick
Developmental Editor: Theresa Collier

PET Clinics (ISSN 1556-8598) is published quarterly by Elsevier Inc., 360 Park Avenue South, New York, NY 10010-1710. Months of issue are January, April, July, and October. Periodicals postage paid at New York, NY, and additional mailing offices. Subscription prices per year are $196.00 (US individuals), $274.00 (US institutions), $97.00 (US students), $223.00 (Canadian individuals), $306.00 (Canadian institutions), $118.00 (Canadian students), $237.00 (foreign individuals), $306.00 (foreign institutions), and $118.00 (foreign students). To receive student and resident rate, orders must be accompanied by name of affiliated institution, date of term, and the signature of program/residency coordinator on institution letterhead. Orders will be billed at individual rate until proof of status is received. Foreign air speed delivery is included in all Clinics subscription prices. All prices are subject to change without notice. POSTMASTER: Send address changes to PET Clinics, Elsevier Health Sciences Division, Subscription Customer Service, 3251 Riverport Lane, Maryland Heights, MO 63043. **Customer service: 1-800-654-2452 (US and Canada). From outside of the US and Canada, call 314-447-8871. Fax: 314-417-8029. E-mail: JournalsCustomerService-usa@elsevier.com (for print support); JournalsOnlineSupport-usa@elsevier.com (for online support).**

Reprints. For copies of 100 or more of articles in this publication, please contact the Commercial Reprints Department, Elsevier Inc., 360 Park Avenue South, New York, NY 10010-1710. Tel.: 212-633-3812; Fax: 212-462-1935; E-mail: reprints@elsevier.com.

Contributors

CONSULTING EDITOR

ABASS ALAVI, MD,
MD (Hon), PhD (Hon), DSc (Hon)
Professor of Radiology, Department of Radiology,
Division of Nuclear Medicine, Hospital of
University of Pennsylvania,
Philadelphia, Pennsylvania

GUEST EDITOR

ROBERT H. MACH, PhD
Professor of Radiology, Division of Radiological
Sciences, Department of Radiology, Mallinckrodt
Institute of Radiology, Washington University
School of Medicine, St. Louis, Missouri

AUTHORS

CAROLYN J. ANDERSON, PhD
Mallinckrodt Institute of Radiology, Washington
University School of Medicine, St. Louis,
Missouri

XIAOYUAN CHEN, PhD
Associate Professor, Department of Radiology
and Bio-X Program, The Molecular Imaging
Program at Stanford, Stanford University School
of Medicine, Stanford, California

FARROKH DEHDASHTI, MD
Professor of Radiology, Department of Radiology,
Division of Radiological Sciences, Mallinckrodt
Institute of Radiology, Washington University
School of Medicine, St. Louis, Missouri

RICCARDO FERDANI, PhD
Mallinckrodt Institute of Radiology, Washington
University School of Medicine, St. Louis,
Missouri

MARK M. GOODMAN, PhD
Professor, Endowed Chair for Imaging Sciences,
Department of Radiology, Center for Systems
Imaging, Emory University School of Medicine,
Atlanta, Georgia

ROBERT J. GROPLER, MD
Professor of Radiology, Medicine and Biomedical
Engineering, Lab Chief, Cardiovascular Imaging
Laboratory, Division of Radiological Sciences,
Edward Mallinckrodt Institute of Radiology,
Washington University School of Medicine,
St. Louis, Missouri

JASON P. HOLLAND, DPhil
Department of Radiology, Memorial Sloan-
Kettering Cancer Center, New York

ANDREW G. HORTI, PhD
Associate Professor, Department of Radiology,
Division of Nuclear Medicine, PET Center, The
Johns Hopkins School of Medicine, Baltimore,
Maryland

SUZANNE E. LAPI, PhD
Assistant Professor, Mallinckrodt Institute of
Radiology, Washington University, St. Louis,
Missouri

JASON S. LEWIS, PhD
Department of Radiology, Memorial
Sloan-Kettering Cancer Center, New York

ROBERT H. MACH, PhD
Professor of Radiology, Department of
Radiology, Division of Radiological Sciences,
Mallinckrodt Institute of Radiology, Washington
University School of Medicine, St. Louis,
Missouri

GANG NIU, PhD
Post Doctoral Fellow, Department of
Radiology and Bio-X Program, The Molecular
Imaging Program at Stanford, Stanford
University School of Medicine, Stanford,
California

JEFFREY S. STEHOUWER, PhD
Assistant Professor, Department of
Radiology, Center for Systems Imaging,
Emory University School of Medicine,
Atlanta, Georgia

THOMAS F. VOLLER, BSc
Research Laboratory Manager, Mallinckrodt
Institute of Radiology, Washington University,
St. Louis, Missouri

MICHAEL J. WELCH, PhD
Professor, Mallinckrodt Institute of Radiology,
Washington University, St. Louis, Missouri

KENNETH T. WHEELER, PhD
Professor of Radiology, Department of Radiology,
Wake Forest University Health Science Center,
Winston-Salem, North Carolina

DEAN F. WONG, MD, PhD
Professor of Radiology, Psychiatry and
Environmental Health Sciences, Radiology Vice
Chair for Research Administration and Training,
The Johns Hopkins School of Medicine, Baltimore,
Maryland

Contents

> Two different strategies have been developed for imaging the proliferative status of solid tumors with the functional imaging technique, PET. The first strategy uses carbon-11 labeled thymidine, or more recently, fluorine-18 labeled thymidine analogs. These agents are a substrate for the enzyme thymidine kinase-1(TK-1) and provide a pulse label of the number of cells in S phase. The second method for imaging the proliferative status of a tumor uses radio-labeled ligands that bind to the sigma-2 receptor which has a 10-fold higher density in proliferating (P) tumor cells versus quiescent (Q) tumor cells. This article compares and contrasts the two different strategies for imaging the proliferative status of solid tumors, and describes the strengths and weaknesses of each approach.

> This article reviews the application of PET in angiogenesis imaging at both the functional and molecular level. Angiogenesis is a highly-controlled process that is dependent on the intricate balance of both promoting and inhibiting factors, involved in various physiologic and pathologic processes. A comprehensive understanding of the molecular mechanisms that regulate angiogenesis has resulted in the design of new and more effective therapeutic strategies. Because of insufficient sensitivity to detect therapeutic effects by using standard clinical end points or by looking for physiologic improvement, a multitude of imaging techniques have been developed to assess tissue vasculature on the structural, functional, and molecular level. All the methods discussed have been successfully used pre-clinically and will hopefully aid in anti-angiogenic drug development in animal studies.

> Hypoxia imaging has applications in functional recovery in ischemic events such as stroke and myocardial ischemia, but especially in tumors in which hypoxia can be predictive of treatment response and overall prognosis. Recently, there has been development of imaging agents using PET for non-invasive imaging of hypoxia. Many of these PET agents have come to the forefront of hypoxia imaging. Halogenated PET nitroimidazole imaging agents labeled with ^{18}F ($t_{1/2}$ = 110 m) and ^{124}I ($t_{1/2}$ = 110 m) have been under investigation for the last 25 years, with radiometal agents (^{64}Cu-ATSM) being developed more recently. This article focuses on these PET imaging agents for hypoxia.

> The positron emitting radionuclide ^{64}Cu has a radioactive half-life of 12.7 hours. The decay characteristics of ^{64}Cu allow for PET images that are comparable in quality to

those obtained using [18]F. Given the longer radioactive half-life of ^{64}Cu compared with ^{18}F and the versatility of copper chemistry, copper is an attractive alternative to the shorter-lived nuclides for PET imaging of peptides, antibodies, and small molecules that may require longer circulation times. This article discusses a number of copper radiopharmaceuticals, such as Cu-ATSM, that have been translated to the clinic and new developments in copper-based radiopharmaceuticals.

Cardiovascular PET provides exquisite measurements of key aspects of the cardiovascular system and as a consequence it plays central role in cardiovascular investigation. Moreover, PET is now playing an ever increasing role in the management of the cardiac patient. Central to the success of PET is the development and use of novel radiotracers that permit measurements of key aspects of cardiovascular health such as myocardial perfusion, metabolism, and neuronal function. Moreover, the development of molecular imaging radiotracers is now permitting the interrogation of cellular and sub cellular processes. This article highlights these various radiotracers and their role in both cardiovascular research and potential clinical applications.

Cerebral nicotinic acetylcholine receptors (nAChR) are linked to various brain functions and disorders. There is a critical necessity for PET imaging of nAChR to study the role of the nicotinic system in the central nervous system. Currently, only two PET radioligands (2-[^{18}F]FA and 6-[^{18}F]FA) for the nAChR imaging are available, but they exhibit substantial drawbacks in imaging quality and potential for quantification. This article summarizes recent progress in the PET imaging of nAChR human subjects and surveys the studies of several research groups whose aim is the development of nAChR PET radioligands with improved imaging properties.

This article focuses on the development of fluorine-18 radiolabeled PET tracers for imaging the dopamine transporter, serotonin transporter, and norepinephrine transporter. All successful dopamine transporter PET tracers reported to date are members of the 3β-phenyltropane class and are synthesized from cocaine. Currently available carbon-11 serotonin transporter PET tracers come from both the diphenylsulfide and 3β-phenylnortropane class, but so far only the nortropanes have found success with fluorine-18 derivatives. Norepinephrine transporter imaging has so far used carbon-11 and fluorine-18 derivatives of reboxetine but because of defluorination of the fluorine-18 derivatives further research is still necessary.

PET Clinics

THE CLINICS ARE NOW AVAILABLE ONLINE!

Access your subscription at:
www.theclinics.com

GOAL STATEMENT

The goal of the *PET Clinics* is to keep practicing radiologists and radiology residents up to date with current clinical practice in positron emission tomography by providing timely articles reviewing the state of the art in patient care.

ACCREDITATION

PET Clinics is planned and implemented in accordance with the Essential Areas and Policies of the Accreditation Council for Continuing Medical Education (ACCME) through the joint sponsorship of the University of Virginia School of Medicine and Elsevier. The University of Virginia School of Medicine is accredited by the ACCME to provide continuing medical education for physicians.

The University of Virginia School of Medicine designates this educational activity for a maximum of 15 AMA PRA Category 1 Credits™ for each issue, 60 credits per year. Physicians should only claim credit commensurate with the extent of their participation in the activity.

The American Medical Association has determined that physicians not licensed in the US who participate in this CME activity are eligible for a maximum of 15 AMA PRA Category 1 Credits™ for each issue, 60 credits per year.

Category 1 credit can be earned by reading the text material, taking the CME examination online at http://www.theclinics.com/home/cme, and completing the evaluation. After taking the test, you will be required to review any and all incorrect answers. Following completion of the test and evaluation, your credit will be awarded and you may print your certificate.

FACULTY DISCLOSURE/CONFLICT OF INTEREST

The University of Virginia School of Medicine, as an ACCME accredited provider, endorses and strives to comply with the Accreditation Council for Continuing Medical Education (ACCME) Standards of Commercial Support, Commonwealth of Virginia statutes, University of Virginia policies and procedures, and associated federal and private regulations and guidelines on the need for disclosure and monitoring of proprietary and financial interests that may affect the scientific integrity and balance of content delivered in continuing medical education activities under our auspices.

The University of Virginia School of Medicine requires that all CME activities accredited through this institution be developed independently and be scientifically rigorous, balanced and objective in the presentation/discussion of its content, theories and practices.

All authors/editors participating in an accredited CME activity are expected to disclose to the readers relevant financial relationships with commercial entities occurring within the past 12 months (such as grants or research support, employee, consultant, stock holder, member of speakers bureau, etc.). The University of Virginia School of Medicine will employ appropriate mechanisms to resolve potential conflicts of interest to maintain the standards of fair and balanced education to the reader. Questions about specific strategies can be directed to the Office of Continuing Medical Education, University of Virginia School of Medicine, Charlottesville, Virginia.

The faculty and staff of the University of Virginia Office of Continuing Medical Education have no financial affiliations to disclose.

The authors/editors listed below have identified no professional or financial affiliations for themselves or their spouse/partner:

Abass Alavi, MD, MD (Hon), PhD (Hon), DSc (Hon) (Consulting Editor); Xiaoyuan Chen, PhD; Farrokh Dehdashti, MD; Barton Dudlick (Acquisitions Editor); Riccardo Ferdani, PhD; Jason P. Holland, DPhil; Andrew G. Horti, PhD; Suzanne E. Lapi, PhD; Jason S. Lewis, PhD; Gang Niu, PhD; Patrice Rehm, MD (Test Author); Jeffrey S. Stehouwer, PhD; Thomas F. Voller, BS; and Michael J. Welch, PhD.

The authors/editors listed below identified the following professional or financial affiliations for themselves or their spouse/partner:

Carolyn J. Anderson, PhD is an industry funded research/investigator for Amgen and Transmolecular, Inc.

Mark Goodman, PhD is a patent holder with Nihon Mediphysics Ltd.

Robert J. Gropler, MD is an industry funded research/investigator for Lantheus and GE-Amersham, serves on the Speakers Bureau for Astellas, and is a consultant for MDS Nordion.

Robert H. Mach, PhD (Guest Editor) owns a patent with Washington University and Wake Forest University, and is an industry funded research/investigator and owns licensed patents with Isotrace Technologies and Bayer-Schering.

Kenneth T. Wheeler, Jr., PhD owns stock in and serves on the Advisory Committee for Sicel Technologies, Inc.

Dean F. Wong, MD, PhD is an industry funded research/investigator for Amgen, Avid, BMS, Intracellular, Lilly, Merck, Orexigen, Otsuka, Philip Morris, Roche, Sanofi Aventis, and Wyeth.

Disclosure of Discussion of Non-FDA Approved Uses for Pharmaceutical Products and/or Medical Devices.

The University of Virginia School of Medicine, as an ACCME provider, requires that all faculty presenters identify and disclose any off-label uses for pharmaceutical and medical device products. The University of Virginia School of Medicine recommends that each physician fully review all the available data on new products or procedures prior to clinical use.

TO ENROLL

To enroll in the PET Clinics Continuing Medical Education program, call customer service at 1-800-654-2452 or visit us online at www.theclinics.com/home/cme. The CME program is available to subscribers for an additional fee of $175.00.

Preface

Over the last 5 years there has been a tremendous growth in the number of PET radiotracers that have shown promise in initial clinical PET imaging studies and in preclinical imaging studies using animal models of disease. In this issue of *PET Clinics*, we provide an update on recent advances in the development of PET radiotracers for imaging different aspects of tumor biology, cardiovascular function, and molecular targets within the central nervous system (CNS).

The first three articles describe imaging strategies for measuring selected properties of tumors, which are important in selecting patients for different types of chemotherapy and radiation therapy. The article by Mach and colleagues presents a review of the different methods for imaging tumor cell proliferation. This includes an update on the current status of imaging the salvage pathway of DNA synthesis, which provides a measure of the S phase fraction of a tumor. This strategy involves the use of ^{18}F-labeled analogs of the DNA precursor thymidine, the only nucleoside incorporated into DNA but not RNA. An update of the clinical studies using [^{18}F]FLT is also provided as well as a comparison of the different methods of data analysis used in [^{18}F]FLT PET studies. The authors also describe an alternative method for imaging cell proliferation, one that uses the sigma-2 receptor as a receptor-based biomarker for imaging the ratio of proliferating to quiescent cells (i.e., the P:Q ratio) of solid tumors. A comparison between the different aspects of proliferation measured by each imaging approach is provided. This comparison discusses the importance of measuring the P:Q ratio of tumors to stratify patients into those who would benefit from cell cycle–specific chemotherapeutics versus non–cell cycle–specific agents, and from conventional versus hyperfractionated radiation therapy.

The second article describes the different strategies developed for imaging angiogenesis. Given the relative high expense and toxicity associated with antiangiogenic drugs, there is a need to develop a sensitive imaging technique that could be used to select patients who will benefit from treatment with anti-angiogenic drugs from those who would not benefit as well as provide a clinical tool both for optimizing the dose of the drug and for monitoring the response to drug treatment. In the article by Niu and Chen of Stanford University, a brief review of the biology of angiogenesis is presented as well as the different strategies that have been used for imaging angiogenesis in murine models of cancer. The rationale for PET imaging versus other modalities for imaging angiogenesis is also provided.

Another aspect of tumor biology that can influence response to both chemotherapy and radiation therapy is the hypoxic environment of the tumor. In the article by Lapi et al. from Washington University, a review of the different imaging agents that have been developed for imaging hypoxia is provided. A comparison is made between the two different classes of hypoxia imaging agents developed to date, the nitroimidazoles including [^{18}F]FMISO, [^{18}F]FAZA, and [^{18}F]EF5 versus the copper-based radiotracer, [$^{64/60}$Cu]ATSM.

The next article in this issue on new PET radiotracers provides an excellent review on the use of copper-64 as a radionuclide for labeling small molecules, peptides, proteins, and nanoparticles. Although carbon-11 and fluorine-18 are often thought of as the principal radionuclides for PET radiotracer development, the authors have provided strong evidence to support the argument that Cu-64 will play a major role in translational PET imaging studies in the future. The relatively long half-life of Cu-64 (t½ = 12.7 hours) is compatible with the pharmacokinetics of agents such as peptides, proteins, and nanoparticles having a slow clearance from blood and tissues serving as a source of nonspecific binding. The low energy of the positron emitted by the decay of Cu-64 also results in PET and micro-PET images that are of similar quality to those obtained with fluorine-18.

The article by Robert Gropler of Washington University provides a comprehensive review of the different PET radiotracers used to study cardiovascular function. This includes a description of the different approaches for imaging myocardial perfusion (Rb-82, [^{13}N]ammonia, [^{15}O]water), and the application of these radiotracers for imaging cardiovascular disease. The second part of this article provides a review of the different metabolic radiotracers developed for studying myocardial metabolism. This includes a review of the clinical data showing the change in myocardial substrate utilization in various diseases such as type I and type II diabetes mellitus, left ventricular hypertrophy, and cardiomyopathy. This review ends with a overview of the different radiotracers developed to image

PET Clin 4 (2009) ix–x
doi:10.1016/j.cpet.2009.06.005

cardiac innervation, with a focus on presynaptic radiotracers including [11C]hydroxyephedrine, [11C]epinephrine, and [18F]dopamine.

The final two articles provide an update on the development of radiotracers for imaging molecular targets within the central nervous system. The article by Horti and Wong of Johns Hopkins School of Medicine provides an interesting description of the many hurdles that needed to be overcome in the development of an optimal ligand for imaging α4β2 nicotinic receptors in the CNS. The development of a clinically useful radiotracer for imaging α4β2 nicotinic receptors is expected to contribute to the study of the loss of cholinergic function in a variety of CNS disorders, including schizophrenia, depression, and age-related cognitive impairment. Finally, the article by Stehouver and Goodman of Emory University provides an excellent review of literature on the development of radiotracers for imaging monoamine transporters for dopamine, serotonin, and norepinephrine. This has been a very active area of research over the last decade, and the authors have provided an excellent comparison of the different radiotracers that have been developed for imaging the dopamine (DAT), serotonin (SERT), and norepinephrine (NET) transporters.

No single issue of *PET Clinics* could adequately cover all of the recent advances in PET radiotracer development in the areas of imaging tumor biology, cardiovascular function, and molecular targets within the CNS. Radiotracers utilizing both standard (F-18 and C-11) and nonstandard (Cu-64) PET radionuclides are discussed. We hope the collection of articles described above provides the readers a strong sense of the outstanding progress that has been achieved in PET radiotracer development in recent years as well as insight regarding potential future applications. Finally, I would like to extend my gratitude to all of the authors for devoting their considerable time and effort in preparing the excellent articles appearing in this issue of *PET Clinics*.

Robert H. Mach, PhD
Washington University School of Medicine
Campus Box 8225
510 South Kingshighway Boulevard
St. Louis, MO 63110

E-mail address:
rhmach@mir.wustl.edu (R.H. Mach)

PET Radiotracers for Imaging the Proliferative Status of Solid Tumors

Robert H. Mach, PhD[a],*, Farrokh Dehdashti, MD[a],
Kenneth T. Wheeler, PhD[b,c]

KEYWORDS

- Cell proliferation • Thymidine analogs
- Sigma-2 receptors • PET imaging • Thymidine Kinase-1

The initiation and progression of tumors involve deregulation of the cell cycle leading to uncontrolled cell proliferation. Consequently, measurement of the proliferative status can provide useful information regarding the prognosis and aggressiveness of tumors, and this information can be used to guide treatment protocols in clinical practice. Frequently, the chemotherapeutic agents and radiotherapy regimens used to treat cancer have serious side effects caused by normal-tissue toxicity that leads to poor patient tolerability. In addition, many of the newer targeted therapies are also limited by resistance, normal-tissue toxicity, and other adverse events that reduce drug efficacy.[1] A measurement of the proliferative status of tumors, which is defined as the fraction of cells progressing through the cell cycle, may identify patients who are at a higher risk of recurrence and can benefit from individual tailoring of radiotherapy, chemotherapy, targeted therapy, or a combination of these modalities. A change in the proliferative status of a tumor during or after treatment also has the potential to serve as a predictor of response and allow further tailoring of therapy.

PET is an imaging technique that provides a means of measuring disease-based changes in cell function at the molecular level. The use of PET in the field of oncology has focused largely on the use of [18F]2-fluorodeoxyglucose ([18F]FDG), a metabolic tracer which measures differences in glucose use between tumors and normal tissue. Although [18F]FDG has proven to be an important PET radiotracer in the diagnosis and staging/restaging of tumors, differences in glucose use do not provide sufficient information to identify an appropriate strategy for treating solid tumors.[2] The uptake of [18F]FDG by solid tumors also does not correlate strongly with their proliferative status because it often simply reflects tumor cell viability.[3] In addition, [18F]FDG uptake is dependent upon the number of infiltrating inflammatory cells, or the oxygenation status of the tumor cells. Therefore, while [18F]FDG is the primary radiotracer typically used for diagnosing and staging/restaging tumors, it is not capable

The sigma-2 receptor studies were funded by a grant, CA102869, awarded by the National Institutes of Health. The sigma-2 receptor radiotracers described in this paper have been licensed from Washington University (RH Mach, inventor) and Wake Forest University (RH Mach and KT Wheeler, inventors) by Isotrace Technologies, Inc., St. Charles, MO and sublicensed to Bayer-Schering Pharma, Berlin, Germany. Dr. Farrokh Dehdashti is currently directing a clinical trial of [18F]6, which is being sponsored by Bayer-Schering Pharma.

[a] Division of Radiological Sciences, Department of Radiology, Mallinckrodt Institute of Radiology, Washington University School of Medicine, 510 South Kingshighway Boulevard, St. Louis, MO 63110, USA
[b] Department of Radiology, Wake Forest University Health Science Center, Medical Center Blvd, Winston-Salem, NC 27157, USA
[c] Wheeler Scientific Consultants, Inc., 2650 Monticello Dr., Winston-Salem, NC 27106, USA
* Corresponding author.
E-mail address: rhmach@mir.wustl.edu (R.H. Mach).

PET Clin 4 (2009) 1–15
doi:10.1016/j.cpet.2009.04.012
1556-8598/09/$ – see front matter © 2009 Elsevier Inc. All rights reserved.

of providing information regarding which chemotherapy regimen or radiation therapy schedule to use based on the proliferative status of the tumor.

Another metabolism-based imaging strategy for assessing a tumor's proliferative status uses the radiolabeled amino acid [^{11}C]methionine, which measures differences in the rates of protein synthesis between normal and tumor cells. Initial studies have shown a good correlation between [^{11}C]methionine uptake and the S-phase fraction of non-small cell lung carcinoma[4] and breast cancer.[5,6] However, the low tumor uptake and low tumor- background ratios indicate that [^{11}C]methionine is not an ideal agent for imaging the proliferative status of these tumors.[7] Recent studies in patients with brain tumors have yielded mixed results. One study in patients with newly diagnosed brain tumors (n = 41) showed no correlation between the [^{11}C]methionine uptake measured by the standardized uptake ratio (SUV) method and the Ki-67 labeling index of the tumor specimen.[8] Another study demonstrated a modest correlation between the [^{11}C]methionine SUV and the Mib-1 labeling index in patients diagnosed with diffuse astrocytoma (n = 21; r = 0.63), but no such correlation for patients diagnosed with oligodendroglioma or oligogastrocytoma.[9] These data indicate that tumor type may be an important factor when seeking a correlation between radiotracer uptake and the proliferative status of brain tumors in PET imaging studies.

Two strategies have emerged for imaging the proliferative status of solid tumors with PET. The first strategy involves the use of radiolabeled thymidine analogs that use the salvage pathway of DNA synthesis for their uptake.[10] This imaging strategy provides a measure of the number of tumor cells in S-phase during the tracer uptake and image acquisition period of a PET scan. The second strategy involves the use of radiotracers that image the sigma-2 receptor status of solid tumors. Previous studies have shown that sigma-2 receptors are expressed in a 10-fold higher density in cycling, proliferating tumor cells versus tumor cells that are driven into quiescence by nutrient deprivation.[11–13] Although not immediately obvious, these two imaging strategies look at two completely different aspects of cell proliferation; radiolabeled thymidine analogs provide a pulse label of the S-phase fraction of a solid tumor, whereas the sigma-2 receptor imaging agents provide a measure of the ratio of cycling, proliferating (P) to quiescent (Q) tumor cells (ie, the P:Q ratio) in a solid tumor.

S-PHASE FRACTION VERSUS PROLIFERATING TO QUIESCENT RATIO

The loss of the ability of a cell to control its progression through the cell cycle, resulting in uncontrolled cell growth, is a hallmark of cancer.[14] As a result, most tumors have a higher S-phase fraction, the phase of the cell cycle where DNA synthesis occurs, than the normal tissue from which they were derived. Historically, measurement of the S-phase fraction of a tumor, or cells growing under culture conditions, has been a reliable method for measuring cell proliferation. The reagents used to measure the S-phase fraction are usually [^{3}H]thymidine, or the thymidine analog 5-bromodeoxyuridine (BrdU). Since the de novo pathway of DNA synthesis involves the conversion of uridine to thymidine by way of the catalytic action of thymidylate synthetase, the incorporation of [^{3}H]thymidine or BrdU into DNA occurs exclusively through the salvage DNA synthesis pathway. The key step in the salvage pathway involves the phosphorylation of the 5-hydroxy position of thymidine by thymidine kinase-1 (TK-1).

Normally, TK-1 is synthesized at the G1/S boundary and consists of 234 amino acids with a monomeric molecular weight of 25.5 kDa. The enzyme exists as a high catalytic-activity tetrameric complex in S phase, and as a lower catalytic activity dimer in the G2/M phases of the cell cycle.[15,16] Phosphorylation of Ser-13 by cyclin-dependent kinases is thought to be a key step in the degradation of TK-1, which declines to near zero in early G_1. There is no expression of the enzyme in quiescent (G_0) cells. Since TK-1 is usually catalytically active only in S phase, tumor cells growing under cell culture conditions or as tumor allografts or xenografts implanted in a laboratory animal must be exposed to [^{3}H]thymidine or BrdU every 8 hours (ie, the average length of S phase) *for at least one and a half to two cell cycle times* if all the cycling cells are to be labeled with a thymidine analog (**Figs.1** and **2**). Consequently, the measurement of tritium- or BrdU-labeled DNA receiving only a single pulse of [^{3}H]thymidine or BrdU will underestimate the total number of cycling, proliferating cells because those cells in the G_1 and G_2/M phases of the cell cycle will not be labeled. In addition, some tumor cells are TK-1 deficient (TK-1$^-$) and rely exclusively on the de novo DNA synthesis pathway. In these tumors, measurements of radiolabeled thymidine, radiolabeled thymidine analogs, or BrdU incorporation will not correlate with their proliferative status.[10]

A number of studies have provided evidence suggesting that there is an altered regulation of TK-1 in tumor cells.[10] For example, TK-1 has been shown to

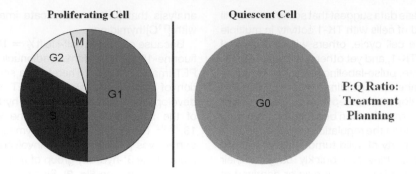

Fig. 1. The characteristics of the P and Q cells in solid tumors. DNA is synthesized in the S phase of the cell cycle. TK-1 is normally synthesized at the G_1/S boundary and is active until early G_2. P cells are Ki-67 positive, whereas Q cells, including Q tumor cells and Q normal cells, are Ki-67 negative.

Within Fig. 1:

Proliferating Cell

Quiescent Cell

P:Q Ratio: Treatment Planning

• P : Q ratio has a profound effect on the outcome of chemotherapy and radiotherapy

• Tumors with a high P:Q ratio respond better to cell cycle specific agents (e.g., 5-FU and Ara-C) and/or hyperfractionated radiation therapy

• A change in the tumor's proliferative status can be used as an indicator of its response to radiation and chemotherapy

be catalytically-active in the S, G2, and M phases of the cell cycle in a number of leukemia cell lines.[17,18] HeLa cervical carcinoma cells have TK-1 activity in all phases of the cell cycle, including G1. Mouse fibroblasts transformed with DNA tumor viruses display a TK-1 activity profile similar to HeLa cells.[17] Truncation of the human TK-1 C-terminus by 30 to 40 amino acids, or changing Ser-13 to an alanine residue that prevents phosphorylation by cyclin-dependent kinases results in a constitutively active

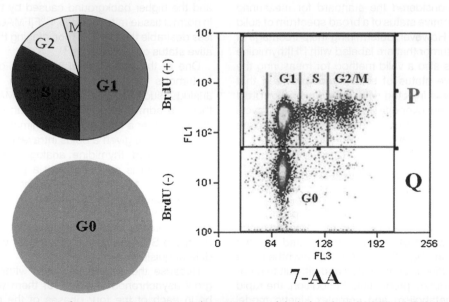

Fig. 2. Flow cytometry of a mouse 66 mammary adenocarcinoma labeled with BrdU (100 mg/kg) every 8 hours over a 48-hour period (ie, ~two tumor cell cycle times). BrdU⁺ cells are P cells. Because the BrdU labeling occurred over two cell cycle times, the cycling P cells in all phases of the cell cycle are labeled. Cells that are BrdU⁻ are Q noncycling cells. The fluorescent probe, 7-AA, distinguishes 66 cells that have a 2C DNA content (G_1/G_0 cells) from cells that have a 4C DNA content (G_2/M). Cells in S phase have an intermediate DNA content and usually are a small fraction of the total cells in a solid tumor.

TK-1.[19,20] These data suggest that some tumors will be comprised of cells with TK-1 activity in multiple phases of the cell cycle, others will have normal regulation of TK-1, and yet others will be TK-1 deficient. Therefore, pulse-labeling studies using either BrdU, radiolabeled thymidine, or a radiolabeled thymidine analog may not represent a true measure of even the S-phase fraction because incorporation is dependent upon the regulation of TK-1.

Another property of solid tumors is that as they increase in size they can quickly outgrow their blood supply and become hypoxic or deprived of nutrients necessary to sustain the high energy requirements for cell proliferation. When this occurs, cycling P cells can exit the cell cycle and enter a prolonged Q state (see **Figs. 1** and **2**).[21–25] A Q- tumor cell is distinct from most Q-normal cells because it remains undifferentiated and can be recruited back into a cycling P-cell state once the conditions of hypoxia or nutrient deprivation are eliminated.[12,13,26,27] All solid tumors, even those as small as 2 to 5 mm in size, contain P and Q cells. The ratio of the P cells to Q cells (the P:Q ratio) is defined as the proliferative status of solid tumors.[11–13] A number of molecular markers have been used to distinguish between the P- and Q- cell populations in a solid tumor, including the presence of Ki-67,[24,28,29] proliferating cell nuclear antigen (PCNA),[29] ribonucleotide reductase M1 subunit (RRM1),[30] and chromatin assembly factor-1 (CAF-1).[31] Of these molecular markers, Ki-67 is considered the standard for measuring the proliferative status of a broad spectrum of solid tumors.[24] However, determining the percentage of cells in a tumor that are labeled with [3H]thymidine or BrdU is also a valid method for measuring the proliferative status of solid tumor provided that the animal is injected with [3H]thymidine or BrdU every 8 hours over one and a half to two cell cycle times to insure that all of the cycling cells are labeled (see **Fig. 2**).[13]

IMAGING THE PROLIFERATIVE STATUS OF TUMORS WITH THYMIDINE AND ITS ANALOGS

The first imaging studies of tumor proliferation used [11C]thymidine labeled in the 5-methyl group and the carbonyl position designated by the asterisks in **Fig. 3**.[32–35] The radiosynthesis of [11C]thymidine is complicated and difficult to automate for routine production. In addition, the rapid in vivo metabolism and complex kinetic model needed to quantify a tumor's proliferative status has limited the utility of [11C]thymidine as a PET radiotracer. The short half-life of carbon-11 ($t\frac{1}{2}$ = 20.4 minutes) also places significant time constraints on image acquisition and metabolite analysis that further complicate imaging studies with [11C]thymidine.

Because of its long half-life ($t\frac{1}{2}$ = 109.8 minutes) fluorine-18 is the preferred radionuclide for clinical PET imaging studies. Therefore, a second generation of thymidine analogs for PET imaging were developed by substitution of the hydroxyl groups of the sugar moiety of thymidine with fluorine-18.[36–39] The first [18F]-labeled thymidine analog reported was [18F]FLT[38] which involved the replacement of the 3'-hydroxy group of thymidine with the [18F] radiolabel (see **Fig. 3**). Since [18F]FLT lacks the 3'-hydroxy group, it is not incorporated into DNA and is trapped in tumor cells following phosphorylation of the 5'-hydroxy group by TK-1 in a manner analogous to the trapping of [18F]FDG in cells by way of phosphorylation by hexokinase.[38,40] Other analogs have been developed by attaching the [18F]-radiolabel to the 2'-beta position of thymidine. Examples of these analogs include the radiotracers [18F]FMAU and [18F]FBAU (see **Fig. 3**).[41–43] Because these analogs contain the 3'-hydroxy group, they can be readily incorporated into DNA and provide a direct measure of DNA synthesis. Of the two, [18F]FMAU has been studied the most in animal tumor models. Although [18F]FMAU is incorporated into DNA, it is a poorer substrate for TK-1 than [18F]FLT. In addition, unlike [18F]FLT, [18F]FMAU is a substrate for the mitochondrial enzyme thymidine kinase-2 (TK-2), which is involved in mitochondrial DNA synthesis. Given its low specificity for TK-1 and the higher background caused by the uptake in normal tissue mitochondria, [18F]FMAU is slightly less desirable than [18F]FLT for imaging the proliferative status of solid tumors.[3]

One of the fundamental limitations of imaging a tumor's proliferative status with thymidine analogs, such as [18F]FLT and [18F]FMAU, is that they are administered as a pulse label. The test subject, either a tumor-bearing animal or a patient with cancer, is given a bolus intravenous injection of the labeled thymidine analog and then the imaging data is acquired over a period ranging from 60 to 120 minutes. Consequently, PET-imaging studies with radiolabeled DNA precursors provide only a snapshot of the small number of cycling, proliferating tumor cells that happen to be in the S phase during radiotracer uptake and data acquisition.

Because the proliferating cells within a tumor grow asynchronously, some of them will always be in each of the four phases of the cell cycle. Therefore, the proliferating cells that are in the G_1-, G_2-, and M-phase of the cell cycle will not be labeled by [18F]FLT or [18F]FMAU, assuming TK-1 is regulated normally. Further complicating the situation, the potential doubling time (ie, the

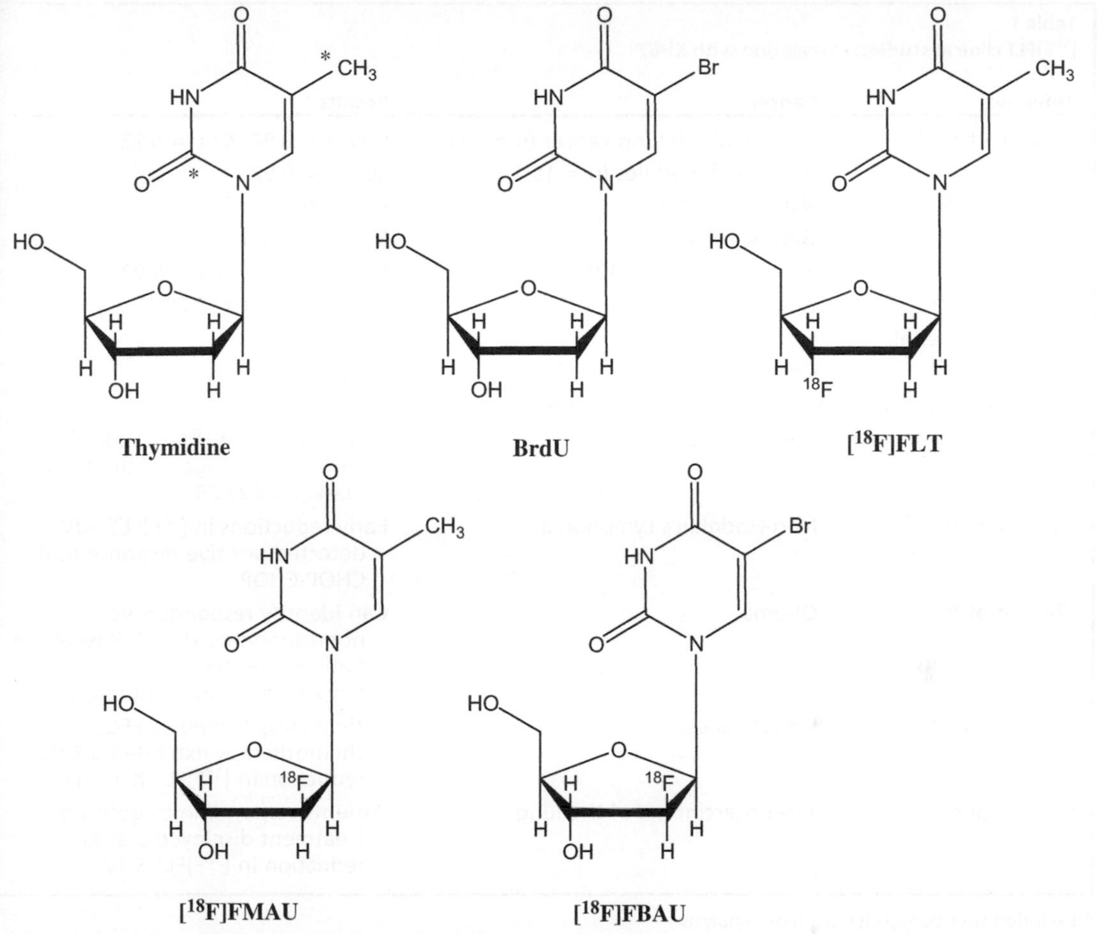

Fig. 3. Structures of thymidine, BrdU, and the ^{18}F-labeled thymidine analogs that have been developed to determine the proliferative status of solid tumors with PET.

cell cycle time) of human tumors is highly variable, typically ranging from 1 to several days. Because the length of the S phase in mammalian cells is constant at 8 to 10 hours, only a small percentage of proliferating tumor cells with long cell-cycle times will be in the S phase during the pulse labeling with a thymidine analog. Thus, the thymidine analogs, such as [^{18}F]FLT and [^{18}F]FMAU, will theoretically underestimate the actual number of cycling, proliferating cells and the P:Q ratio in a solid tumor, if TK-1 is catalytically active only during the S phase.

Despite these potential limitations, a number of clinical imaging studies have shown a good correlation and a steep slope in plots of the uptake of [^{18}F]FLT versus the Ki-67- labeling index in breast,[40] lung,[44–46] brain,[8,9,47–50] and colon tumors.[51,52] A key requirement for obtaining a high correlation between [^{18}F]FLT uptake and the Ki-67- labeling index involves the method used for analyzing the PET data. Although most

imaging studies reported to date have used SUV for measuring [^{18}F]FLT uptake in tumors, a number of more recent studies have shown that a graphical (ie, Patlak) analysis is needed to give a high correlation between the tracer uptake and the Ki-67-labeling index. This Patlak analysis requires the measurement of metabolite-corrected arterial blood samples (ie, the input function) in addition to a 45- to 95-minute dynamic acquisition scan to quantify the [^{18}F]FLT uptake.[40,46,48,49] This imaging protocol is considerably more complicated than the typical intravenous injection of [^{18}F]FLT followed be a 15-minute emission scan acquired at 60 minutes after injection of the radiotracer. A summary of the clinical studies reported to date using [^{18}F]FLT to image a tumor's proliferative status is provided in **Table 1**.

Finally, the uptake of [^{18}F]FLT in normal tissues can also place limitations on the type of clinical imaging studies conducted with this radiotracer. [^{18}F]FLT is metabolized by forming glucuronide

Table 1
[¹⁸F]FLT clinical studies: correlation with Ki-67

Reference	Cancer	Results
Vesselle et al.[44]	Non-small cell lung cancer (n = 11)	SUV: r = 0.84; K_I: r = 0.92
Buck et al.[45]	Pulmonary nodules (n = 15)[a]	SUV: r = 0.92
Muzi ett al.[46]	NSCLC (n = 17)	K_I: r = 0.92
Choi et al.[47]	Glioma (n = 9)	SUV: r = 0.817
Kenny et al.[40]	Breast cancer (n = 12)	SUV: r = 0.79; K_I: r = 0.92
Ullrich et al.[48]	Glioma (n = 11)	SUV: NC[b]; K_I: r = 0.88[c]
Hatakeyama et al.[8]	Glioma (n = 18)	SUV: r = 0.89
Francis et al.[51]	Colorectal cancer (n = 10)	SUV: r = 0.8
[¹⁸F]FLT clinical studies monitoring response to therapy		
Pio et al.[54]	Breast cancer	Early changes in [¹⁸F]FLT correlated with later changes of the tumor marker, CA27.29
Herrmann et al.[57]	Non-Hodgkin's Lymphoma	Early reductions in [¹⁸F]FLT SUV detected positive response to R-CHOP/CHOP
Chen et al.[56]	Glioma	Can identify responders vs nonresponders after 1–2 weeks in patients treated with bevacizumab and irinotecan
Kenny et al.[40,53]	Breast cancer	Patients responding to FEC[d] chemotherapy exhibited a 53% reduction in [¹⁸F]FLT K_I value
Sohn et al.[55]	Adenocarcinoma of the lung	Patients responding to gefitnib treatment displayed a 36% reduction in [¹⁸F]FLT SUV

[a] Excluded four benign lesions from analysis.
[b] no correlation.
[c] compartmental modeling showed a correlation of r = 0.88 for k3 versus Ki-67 expression.
[d] 5-fluorouracil/epirubicin/cyclophosphamide.

that is excreted by way of the hepatobiliary system. The high uptake of [¹⁸F]FLT and its glucuronide metabolite by the liver usually limits its ability to image tumors in the abdominal cavity. There is also a high uptake of [¹⁸F]FLT in bone that reflects the high proliferative activity of hematopoietic cells in bone marrow (**Fig. 4**).[3] Consequently, the high uptake of [¹⁸F]FLT in bone can limit the ability of this radiotracer to define the extent of tumors near, or invading bony structures.

Recent studies have also demonstrated that [¹⁸F]FLT PET imaging can be used to assess the response to chemotherapy.[36] For example, Kenny and colleagues[53] reported that serial imaging studies in patients with breast cancer demonstrated a reduction in [¹⁸F]FLT uptake at 1 week after combination chemotherapy with 5-fluorouracil, epirubicin, and cyclophosphamide (FEC). This reduction in uptake exceeded test/retest variability, and preceded any physical change in tumor diameter. This reduction in [¹⁸F]FLT uptake was observed using the Patlak compartmental modeling and SUV methods. An earlier study by Pio and colleagues[54] demonstrated that a change in [¹⁸F]FLT SUV values after a single dose of chemotherapy in patients with breast cancer had a higher correlation with posttreatment changes in the glycoprotein cancer antigen 27.29 (CA27.29), than with the change in [¹⁸F]FDG SUV values. The relative change in [¹⁸F]FLT SUV values at 1 week after treatment with gefitnib clearly delineates between the responders and nonresponders who have lung tumors.[55] Similar results have been reported for patients with: (1) glioma treated with bevacizumab and irinotecan,[56] and (2) lymphoma treated with cyclophosphamide, doxorubicin, vincristine, and prednisone chemotherapy (CHOP).[57] These data clearly demonstrate the potential utility of [¹⁸F]FLT in determining a positive response to chemotherapy.

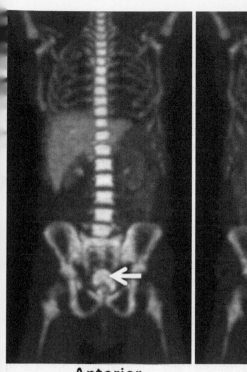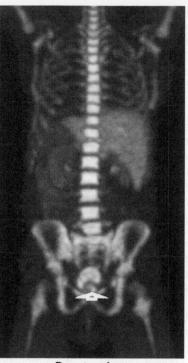

Anterior **Posterior**

Fig. 4. [^{18}F]FLT-PET in a patient with locally advanced rectal cancer. Anterior and posterior projection images demonstrate intense [^{18}F]FLT uptake in bone that reflects the proliferation of cells in the bone marrow. There is increased accumulation of [^{18}F]FLT in the rectal cancer (arrowhead in right panel). In addition, there is increased accumulation of [^{18}F]FLT in the urinary bladder (arrow in the left panel), which is a normal finding.

THE SIGMA-2 RECEPTOR AS A BIOMARKER FOR IMAGING THE PROLIFERATIVE STATUS OF TUMORS

Another potential method for measuring a tumor's proliferative status with PET is to devise a way to image Ki-67 expression (see **Fig. 1**). Unfortunately, there are no small molecules having a high affinity for Ki-67 which can serve as lead compounds for PET radiotracer development. In lieu of imaging Ki-67, another option would be to identify a protein that behaves in a similar manner and has small molecules that bind to this protein. These molecules could then serve as lead compounds for PET radiotracer development. Over the past decade our group has shown that the sigma-2 receptor is regulated in a manner similar to Ki-67 and is a receptor-based biomarker of cell proliferation.[11–13] Therefore, PET radiotracers that can image the sigma-2 receptor may provide an alternative strategy to the radiolabeled DNA analogs for imaging the proliferative status of tumors.

Sigma receptors are a class of proteins that were originally thought to be a subtype of the opiate receptors.[58] Subsequent studies revealed that sigma binding sites represent a distinct class of receptors. There are two well-characterized subtypes of sigma receptors, sigma-1 and sigma-2. Sigma-1 receptors have a molecular weight of approximately 25 kDa, whereas the sigma-2 receptor has a molecular weight of approximately 21.5 kDa. The sigma-1 receptor gene has been cloned from guinea pig liver, human placental choriocarcinoma, rat brain, and mouse kidney.[59,60] The sigma-2 receptor has not been sequenced or cloned. Historically, the differentiation of the sigma-2 receptor from the sigma-1 receptor has been based on the in vitro binding properties of two different radioligands, [^{3}H](+)-pentazocine and [^{3}H]1,3-di-o-tolylguanidine ([^{3}H]DTG). [^{3}H](+) pentazocine has a high (~3 nM) affinity for the sigma-1 receptor and a low (>1000 nM) affinity for the sigma-2 receptor, whereas [^{3}H]DTG has a modest affinity (~25 nM) for the sigma-1 and sigma-2 receptors.[58,61]

The role of the sigma receptors as potential biomarkers for breast cancer became apparent when it was shown that the radiotracer [^{125}I]N-(N-benzylpiperidin-4-yl)-4-iodobenzamide, which possesses a high affinity for both sigma-1 and sigma-2 receptors, labeled MCF-7 human breast tumor cells in vitro.[62,63] A subsequent study revealed that MCF-7 cells possess a high density of sigma-2 receptors, as measured by [^{3}H]DTG in the presence of dextrallorphan to mask sigma-1 sites.[64] There was no detectable binding of the sigma-1 radiotracer, [^{3}H](+)-pentazocine, to MCF-7 cells.[64] Further studies indicated that many murine and human tumor cells possess a high density of sigma-2 receptors when grown under cell culture conditions. With the exception of LNCaP human prostate-tumor cells, which have an equal density of sigma-1 and sigma-2 receptors, and ThP-1 leukemia cells, which have a higher density of sigma-1 versus sigma-2 receptors, the sigma-2 receptors density is much higher than the sigma-1 receptor density in all of the tumor cells evaluated to date.[65]

Although in vitro binding studies suggest that the sigma-2 receptor is a potential target for imaging solid tumors,[65] these studies do not address whether or not there is a difference in the sigma-2 receptor density between proliferating and quiescent tumor cells. This issue was investigated in a series of in vitro and in vivo studies reported by Wheeler and colleagues.[11–13] These studies used the well-characterized in vitro and in vivo mouse mammary adenocarcinoma model, 66, in which pure (>97%) populations of proliferative (66 P) and quiescent (66 Q) cells can be obtained under tissue culture conditions.[26,27] The 66 P cells have a cell cycle distribution and a tritiated thymidine labeling index characteristic of a mammalian cell line with a 13.8-hour doubling time.[26,27] The 66 Q cells have predominantly a G_1 DNA content (>90%), a reduced cell volume (~50%), a mitotic and tritiated thymidine labeling index of virtually zero (<1%), and a reduced RNA content (~50%). 66 Q cells are viable (>98% trypan blue excluding) and can be recruited back into the P-cell compartment.[26,27] Therefore, these 66 mouse breast-tumor cells have all of the properties needed to determine if there is a difference in the sigma-2 receptor density between P and Q tumor cells.

In the initial study,[11] the sigma-2 receptor density was measured in 3-day 66 P cells and in 7-, 10-, and 12-day 66 Q cells. Since the transition from 66 P cells to a pure population of 66 Q cells is not complete until day 7 in this in-vitro model, the Q-cell populations in this study corresponded to about 1, 3, and 5 days into quiescence. The results of Scatchard studies revealed a receptor density of approximately 180,000 sigma-2 receptors per cell in 7-day 66 Q cells and approximately 510,000 sigma-2 receptors per cell in the corresponding 3-day 66 P cells to give a 7-day P/Q ratio of approximately 2.8:1. The sigma-2 receptor density of 10-day 66 Q cells was approximately 88,000 receptors per cell. The sigma-2 receptor density in the corresponding 3-day 66 P cells was approximately 840,000 receptors cell, resulting in a P:Q ratio of approximately 9.5:1. The 12-day results were not statistically different from the 10-day results. These data suggest that at least a 3-day period in quiescence is required to maximize the loss of sigma-2 receptors from 66 cells; kinetics identical to those for the loss of

Ki-67 during the 66 cell P to Q transition. Although the number of sigma-2 receptors in the 3-day 66 P cells appears to be exceptionally high (510,000–840,000 receptors/cell), this number is consistent with the number of sigma-2 receptors per cell reported in other tumor cell lines.[65]

In a follow-up study, these investigators measured the density of sigma-2 receptors during the P to Q and Q to P transitions.[12] When 10-day 66 Q cells were recultured, the Q cells rapidly entered the P-cell compartment with little or no delay (**Fig. 5**A). The kinetics of the expression of sigma-2 receptors in 66 cells followed the population growth curve as expected. There was a rapid increase in the sigma-2 receptor density during the exponential growth phase that leveled off during early plateau phase. This represents the initial P to Q transition. The sigma-2 receptor density remained stable for 3 days, and then decreased during late-plateau phase. The decrease in the sigma-2 receptor density in late-plateau phase did not start until 5 days following reentry into quiescence. Therefore, the sigma-2 receptor density, like many membrane-bound receptors, is up-regulated and down-regulated over a 2- to 3- day period instead of the few hours for TK-1 and the cell cycle checkpoint proteins.

Finally, the sigma-2 receptor density of tumor xenografts derived from 66 cells correlated with the P:Q ratio determined by flow cytometry after labeling the proliferative cells with BrdU for approximately two cell cycles.[13] In this study, tumor-bearing mice were injected with a dose of BrdU (100 mg/kg, intraperitoneal) every 8 hours over a 48-hour period, and Scatchard studies were conducted on membrane preparations from one half of the tumor while flow cytometry studies were conducted on the dissociated tumor cells obtained from the other half (**Fig. 5**B). A mathematical equation was derived that determined the P:Q ratio from a plot of the dpm/mg of tumor obtained at saturation from the Scatchard studies divided by the fraction of Q cells obtained from the flow cytometry studies against the P:Q ratio obtained from the flow cytometry studies. The sigma-2 receptor density P:Q ratio is estimated by calculating the ratio of the slope to the intercept determined from a linear regression analysis of the data (see **Fig. 5**B).[13] The results indicated that there is excellent agreement between the in vivo sigma-2 receptor density P:Q ratio (10.6) and the in vitro sigma-2 receptor density P:Q ratio (9.5).

The above studies demonstrate that the sigma-2 receptor is a good biomarker for measuring the P:Q ratio of solid tumors in vivo. That is, it is a protein that possesses kinetic properties similar to Ki-67 and other protein-based biomarkers of

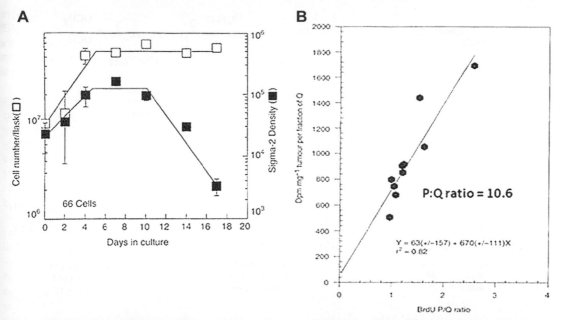

Fig. 5. Validation of the sigma-2 receptor as a biomarker for imaging the proliferative status of solid tumors. (A) Up-regulation and down-regulation of the sigma-2 receptors in 66 cells during the P to Q and the Q to P transitions. (B) Determination of the sigma-2 receptor density P:Q ratio in solid 66 tumor xenografts grown in nude mice.

proliferation.[24,28] The 10-fold higher density of sigma-2 receptors in P versus Q cells indicates that it should be possible to differentiate between tumors having a high proliferative status (ie, high P:Q ratio) versus a low proliferative status (ie, low P:Q ratio). Furthermore, the high density of sigma-2 receptors in Q cells (~88,000 receptor/cell) also suggests that the sigma-2 receptor may be a useful biomarker for differentiating between Q tumor cells and normal cells since the density of sigma-2 receptors in normal tissues has been reported to be even lower than Q tumor cells.[65] In this regard, the sigma-2 receptor may be a more reliable marker than Ki-67 for determining the proliferative status of solid tumors since quiescent tumors and quiescent normal cells are Ki-67 negative. However, further studies are needed to validate this hypothesis.

DEVELOPMENT OF RADIOTRACERS FOR IMAGING THE SIGMA-2 RECEPTOR WITH PET

A class of compounds that has proven useful for developing PET radiotracers for imaging sigma-2 receptors is the conformationally flexible benzamide analogs. The identification of this class of compounds as PET radiotracers for imaging sigma-2 receptors was a serendipitous discovery resulting from a structure-activity relationship study aimed at developing probes for imaging

the dopamine D_3 receptor.[66,67] The lead compound for the D_3 studies was the benzamide analog, 1, which has high affinity and modest selectivity for the D_3 versus D_2 receptors, but a log P that suggests it is not capable of readily crossing the blood-brain barrier (**Fig. 6**). To prepare D_3 selective compounds having a lipophilicity that would more readily cross the blood-brain barrier, the 2,3-dichloropiperazine moiety of 1 was replaced with a 6,7-dimethoxytetrahydroisoquinoline ring to give compound 2 (see **Fig. 6**). Although this substitution increased the overall lipophilicity of the compound, it also resulted in an undesired reduction in affinity for the dopamine D_3 receptor. However, an unexpected observation was the dramatic increase in affinity for the sigma-2 receptors, and the unusually high selectivity for sigma-2 versus sigma-1 receptors. Consequently, compound 2 served as the lead compound for the development of carbon-11,[68] fluorine-18,[69] and bromine-76[70] labeled probes for imaging the sigma-2 receptor with PET.

The first PET radiotracers based on the conformationally flexible benzamide analogs were [^{11}C]2 to 5, whose synthesis involves labeling the corresponding ortho-hydroxy group with [^{11}C]methyl iodide. Although the affinities of [^{11}C]2, [^{11}C]3, [^{11}C]4, and [^{11}C]5 for the sigma-2 receptor are similar, in vivo studies indicated that [^{11}C]4 has the highest tumor uptake at all time points.[71] One

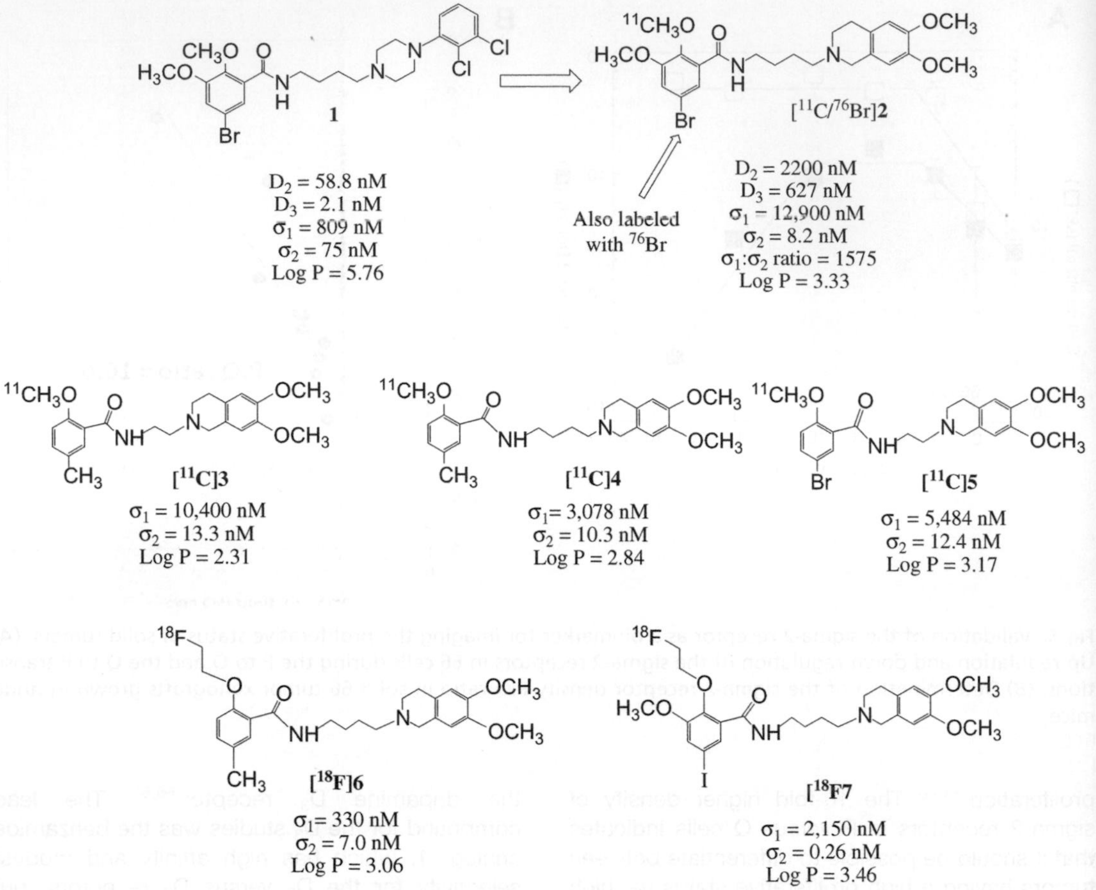

CH3O
H3CO
O
N
H
N
N
Cl
Cl
Br
1
D2 = 58.8 nM
D3 = 2.1 nM
σ1 = 809 nM
σ2 = 75 nM
Log P = 5.76
11CH3O
H3CO
Br
OCH3
OCH3
[11C/76Br]2
Also labeled with 76Br
D2 = 2200 nM
D3 = 627 nM
σ1 = 12,900 nM
σ2 = 8.2 nM
σ1:σ2 ratio = 1575
Log P = 3.33
[11C]3
σ1 = 10,400 nM
σ2 = 13.3 nM
Log P = 2.31
[11C]4
σ1= 3,078 nM
σ2 = 10.3 nM
Log P = 2.84
[11C]5
σ1 = 5,484 nM
σ2 = 12.4 nM
Log P = 3.17
18F
[18F]6
σ1= 330 nM
σ2 = 7.0 nM
Log P = 3.06
[18F7
σ1 = 2,150 nM
σ2 = 0.26 nM
Log P = 3.46

Fig. 6. Structures of the conformationally flexible benzamide analogs for imaging sigma-2 receptors with PET.

explanation for this observation is that [^{11}C]4 may have the optimal lipophilicity for tumor uptake since a parabolic relationship was observed between the percent injected dose per gram (% I.D./g) of tumor and the calculated log P of the radiotracer (**Fig. 7**). These data suggest that the receptor affinity and lipophilicity are important properties that one must factor into the design of receptor-based tumor-imaging agents. MicroPET and MicroCT imaging studies of [^{11}C]4 in the human melanoma tumor MDA-MB-435 are shown in **Fig. 8**A and clearly demonstrate its potential as a radiotracer for imaging the sigma-2 receptor status of solid tumors with PET. The presence of the bromine atom in the benzamide ring of compound 2 led to the preparation of [^{76}Br]2.[63] Although [^{76}Br]2 displayed high-tumor uptake and excellent tumor-to-background ratios, the limited availability and high positron energy of Br-76, which degrades image resolution, limits the utility of [^{76}Br]2 as a potential radiotracer in clinical PET studies.

Although the preclinical microPET imaging and tumor-uptake studies of [^{11}C]4 have shown promising results, the short half-life of carbon 11 ($t_{1/2}$ = 20.4 minutes) is not ideal for the development of radiotracers that would have a widespread use in clinical PET imaging studies. The longer half-life of ^{18}F ($t_{1/2}$ = 109.8 minutes) compared

Tumor Uptake versus Log P
%I.D./g Tumor
1.5
1.25
1
0.75
0.5
0.25
2.25
2.5
2.75
3
3.25
3.5
[11C]4
[11C]5
[11C]3
[11C]2

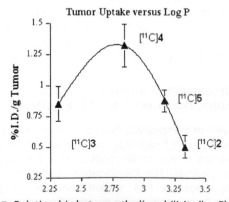

Fig. 7. Relationship between the lipophilicity (log P) and tumor uptake of the ^{11}C-labeled conformationally flexible benzamide analogs shown in **Fig. 6**.

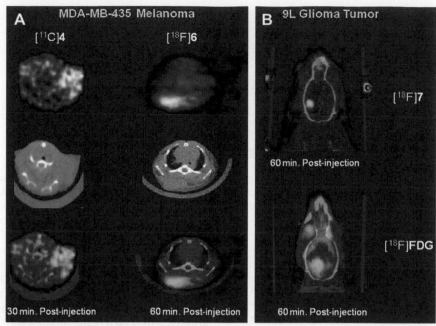

Fig. 8. PET and CT images of solid tumors with sigma-2 radiotracers and [^{18}F]FDG. (*A*) MicroPET, microCT, and coregistered images of MDA-MB-435 melanoma tumors obtained 30 minutes after intravenous (IV) injection of [^{11}C]4 and 60 minutes after IV injection of [^{18}F]6. (*B*) Coregistered microPET and microCT images of a rat intracranial 9L brain tumor obtained 60 minutes after IV injection of [^{18}F]7 (top) or 60 minutes after IV injection of [^{18}F]FDG (bottom).

with ^{11}C places fewer time constraints on tracer synthesis, enables distribution to PET scanners within 2 hours of the cyclotron, and permits longer scan sessions that usually give higher tumor-to-normal-tissue ratios. Therefore, the development of an ^{18}F-labeled radiotracer was important for the clinical translation of imaging the σ_2 receptor status of human solid tumors with PET.

A limited number of ^{18}F-labeled radiotracers based on the conformationally flexible benzamide analogs have been evaluated in murine tumor models.[69] The strategy involved replacement of the 2-methoxy group in the benzamide ring with a 2-fluoroethoxy group (see **Fig. 6**). The 2-fluoroethoxy- for -methyl substitution is a common method for incorporating a fluorine-18 into a receptor-based imaging agent.[69] In vivo tumor-uptake and microPET imaging studies indicate that [^{18}F]6 and [^{18}F]7 are potential probes for imaging the sigma-2 receptor status of solid tumors with PET (see **Fig. 6**).[69] Although most of the initial preclinical evaluation of these probes involves imaging murine models of melanoma (see **Fig. 8A**), an important clinical use of these radiotracers may be determining the tumor margins and proliferative status of brain tumors to select appropriate radiotherapy regimens. For example, microPET studies of an intracranial 9L

brain tumor demonstrated a higher tumor uptake and more favorable differentiation of tumor versus normal brain tissue with [^{18}F]7 than observed with [^{18}F]FDG, the metabolic tracer used routinely in the diagnosis and staging of brain tumors (**Fig. 8B**). The low tumor to background ratio of [^{18}F]FDG is attributed to the high uptake of the radiotracer in normal brain tissue because glucose is the major energy source for the brain.

A limited number of studies have been conducted comparing the sigma-2 receptor imaging approach to the [^{18}F]FLT approach. Studies with the ^{11}C-labeled radiotracer, [^{11}C]4, displayed higher tumor to blood and tumor to muscle ratios for the sigma-2 receptor-based imaging agent compared with those for [^{18}F]FLT, whereas the tumor to fat ratios for the two radiotracers were similar.[68] A microPET-imaging study comparing [^{76}Br]2 and [^{18}F]FLT also showed a much greater visualization of the tumor and higher tumor to background ratios for the sigma-2 receptor imaging agent (**Fig. 9**).[70] Clinical trials of [^{18}F]6 are ongoing at Washington University in St. Louis. These trials will compare the images obtained with [^{18}F]6 to those obtained with [^{18}F]FLT, and determine if the relationship between each radiotracer and the Ki-67 labeling index is similar to that obtained with animal models.

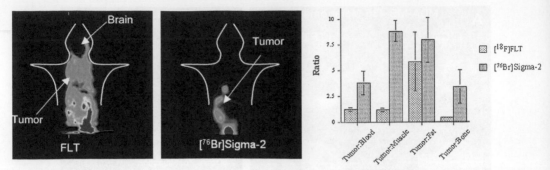

Fig. 9. Comparison of the sigma-2 receptor imaging strategy (right) with the DNA precursor, [^{18}F]FLT (left) in EMT-6 tumors. Note the high contrast and high signal to noise ratio of the sigma-2 imaging agent, [^{76}Br]**2**, relative to [^{18}F]FLT. The tumor to background ratios of both tracers from biodistribution studies are shown in the graph.

SUMMARY

The development of radiotracers for imaging the proliferative status of solid tumors has been an active area of research over the past decade. A noninvasive imaging measurement of a tumor's proliferative status may provide information that can be used for the identification of an appropriate treatment strategy for individual patients. For example, highly proliferative tumors are generally aggressive with a high metastatic potential that requires an aggressive initial treatment. Thus, they usually respond better to cell-cycle specific agents (eg, Ara-C and 5-fluorouracil) or hyperfractionated radiotherapy. In contrast, slowly proliferative tumors respond better to cell-cycle nonspecific agents (eg, cyclophosphamide and BCNU) or conventional radiation therapy. Furthermore, when imaging is conducted both pre- and posttreatment, a reduction in the proliferative status of a tumor has the potential to be used as an early indicator of the tumor's response to therapy.

Two strategies, radiolabeled thymidine analogs and sigma-2 receptor radiotracers, have been developed for imaging the proliferative status of solid tumors with PET. Radiolabeled thymidine analogs, such as [^{18}F]FLT, provide an image that depends on the level of TK-1 activity in tumor cells. The uptake of [^{18}F]FLT and its structural analogs reflects a pulse label of the number of cycling, proliferating cells that are in S phase during the uptake and data-acquisition period. However, since the regulation of TK-1 can be altered in many tumors, thymidine analogs only provide: (1) an estimate of the number of cycling tumor cells in the S-phase fraction if the cells regulate TK-1 similar to normal cells, (2) an estimate of the number of cycling tumor cells in the S/G$_2$/M phases if TK-1 is active through M phase, and (3) no estimate of the number of cycling tumor cells if the tumor cells are

TK-1 deficient. Because TK-1 is low or nonexistent in the G$_1$ phase, thymidine analogs cannot differentiate among cycling, P tumor cells in G$_1$, Q tumor cells in G$_0$, and normal cells which are predominantly in G$_0$. Consequently, the sigma-2 imaging approach may be a better strategy for: (1) differentiating normal tissue from tumor tissue, and (2) estimating the P to Q ratio of a tumor than the radiolabeled analogs of thymidine. Although the sigma-2 receptor imaging strategy has shown great promise in animal models, clinical-imaging studies must be conducted in patients with cancer to validate it as a viable alternative to radiolabeled thymidine analogs for determining the proliferative status of human solid tumors.

ACKNOWLEDGMENTS

The MDA-MB-435 cell line was a gift from Dr. Janet Price of the MD Anderson Cancer Center, University of Texas, Houston. The EMT-6 cell line was a gift from Drs. Ronald S. Pardini and Sandra Johnson of the Department of Biochemistry, University of Nevada, Reno. The authors would like to thank Ms. Lynne Jones for her excellent editorial assistance and Dr. Ryuji Higashikubo for providing the flow cytometry data used in **Fig. 2**.

REFERENCES

1. Penas-Prado M, Gilbert MR. Molecularly targeted therapies for malignant gliomas: advances and challenges. Expert Rev Anticancer Ther 2007;7(5): 641–61.
2. Bastiaannet E, Groen H, Jager PL, et al. The value of FDG-PET in the detection, grading and response to therapy of soft tissue and bone sarcomas; a systematic review and meta-analysis. Cancer Treat Rev 2004;30(1):83–101.

3. Bading JR, Shields AF. Imaging of cell proliferation: status and prospects. J Nucl Med 2008;49(Suppl 2):64S–80S.

4. Miyazawa H, Arai T, Iio M, et al. PET imaging of non-small-cell lung carcinoma with carbon-11-methionine: relationship between radioactivity uptake and flow-cytometric parameters. J Nucl Med 1993; 34(11):1886–91.

5. Leskinen-Kallio S, Nagren K, Lehikoinen P, et al. Uptake of 11C-methionine in breast cancer studied by PET. An association with the size of S-phase fraction. Br J Cancer 1991;64(6):1121–4.

6. Jansson T, Westlin JE, Ahlstrom H, et al. Positron emission tomography studies in patients with locally advanced and/or metastatic breast cancer: a method for early therapy evaluation? J Clin Oncol 1995;13(6):1470–7.

7. Amano S, Inoue T, Tomiyoshi K, et al. In vivo comparison of PET and SPECT radiopharmaceuticals in detecting breast cancer. J Nucl Med 1998;39(8):1424–7.

8. Hatakeyama T, Kawai N, Nishiyama Y, et al. 11C-methionine (MET) and 18F-fluorothymidine (FLT) PET in patients with newly diagnosed glioma. Eur J Nucl Med Mol Imaging 2008;35(11):2009–17.

9. Kato T, Shinoda J, Oka N, et al. Analysis of 11C-methionine uptake in low-grade gliomas and correlation with proliferative activity. AJNR Am J Neuroradiol 2008;29(10):1867–71.

10. Schwartz JL, Tamura Y, Jordan R, et al. Monitoring tumor cell proliferation by targeting DNA synthetic processes with thymidine and thymidine analogs. J Nucl Med 2003;44(12):2027–32.

11. Mach RH, Smith CR, al-Nabulsi I, et al. Sigma 2 receptors as potential biomarkers of proliferation in breast cancer. Cancer Res 1997;57(1):156–61.

12. Al-Nabulsi I, Mach RH, Wang LM, et al. Effect of ploidy, recruitment, environmental factors, and tamoxifen treatment on the expression of sigma-2 receptors in proliferating and quiescent tumour cells. Br J Cancer 1999;81(6):925–33.

13. Wheeler KT, Wang LM, Wallen CA, et al. Sigma-2 receptors as a biomarker of proliferation in solid tumours. Br J Cancer 2000;82(6):1223–32.

14. Hanahan D, Weinberg RA. The hallmarks of cancer. Cell 2000;100(1):57–70.

15. Munch-Petersen B, Cloos L, Jensen HK, et al. Human thymidine kinase 1. Regulation in normal and malignant cells. Adv Enzyme Regul 1995;35:69–89.

16. Birringer MS, Perozzo R, Kut E, et al. High-level expression and purification of human thymidine kinase 1: quaternary structure, stability, and kinetics. Protein Expr Purif 2006;47(2):506–15.

17. Hengstschlager M, Knofler M, Mullner EW, et al. Different regulation of thymidine kinase during the cell cycle of normal versus DNA tumor virus-transformed cells. J Biol Chem 1994; 269(19):13836–42.

18. Chiba P, Tihan T, Eher R, et al. Effect of cell growth and cell differentiation on 1-beta-D-arabinofuranosylcytosine metabolism in myeloid cells. Br J Haematol 1989;71(4):451–5.

19. Sutterluety H, Bartl S, Karlseder J, et al. Carboxy-terminal residues of mouse thymidine kinase are essential for rapid degradation in quiescent cells. J Mol Biol 1996;259(3):383–92.

20. Chang ZF, Huang DY, Hsue NC. Differential phosphorylation of human thymidine kinase in proliferating and M phase-arrested human cells. J Biol Chem 1994;269(33):21249–54.

21. Shackney SE, Shankey TV. Cell cycle models for molecular biology and molecular oncology: exploring new dimensions. Cytometry 1999;35(2):97–116.

22. Wilson GD. A new look at proliferation. Acta Oncol 2001;40(8):989–94.

23. Wilson GD. Proliferation models in tumours. Int J Radiat Biol 2003;79(7):525–30.

24. Keng PC, Siemann DW. Measurement of proliferation activities in human tumor models: a comparison of flow cytometric methods. Radiat Oncol Investig 1998;6(3):120–7.

25. Carroll JS, Prall OW, Musgrove EA, et al. A pure estrogen antagonist inhibits cyclin E-Cdk2 activity in MCF-7 breast cancer cells and induces accumulation of p130-E2F4 complexes characteristic of quiescence. J Biol Chem 2000;275(49):38221–9.

26. Wallen CA, Higashikubo R, Dethlefsen LA. Murine mammary tumour cells in vitro. I. The development of a quiescent state. Cell Tissue Kinet 1984;17(1):65–77.

27. Wallen CA, Higashikubo R, Dethlefsen LA. Murine mammary tumour cells in vitro. II. Recruitment of quiescent cells. Cell Tissue Kinet 1984;17(1):79–89.

28. Quinones-Hinojosa A, Sanai N, Smith JS, et al. Techniques to assess the proliferative potential of brain tumors. J Neurooncol 2005;74(1):19–30.

29. Celis JE, Madsen P, Nielsen S, et al. Nuclear patterns of cyclin (PCNA) antigen distribution subdivide S-phase in cultured cells–some applications of PCNA antibodies. Leuk Res 1986;10(3):237–49.

30. Mann GJ, Musgrove EA, Fox RM, et al. Ribonucleotide reductase M1 subunit in cellular proliferation, quiescence, and differentiation. Cancer Res 1988; 48(18):5151–6.

31. Polo SE, Theocharis SE, Klijanienko J, et al. Chromatin assembly factor-1, a marker of clinical value to distinguish quiescent from proliferating cells. Cancer Res 2004;64(7):2371–81.

32. Shields AF, Lim K, Grierson J, et al. Utilization of labeled thymidine in DNA synthesis: studies for PET. J Nucl Med 1990;31(3):337–42.

33. Vander Borght T, Labar D, Pauwels S, et al. Production of [2-11C] thymidine for quantification of cellular proliferation with PET. Int J Rad Appl Instrum [A] 1991;42(1):103–4.

34. Vander Borght T, Pauwels S, Lambotte L, et al. Brain tumor imaging with PET and 2-[carbon-11] thymidine. J Nucl Med 1994;35(6):974–82.

35. Goethals P, Lameire N, van Eijkeren M, et al. [Methyl-carbon-11] thymidine for in vivo measurement of cell proliferation. J Nucl Med 1996;37(6): 1048–52.

36. Krohn KA, Mankoff DA, Eary JF. Imaging cellular proliferation as a measure of response to therapy. J Clin Pharmacol Jul 2001;41:96S–103S.

37. Mankoff DA, Shields AF, Krohn KA. PET imaging of cellular proliferation. Radiol Clin North Am 2005; 43(1):153–67.

38. Shields AF, Grierson JR, Dohmen BM, et al. Imaging proliferation in vivo with [F-18]FLT and positron emission tomography. Nat Med 1998; 4(11):1334–6.

39. Krohn KA, Mankoff DA, Muzi M, et al. True tracers: comparing FDG with glucose and FLT with thymidine. Nucl Med Biol 2005;32(7):663–71.

40. Kenny LM, Vigushin DM, Al-Nahhas A, et al. Quantification of cellular proliferation in tumor and normal tissues of patients with breast cancer by [18F]fluorothymidine-positron emission tomography imaging: evaluation of analytical methods. Cancer Res 2005;65(21):10104–12.

41. Mangner TJ, Klecker RW, Anderson L, et al. Synthesis of 2'-deoxy-2'-[18F]fluoro-beta-D-arabinofuranosyl nucleosides, [18F]FAU, [18F]FMAU, [18F]FBAU and [18F]FIAU, as potential PET agents for imaging cellular proliferation. Synthesis of [18F]labeled FAU, FMAU, FBAU, FIAU. Nucl Med Biol 2003;30(3):215–24.

42. Nimmagadda S, Mangner TJ, Sun H, et al. Biodistribution and radiation dosimetry estimates of 1-(2'-deoxy-2'-(18)F-Fluoro-1-beta-D-arabinofuranosyl)-5-bromouracil: PET imaging studies in dogs. J Nucl Med 2005;46(11):1916–22.

43. Sun H, Mangner TJ, Collins JM, et al. Imaging DNA synthesis in vivo with 18F-FMAU and PET. J Nucl Med 2005;46(2):292–6.

44. Vesselle H, Grierson J, Muzi M, et al. In vivo validation of 3 deoxy-3-[(18)F]fluorothymidine ([(18)F]FLT) as a proliferation imaging tracer in humans: correlation of [(18)F]FLT uptake by positron emission tomography with Ki-67 immunohistochemistry and flow cytometry in human lung tumors. Clin Cancer Res 2002;8(11):3315–23.

45. Buck AK, Halter G, Schirrmeister H, et al. Imaging proliferation in lung tumors with PET: 18F-FLT versus 18F-FDG. J Nucl Med 2003;44(9):1426–31.

46. Muzi M, Vesselle H, Grierson JR, et al. Kinetic analysis of 3'-deoxy-3'-fluorothymidine PET studies: validation studies in patients with lung cancer. J Nucl Med 2005;46(2):274–82.

47. Choi SJ, Kim JS, Kim JH, et al. [18F]3'-deoxy-3'-fluorothymidine PET for the diagnosis and grading of brain tumors. Eur J Nucl Med Mol Imaging 2005; 32(6):653–9.

48. Ullrich R, Backes H, Li H, et al. Glioma proliferation as assessed by 3-fluoro-3-deoxy-L-thymidine positron emission tomography in patients with newly diagnosed high-grade glioma. Clin Cancer Res 2008;14(7):2049–55.

49. Muzi M, Spence AM, O'Sullivan F, et al. Kinetic analysis of 3'-deoxy-3'-18F-fluorothymidine in patients with gliomas. J Nucl Med 2006;47(10):1612–21.

50. Schiepers C, Chen W, Dahlbom M, et al. 18F-fluorothymidine kinetics of malignant brain tumors. Eur J Nucl Med Mol Imaging 2007;34(7):1003–11.

51. Francis DL, Freeman A, Visvikis D, et al. In vivo imaging of cellular proliferation in colorectal cancer using positron emission tomography. Gut 2003; 52(11):1602–6.

52. Francis DL, Visvikis D, Costa DC, et al. Potential impact of [18F]3'-deoxy-3'-fluorothymidine versus [18F]fluoro-2-deoxy-D-glucose in positron emission tomography for colorectal cancer. Eur J Nucl Med Mol Imaging 2003;30(7):988–94.

53. Kenny L, Coombes RC, Vigushin DM, et al. Imaging early changes in proliferation at 1 week post chemotherapy: a pilot study in breast cancer patients with 3'-deoxy-3'-[18F]fluorothymidine positron emission tomography. Eur J Nucl Med Mol Imaging 2007; 34(9):1339–47.

54. Pio BS, Park CK, Pietras R, et al. Usefulness of 3-[F-18]fluoro-3'-deoxythymidine with positron emission tomography in predicting breast cancer response to therapy. Mol Imaging Biol 2006;8(1):36–42.

55. Sohn HJ, Yang YJ, Ryu JS, et al. [18F]Fluorothymidine positron emission tomography before and 7 days after gefitinib treatment predicts response in patients with advanced adenocarcinoma of the lung. Clin Cancer Res 2008;14(22):7423–9.

56. Chen W, Delaloye S, Silverman DH, et al. Predicting treatment response of malignant gliomas to bevacizumab and irinotecan by imaging proliferation with [18F] fluorothymidine positron emission tomography: a pilot study. J Clin Oncol 2007;25(30): 4714–21.

57. Herrmann K, Wieder HA, Buck AK, et al. Early response assessment using 3'-deoxy-3'-[18F]fluorothymidine-positron emission tomography in high-grade non-Hodgkin's lymphoma. Clin Cancer Res 2007;13(12):3552–8.

58. Walker JM, Bowen WD, Walker FO, et al. Sigma receptors: biology and function. Pharmacol Rev 1990;42(4):355–402.

59. Hanner M, Moebius FF, Flandorfer A, et al. Purification, molecular cloning, and expression of the mammalian sigma1-binding site. Proc Natl Acad Sci U S A 1996;93(15):8072–7.

60. Kekuda R, Prasad PD, Fei YJ, et al. Cloning and functional expression of the human type 1 sigma

receptor (hSigmaR1). Biochem Biophys Res Commun 1996;229(2):553–8.

61. Hellewell SB, Bruce A, Feinstein G, et al. Rat liver and kidney contain high densities of sigma 1 and sigma 2 receptors: characterization by ligand binding and photoaffinity labeling. Eur J Pharmacol 1994;268(1):9–18.

62. John CS, Bowen WD, Saga T, et al. A malignant melanoma imaging agent: synthesis, characterization, in vitro binding and biodistribution of iodine-125-(2-piperidinylaminoethyl)4-iodobenzamide. J Nucl Med 1993;34(12):2169–75.

63. John CS, Gulden ME, Li J, et al. Synthesis, in vitro binding, and tissue distribution of radioiodinated 2-[125I]N-(N-benzylpiperidin-4-yl)-2-iodo benzamide, 2-[125I]BP: a potential sigma receptor marker for human prostate tumors. Nucl Med Biol 1998;25(3):189–94.

64. John CE, Budygin EA, Mateo Y, et al. Neurochemical characterization of the release and uptake of dopamine in ventral tegmental area and serotonin in substantia nigra of the mouse. J Neurochem 2006; 96(1):267–82.

65. Vilner BJ, John CS, Bowen WD. Sigma-1 and sigma-2 receptors are expressed in a wide variety of human and rodent tumor cell lines. Cancer Res 1995;55(2):408–13.

66. Mach RH, Huang Y, Freeman RA, et al. Conformationally-flexible benzamide analogues as dopamine D3 and sigma 2 receptor ligands. Bioorg Med Chem Lett 2004;14(1):195–202.

67. Chu W, Tu Z, McElveen E, et al. Synthesis and in vitro binding of N-phenyl piperazine analogs as potential dopamine D3 receptor ligands. Bioorg Med Chem 2005;13(1):77–87.

68. Tu Z, Dence CS, Ponde DE, et al. Carbon-11 labeled sigma2 receptor ligands for imaging breast cancer. Nucl Med Biol 2005;32(5):423–30.

69. Tu Z, Xu J, Jones LA, et al. Fluorine-18-labeled benzamide analogues for imaging the sigma(2) receptor status of solid tumors with positron emission tomography. J Med Chem 2007;50(14):3194–204.

70. Rowland DJ, Tu Z, Xu J, et al. Synthesis and in vivo evaluation of 2 high-affinity 76Br-labeled sigma2-receptor ligands. J Nucl Med 2006;47(6):1041–8.

71. Seth P, Leibach FH, Ganapathy V. Cloning and structural analysis of the cDNA and the gene encoding the murine type 1 sigma receptor. Biochem Biophys Res Commun 1997;241(2):535–40.

PET Imaging
of Angiogenesis

Gang Niu, PhD, Xiaoyuan Chen, PhD*

KEYWORDS

- Angiogenesis • Molecular imaging
- Integrin • VEGFR • MMP

Angiogenesis refers to the process by which new blood vessels are formed and is involved in various physiologic as well as pathologic processes, including physical development, wound repair, reproduction, response to ischemia, arthritis, psoriasis, retinopathies, solid tumor growth, and metastatic tumor spread.[1] Angiogenesis is a highly controlled process that is dependent on the intricate balance of both promoting and inhibiting factors.

Antiangiogenic and antivascular agents are intensively investigated for tumor therapy and can be potentially used to control eye diseases and arthritis. Proangiogenic therapy are also undergoing clinical trials in human patients suffering from ischemic heart disease, peripheral vascular disease, chronic wounds, or stroke.[2] A comprehensive understanding of the molecular mechanisms that regulate angiogenesis has resulted in the design of new and more effective therapeutic strategies.[3] Although preclinical animal studies have demonstrated the benefit of proangiogenic therapy, recent clinical trials focused on the stimulation of myocardial or peripheral angiogenesis by the local delivery of growth factors were somewhat disappointing, showing no clear benefit over placebo in subjects with severe ischemia.[4] Most of these studies evaluated angiogenesis by using standard clinical endpoints or by looking for a physiologic improvement (ie, improvement in perfusion). These approaches may have insufficient sensitivity to detect a therapeutic benefit.

For tumor therapy, bevacizumab, a humanized monoclonal antibody directed against vascular endothelial growth factor (VEGF), is the first drug developed as an inhibitor of angiogenesis approved by the Food and Drug Administration (FDA).[5–7] Sorafenib and sunitinib that target multiple receptor tyrosine kinases (VEGF receptors and platelet-derived growth factor—PDGF—receptors), have also been approved by the FDA as antiangiogenic drugs.[8] Traditionally, the gold standard to evaluate therapeutic response is tumor volume change. Clinical trials with conventional cytotoxic chemotherapeutic agents have mainly used morphologic imaging to provide indices of therapeutic response, mostly CT or MR imaging according to the Response Evaluation Criteria in Solid Tumors introduced in 2000.[9] However, antiangiogenic agents are typically cytostatic rather than cytotoxic and lead to a stop or delay of tumor progression rather than tumor shrinkage. Thus, it is not sensitive to use tumor volume as an indicator for therapeutic efficacy evaluation and it might take months or years to assess.

Both the success and setback in angiogenesis-related therapies spur the need for the development of noninvasive imaging strategies for the direct noninvasive evaluation of molecular events associated with angiogenesis. Imaging is

Some of the research presented in this article was supported in part by the National Institute of Biomedical Imaging and Bioengineering (R21 EB001785), National Cancer Institute (R21 CA102123, P50 CA114747, U54 CA119367, and R24 CA93862), Department of Defense (W81XWH-04-1-0697, W81XWH-06-1-0665, W81XWH-06-1-0042, and DAMD17-03-1-0143), and a Department of Defense Prostate Postdoctoral Fellowship from Department of Defense (to G.N.)

The Molecular Imaging Program at Stanford, Department of Radiology and Bio-X Program, Stanford University School of Medicine, 1201 Welch Road, P095, Stanford, CA 94305-5484, USA

* Corresponding author.

E-mail address: shawchen@stanford.edu (X. Chen).

PET Clin 4 (2009) 17–38

doi:10.1016/j.cpet.2009.04.011

expected to provide a novel approach to noninvasively monitor angiogenesis, to optimize the dose of new antiangiogenic agents, and to assess the efficacy of therapies directed at modulation of the angiogenic process.[10–13] This article, after brief introduction of angiogenesis biology and structure and functional imaging of angiogenesis with various imaging modalities, focuses on the application of PET in angiogenesis imaging at both the functional and molecular level.

BIOLOGY OF ANGIOGENESIS

The whole angiogenesis process involves several steps, including the growth of endothelial sprouts from pre-existing postcapillary venules and following the growth and remodeling process of the primitive network into a complex network.[14] The cellular and molecular mechanisms of angiogenesis differ in various tissues and physiologic or pathologic angiogenesis.[15] This section gives a brief introduction of tumor angiogenesis.

Each solid malignancy starts as a small population of transformed cells that do not initially have a blood supply of their own. Tumor cells are initially supplied by diffusion and tumor growth is limited by the lack of access to growth factors, circulating oxygen, and nutrients.[16] Without angiogenesis, the growth of solid tumors remains restricted to 2 mm to 3 mm in diameter.[17] Tumor angiogenesis occurs as a series of events.[18,19] First, diseased tissues produce and release angiogenic growth factors that diffuse into the nearby tissues in response to tumor hypoxia, such as the VEGF, the acidic and basic fibroblast growth factors (aFGF, bFGF), and the platelet-derived endothelial cell growth factor.[20] When the angiogenic growth factors bind to their corresponding specific receptors located on the endothelial cells of pre-existing blood vessels, various signal transduction pathways are activated, for example phosphorylation of tyrosine kinases, protein kinases, and MAP kinases, and consequently to the activation of endothelial cells.[21,22] Consequently, the original vessels undergo characteristic morphologic changes, including enlargement of the diameter, basement membrane degradation, a thinned endothelial cell lining, increased endothelial number, decreased pericyte number, and pericyte detachment.[23] In the next step, several different mechanisms may lead to the formation of new tumor blood vessels.[24,25] The original vessels may retain their large diameter and evolve into medium-sized arteries and veins by acquiring a smooth muscle and internal elastica. Alternatively, the endothelium of a mother vessel may form smaller, separate, well-differentiated vessel channels by projecting cytoplasmic structures into the lumen, which form translumenal bridges. A third process is called "intussusception" and involves focal invagination of connective tissue pillars from within the mother vessel. Finally, endothelial cell-sprouting may occur, which requires the focal dissolution of the basement membrane surrounding mother vessels.[26] This is achieved by a number of proteolytic enzymes, including matrix metalloproteinases (MMPs) and plasminogen activator, which enable endothelial cells to exit the vessel. Activated angiogenic endothelial cells proliferate rapidly and migrate into the extracellular matrix toward the angiogenic stimulus.[27] Cell surface-adhesion molecules, such as integrins, play an important role in endothelial cell migration and in contact with the extracellular tumor matrix, facilitate cell survival.[28,29] At the sprouting tips of growing vessels, endothelial cells secrete MMPs that facilitate degradation of the extracellular matrix and cell invasion.[30] Next, a lumen within an endothelial cell tubule has to be formed, which requires interactions between the extracellular matrix and cell-associated surface proteins, among them are galectin-2, PECAM-1, and VE-cadherin.[31] Finally, newly formed vessels are stabilized through the recruitment of smooth muscle cells and pericytes.

STRUCTURAL IMAGING OF VASCULATURE/ ANGIOGENESIS

All imaging modalities can provide structural information, although they have different spatial resolution. The old-fashioned way for vascular structure imaging is X-ray angiography. However, it is difficult to provide microvasculature information. Following the steps of improvement of imaging equipments, contrast agents, and data acquisition and analysis techniques, more detailed vascular structure was deciphered. Several modalities are available for tumor microvascular imaging, including intravital microscope, CT angiography, contrast-enhanced ultrasound (US), and high-resolution MR angiography.[32] Ex vivo structural imaging of tumor vasculature can be achieved by various techniques, such as vascular casts,[33,34] immunohistochemic staining of endothelial cell markers such as CD31 and von Willebrand factor,[35,36] labeling the endothelial cells by fluorescent reporters expressed in transgenic mice,[37,38] and intravital labeling.[39,40] Tumor macrovasculature imaging can be performed clinically by various imaging modalities, such as CT,[41,42] MR imaging,[43,44] and US.[45] However, visualization of the microvasculature is very challenging even after administration of intravascular contrast agents.

Scanners dedicated to small-animal imaging studies, such as microCT, have better spatial resolution in preclinical models but with poor temporal resolution and large radiation exposure.[46]

Intravital microscopy of tumors growing in window chambers in animal models can directly investigate tumor angiogenesis and vascular response to treatment, in terms of both the morphology of the vascular networks and the function of individual vessels.[47] This technique allows for repeated measurements of the same tumor with very high resolution (down to submicrometer level). Multiphoton fluorescence microscopy techniques have also been applied to these model systems to obtain three-dimensional images of the tumor vasculature.[47]

FUNCTIONAL IMAGING OF VASCULATURE

The major consequence of angiogenesis is to perfuse and oxygenate surrounding tissue; therefore, the angiogenic process can be assessed by the evaluation of standard physiologic parameters, such as regional perfusion, function, and metabolism. During antiangiogenic or proangiogenic therapies, the changes in hemodynamic parameters can also be promising biomarkers for evaluating the therapeutic effect along with morphologic changes. Traditionally, tumor angiogenesis and antiangiogenic therapy have been evaluated by methods such as measurement of circulating angiogenic markers and histologic estimate of microvascular density. Various imaging modalities, including dynamic contrast-enhanced (DCE) MR imaging, US, PET (especially with [^{15}O]water), and DCE-CT are currently employed to provide functional information of the vasculature.[48]

DCE-MR imaging has been well established to investigate angiogenesis within tumors, and in particular the response to antiangiogenic therapy. DCE-MR imaging works by tracking the pharmacokinetics of injected contrast agents as they pass through the tumor vasculature, which represents a complex summation of vascular permeability, blood flow, vascular surface area, and interstitial pressure.[49,50]

DCE-MR imaging can be performed with low-molecular-weight contrast media (LMCM) such as Gd-diethylenetriamine pentaacetic acid (Gd-DTPA) or macromolecular contrast media (MMCM), such as Gd conjugated human serum albumin.[51] It has been shown that DCE-MR imaging can detect responses to PTK/ZK (a VEGF receptor-tyrosine kinase inhibitor) therapy as early as 2 days after therapy with significant reductions in area under gadolinium-contrast-medium curve[52]

or permeability parameters,[53] which also predict subsequent response. LMCM DCE-MR imaging has also shown significant reductions in permeability values in patients treated with the antivascular agents AG-013,736 (an inhibitor of the VEGF, PDGF, and c-Kit receptor tyrosine kinases) and SU5416 (a selective inhibitor of VEGFR-2 tyrosine kinase) activity.[54] Although consensus is still lacking on the exact kinetic model to be used in analyzing DCE-MR imaging data, the differences among the various methods are often marginal. Therefore, DCE-MR imaging is rapidly emerging as the imaging technique of choice for monitoring clinical response in trials of new antiangiogenic and antivascular therapies. Unlike LMCM, the increased size of MMCMs makes them less diffusible, and K^{trans} values may reflect permeability within tumors more accurately.[55] MMCMs can also give more accurate estimates of tumor blood volume because they are excellent blood-pool agents. For example, SU6668 is an oral, small-molecule inhibitor of angiogenic receptor tyrosine kinases, such as VEGFR-2 (Flk-1/KDR), PDGFR, and FGF receptor. DCE-MR imaging clearly detected the early effect (after 24 hours of treatment) of SU6668 on tumor vasculature as a 51% and 26% decrease in the average vessel permeability measured in the tumor rim and core, respectively. A substantial decrease was also observed in average fractional plasma volume in the rim (59%) and core (35%) of the tumor.[56,57] In addition to DCE-MR imaging, other MR imaging techniques have also been developed to retrieve functional information of the vasculature. In arterial spin labeling, water molecules can be labeled for MR imgaging by inverting the nuclear spin of their hydrogen atoms with a radiofrequency pulse directed at the arterial blood before it enters the regions of interest (ROIs).[50,60] An absolute value of blood flow is determined by the change in the MR signal as the labeled water in the arterial bloodstream arrives in the ROI.[60] Blood-oxygen-level dependent MR imaging can detect the changes in oxygen saturation of the blood and this effect can be enhanced by increasing the amount of oxygen in the breathed air.[61,62]

US is also well established as a means of measuring blood flow or, more precisely, blood velocity using the Doppler principle or microbubbles as contrast agent.[63–66] Power Doppler can be quantified to give an estimate of the relative fractional vascular volume, while microbubbles can show blood flow down to the microcirculation level by raising the signal from smaller vessels.[67,68] Specialized contrast-specific US techniques have been developed for improving image qualities, such as pulse inversion[69,70] and power modulation.[71] Given the fundamental assumption that the relation between microbubble-concentration video intensity is linear up to the achievement of a plateau phase,[72] in animal models contrast-enhanced US can quantify tumor vascularity determined by neoangiogenesis.[73,74] The use of US contrast agents and nonlinear processing provide access to the bulk properties of the microvascular compartment but they do not offer sufficient resolution to observe the morphology and detailed flow characteristics of the microvasculature. With high-frequency US, it is possible to achieve resolution ranging from 15 μm to 100 μm in the 20-MHz to 100-MHz range.[45] However, it is subject to an inherent trade-off between image resolution and imaging depth.[75] US (particularly microbubble contrast-enhanced US) is a valuable imaging modality to determine the tumor microvascular-blood volume and blood velocity.[76] DCE-US allows repeated examinations and provides both morphologic and functional analyses. US modes, based on the second harmonic signal generated by the nonlinear properties of contrast agents, have provided access to tumor blood flow with the quantification of the contrast-uptake kinetics within tumors after a bolus injection of contrast agent.[77] Several quantitative parameters considered as indicators of tumor flow, such as the peak intensity or time-to-peak intensity, can be extracted from the time-intensity curves of contrast uptake.[78] Using DCE-US, the antitumor efficacy of AVE8062, a tumor vasculature-disruptive agent, has been assessed in melanoma-bearing nude mice.[79]

Many other imaging modalities can also reveal the functional properties of the vasculature. DCE-CT is analogous to DCE-MR imaging.[80,81] To minimize the exposure to ionizing radiation and the nephrotoxicity of CT contrast agents, DCE-CT studies are typically quite brief, using only a low dose of contrast agent. Optical imaging can also be applied to evaluate important functional indexes of blood vessels, such as vascular permeability, vessel size, and blood flow.[82] Multiphoton microscopy in combination with fluorescently labeled molecules can be used to quantify the permeability of individual tumor blood vessels noninvasively deep inside living animals.[83] Fluorescence-mediated tomography has been applied to measure angiogenesis in superficial tissue by using fluorescent nanoparticles.[84] However, optical imaging is still limited to tissue and animal models.

PET IMAGING

So far, PET is the most sensitive and specific technique for imaging molecular pathways in vivo in humans.[85] PET radiotracers are physiologically and pharmacologically relevant compounds labeled with positron-emitting radioisotopes (such as fluoride-18 or carbon-11). After internalization by injection or inhalation, the tracer reaches the target and the location and the quantity is then detected with a PET scanner. With a ring-shaped array of photoelectric crystals, PET detectors capture "coincidentally" a pair of 511 keV photons at almost 180° separation emitted by interaction of a positron with negatively charged electrons. The raw PET-scan data are the set of coincidental photoelectric events, logged for time and location, which indicate the position of the molecule spatiotemporally. Using reconstruction algorithms, images can then be constructed tomographically and regional time activities can be derived.[86]

The inherent sensitivity and specificity of PET is the major strength of this technique. Isotopes can be detected down to the 100-picomolar level in the target tissues. At this low level, the compounds often have little or no physiologic effect on the patient or the test animal, which permits studying the mechanism of action or biodistribution independent of any physiologic consequences.[87,88] The spatial resolution of PET down to the millimeter level permits applications not only to human beings for diagnosis and drug development but also to animals for preclinical studies. The ability of PET to translate studies from animals to human beings adds to its appeal.

Compared with single-photon emission computed tomography (SPECT), PET offers increased spatial information and permits more accurate attenuation correction. Many PET radiotracers have a short half-life, which allows for repetitive imaging over time. However, the anatomic resolution of PET (approximately 4 mm^3–8 mm^3 in clinical and 1 mm^3–2 mm^3 in small-animal imaging systems) is noticeably poorer than that achieved by CT or MR imaging.[89] The variable movement of positrons before annihilation, and the deviation of the generated 511 keV photons from the exact 180° angular separation, can limit the resolution. To overcome this limitation, hybrid systems such as PET-CT have been introduced.[90] The CT component of the hybrid system is used to improve anatomic definition of the ROIs for analysis and to create radiation-attenuation maps to correct for nonuniform attenuation.[91] With the development of microPET or microPET/CT scanners dedicated to small-animal imaging studies, PET can provide a similar in vivo imaging capability in mice, rats, monkeys, and human beings, so one can readily transfer knowledge and molecular measurements between species.[92,93] Initial experiments with PET/MR imaging prototypes also showed very promising results, indicating its great potential for clinical and preclinical imaging.[94]

Functional Imaging of Angiogenesis with PET

A major advantage of the nuclear medicine techniques especially using PET tracers is that they are truly quantitative and that the tissue concentration C_t can be measured noninvasively.[95] ^{133}Xe has been used to measure regional cerebral blood flow[96] and ^{11}C-microspheres of approximately 10-μm diameter have been used as the gold standard for perfusion measurements or for validation of new imaging methods for perfusion measurement.[97]

Today, most PET-perfusion measurements are performed using ^{15}O-H$_2$O, using either static or dynamic PET imaging.[98] ^{15}O-H$_2$O satisfies all the requirements for a perfusion tracer in Fick's model[99] (1) because it is biologically and metabolically inert, and freely diffusible into and out of tissue water.

$$C_t = P^* \int (C_i - C_e) d_t \qquad (1)$$

C_t = tissue concentration, mol*ml$_{tissue}$$^{-1}$; C_i = Influx concentration, mol*ml$_{carrier}$$^{-1}$

C_e = eflux concentration, mol*ml$_{carrier}$$^{-1}$; P = Perfusion, ml$_{carrier}$ * min^{-1}* ml$_{tissue}$$^{-1}$

Thus, "tissue water" can be modeled as a single compartment including both tissue and its draining fluids (lymphatics and veins). Two methods can be used for measuring perfusion with [^{15}O]H$_2$O, the steady-state method, and the ^{15}O-dynamic water method.[100,101] The latter is currently used most often for perfusion studies because of improved PET scanner technology. The tracer is administered by inhalation or by peripheral venous bolus injection. Continuous arterial data are obtained either by image-based arterial input functions (a large vessel like the aorta or the left ventricle) or by peripheral sampling to a well-counter device. The data are compatible with those from diseases investigated with other methods, and the values reported by PET for tumors are within the reported range for PET in other tissues.[102,103] In locally advanced breast cancer, first results with dynamic ^{15}O-H$_2$O PET are promising, as tumor blood flow decreased in the responder group after chemotherapy, whereas it increased in the nonresponder group.[104]

PET imaging can also be used to derive data on blood volume and vascular permeability. Blood volume imaging with PET uses ^{15}O-CO or ^{11}C-CO carbon monoxide. ^{15}O-CO binds irreversibly with hemoglobin to form ^{15}O-CO-Hb carboxyhemoglobin.[86] Because ^{15}O-CO-Hb remains exclusively within the vasculature, it can be used as a tracer of vascular volume. A tissue concentration dataset is obtained over a further 5 to 6 minutes and an arterial ^{15}O-CO-Hb concentration curve is derived from a series of arterial blood samples over the same interval. Another method for blood volume imaging is labeling red blood cells or albumin with radionuclides, because both are too large to leave normal blood vessels and are retained in the blood pool. In tumor vessels, leakage of these contrast agents into the tumor will occur, but this effect can be used to calculate the tumor vessel permeability when dynamic imaging is performed. For PET, the tracer ^{68}Ga-DOTA-albumin has been developed and showed favorable results in first animal studies.[105]

Imaging of Molecular Markers of Vasculature

Even though structural and functional imaging of the vasculature can reveal potentially useful information before, during, and after therapeutic intervention, they do not convey enough knowledge about the biologic changes upon therapy at the molecular level, which may occur long before any structural or functional changes can be detected. While techniques such as DCE-MR imaging and ^{15}O-H$_2$O PET for the assessment of hemodynamic parameters are widely used, the interpretation of the results with regard to their physiologic meaning often remains difficult. Therefore, more specific markers of angiogenic activity are necessary for pretherapeutic assessment of angiogenesis and response evaluation during therapy. One approach is to identify molecular markers of angiogenesis—such as receptors, enzymes, or extracellular matrix proteins—and to use specific ligands to these targets conjugated with imaging probes for PET, SPECT, MR imaging, optical imaging, or US.[106–108] Several molecular imaging makers including integrins, VEGF/VEGFR, MMPs, and Hypoxia/HIF1 are angiogenesis-related and PET imaging targeting to these markers is discussed in the following sections.

PET imaging of integrins

Integrins, a family of cell-adhesion molecules, are involved in a wide range of cell-extracellular matrix and cell-cell interactions.[28,109] Integrins are heterodimeric transmembrane glycoproteins consisting of different α- and β-subunits, which play an important role in cell-cell- and cell-matrix-interactions.[110] In mammals, 18-α and 8-β subunits assemble into at least 24 different receptors.[111] Integrins expressed on endothelial cells modulate cell migration and survival during angiogenesis, while integrins expressed on carcinoma cells potentiate metastasis by facilitating invasion and movement across the blood vessels. The $\alpha_v\beta_3$ integrin, which binds to Arginine-Glycine-Aspartic acid (RGD)-containing components of the interstitial matrix, such as vitronectin, fibronectin, and thrombospondin,[112,113] is expressed in a number of tumor types, such as melanoma, late-stage glioblastoma, ovarian, breast, and prostate cancer.[114–116] The critical role of integrin $\alpha_v\beta_3$ in tumor invasion and metastasis arises from its ability to recruit and activate MMP-2 and plasmin, which can degrade components of the basement membrane and interstitial matrix.[117] Among all 24 integrins discovered to date, integrin $\alpha_v\beta_3$ is the most intensively studied, though many other integrins, such as $\alpha_v\beta_1$, $\alpha_v\beta_5$, $\alpha_5\beta_1$, and $\alpha_4\beta_1$ also play important roles in regulating angiogenesis.[29,118–121]

Several extracellular matrix proteins like vitronectin, fibrinogen, and fibronectin interact via the RGD tripeptide sequence with the integrins.[113] Based on these findings, linear as well as cyclic RGD peptides have been introduced and showed high affinity and selectivity for $\alpha_v\beta_3$.[122,123] The first in vivo application of radioiodinated RGD peptides revealed the receptor-specific tumor uptake but also predominantly hepatobiliary elimination, resulting in high activity concentration in the liver and small intestine.[124] Consequently, several strategies to improve the pharmacokinetics of radiohalogenated peptides have been studied, including conjugation with sugar moieties, hydrophilic amino acids and polyethylene glycol (PEG).[125–128] Besides radiohalogenated RGD peptides, a variety of radiometalated tracers have been developed as well, including peptides labeled with ^{111}In, ^{99m}Tc, ^{64}Cu, ^{90}Y, ^{188}Re, and ^{68}Ga.[129–132] Most of them are based on the cyclic pentapeptide and are conjugated via the γ-amino function of a lysine with different chelator systems, like DTPA, the tetrapeptide sequence H-Asp-Lys-Cys-Lys-OH, 1, 4, 7, 10-tetraazacyclododecane-N-N''-N''-N'''-tetraacetic acid (DOTA), and 1,4,7-triazacyclononane-1,4,7-triacetic acid. While all these compounds have shown high receptor affinity and selectivity and specific tumor accumulation, the pharmacokinetics of most of them still have to be improved.[133] Among them, the compound ^{99m}Tc-NC100692 by GE Healthcare has been used for SPECT imaging in preclinical and clinical studies.[134]

In a human melanoma M21 model, ^{18}F-Galacto-RGD showed a tumor uptake of 1.5%ID/g at 120 minutes after injection.[135,136] Integrin receptor-specific accumulation was demonstrated by blocking experiments injecting c(RGDfV) 10 minutes before tracer injection, which reduced

tumor accumulation to approximately 35% of control. A correlation between integrin expression and tracer accumulation was observed in imaging studies with mice bearing melanoma tumors with increasing amounts of $\alpha_v\beta_3$-positive cells.[137] These data demonstrate that noninvasive determination of $\alpha_v\beta_3$ expression and quantification with radiolabeled RGD peptides is feasible with PET scans. ^{18}F-Galacto-RGD has also been applied to patients and successfully imaged $\alpha_v\beta_3$ expression in human tumors with good tumor-background ratios.[138] Rapid clearance of ^{18}F-Galacto-RGD from the blood pool and primarily renal excretion was confirmed by following biodistribution and dosimetry studies. Background activity in lung and muscle tissue was low and the calculated effective dose is very similar to an ^{18}F-FDG scan (**Fig. 1**).[138] Results from dynamic emission scans over 60 minutes and kinetic modeling studies suggested that standardized uptake values (SUVs) derived from static emission scans at approximately 60 minutes after injection can be used for the assessment of $\alpha_v\beta_3$ receptor density with reasonable accuracy.[139] SUVs and tumor-blood ratios based on PET imaging using ^{18}F-Galacto-RGD were also found to correlate with the intensity of immunohistochemical staining of $\alpha_v\beta_3$ expression, as well as with the microvessel density.[140] Good tumor-background ratios with ^{18}F-Galacto-RGD PET also have been demonstrated in squamous cell carcinoma of the head and neck with a widely varying intensity of tracer uptake. Immunohistochemistry demonstrated predominantly vascular $\alpha_v\beta_3$ expression, thus in squamous cell carcinoma of the head and neck, ^{18}F-Galacto-RGD PET might be used as a surrogate parameter of angiogenesis.[141] Moreover, there was no obvious correlation between the tracer uptake of ^{18}F-FDG and ^{18}F-Galacto-RGD in patients with various tumors, indicating that $\alpha_v\beta_3$ expression and glucose metabolism are not closely correlated in tumor lesions and that consequently ^{18}F-FDG cannot provide similar information as ^{18}F-Galacto-RGD.[142]

Within physiologic ^{18}F-Galacto-RGD uptake areas, such as liver, spleen, and intestine, lesion identification is still problematic. Therefore, multimeric RGD peptides have been developed to provide more effective antagonists with better targeting capability and higher cellular uptake through the integrin-dependent binding.[143] The underlying rationale is that the interaction between integrin $\alpha_v\beta_3$ and RGD-containing extracellular matrix-proteins involves multivalent binding sites with clustering of integrins. A series of multimeric RGD peptides labeled with ^{18}F or ^{64}Cu for PET imaging to improve the tumor-targeting

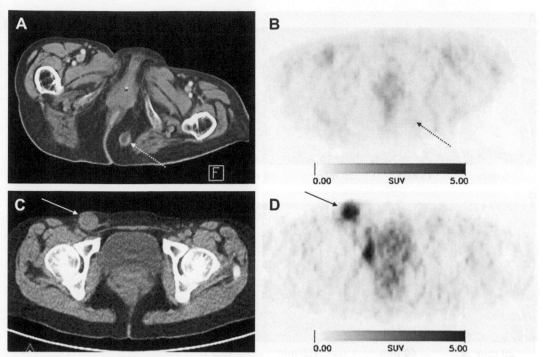

Fig. 1. ^{18}F-Galacto-RGD scans of two patients with metastases from malignant melanoma and different tracer uptake. (*Upper row*) An 89-year-old female patient with metastasis in subcutaneous fat in gluteal area on left side (*arrow with dotted line*). Tumor can be clearly delineated in CT scan (*A*), whereas it shows no significant uptake in ^{18}F-Galacto-RGD PET scan (*B*) (60 minutes after injection). (*Lower row*) A 36-year-old female patient with lymph node metastasis in right groin (*arrow*). Again, tumor is clearly visualized in CT scan (*C*) but also shows intense tracer uptake in ^{18}F-Galacto-RGD PET scan (*D*) (89 minutes after injection; SUV, 6.8). (*From* Beer AJ, Haubner R, Goebel M, et al. Biodistribution and pharmacokinetics of the $\alpha_v\beta_3$-selective tracer ^{18}F-galacto-RGD in cancer patients. J Nucl Med 2005;46(8):1340; with permission.)

efficacy and pharmacokinetics have been reported.[130,144–148] ^{18}F-FB-E[c(RGDyK)]$_2$ (abbreviated as ^{18}F-FRGD2) showed predominantly renal excretion and almost twice as much tumor uptake in the same animal model when compared with the monomeric tracer ^{18}F-FB-c(RGDyK).[144,145] Tumor uptakes quantified by microPET scans in six tumor xenograft models correlated well with integrin $\alpha_v\beta_3$ expression level measured by sodium dodecyl sulfate-polyacrylamide gel electrophoresis autoradiography. The tetrameric RGD peptide-based tracer, ^{18}F-E[E[c(RGDfK)]$_2$]$_2$, showed significantly higher receptor binding affinity than the corresponding monomeric and dimeric RGD analogs and demonstrated rapid blood clearance, high metabolic stability, predominant renal excretion, and significant receptor-mediated tumor uptake with good contrast in xenograft-bearing mice (**Fig. 2**).[148] Therefore, ^{18}F-E[E[c(RGDfK)]$_2$]$_2$ is a promising agent for peptide receptor radionuclide imaging as well as targeted internal radiotherapy of integrin $\alpha_v\beta_3$-positive tumors. Compared with tetramer, RGD octamer further increased the integrin avidity by another threefold.

In vivo microPET imaging showed that ^{64}Cu-DOTA-RGD octamer had slightly higher initial tumor uptake and much longer tumor retention in U87MG tumor that express high levels of integrin.[149] However, compared with tetramers, higher renal uptake of the octamer was observed, which was attributed mainly to the integrin positivity of the kidneys. Wester and Kessler groups have also synthesized a series of monomeric, dimeric, tetrameric, and octameric RGD peptides. These compounds contain different numbers of c(RGDfE) peptides connected via PEG linker and lysine moieties, which are used as branching units.[150,151]

Besides RGD peptides, in vivo imaging using etaracizumab, a humanized monoclonal antibody against human integrin $\alpha_v\beta_3$, has been performed after DOTA conjugation and ^{64}Cu labeling. MicroPET studies revealed that ^{64}Cu-DOTA-etaracizumab had a high tumor-activity accumulation up to 49.41% plus or minus 4.54% injected dose per gram at 71 hours after injection for U87MG tumors.[152] Not only in malignant diseases: the integrin expression after myocardial infarction has also been monitored with ^{18}F-Galacto-RGD

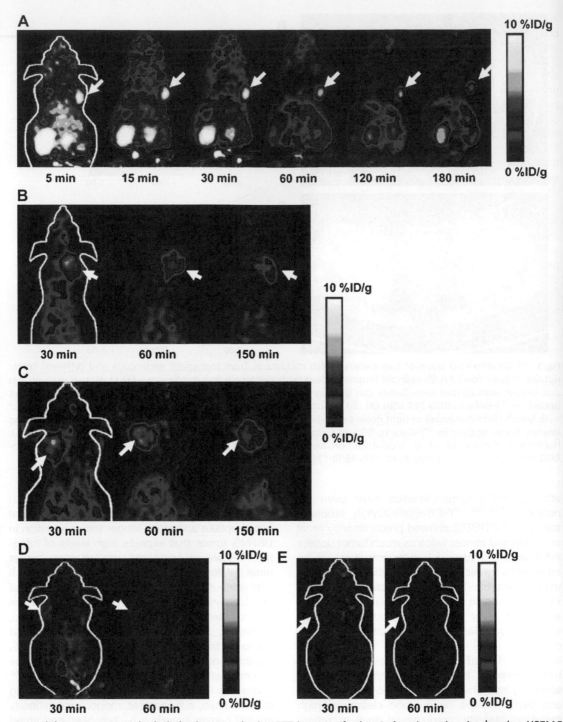

Fig. 2. (A) Decay-corrected whole-body coronal microPET images of athymic female nude mice bearing U87MG tumor at 5, 15, 30, 60, 120, and 180 minutes after injection of ^{18}F-FPRGD4 [3.7 MBq (100 μCi)]. (B) Decay-corrected whole-body coronal microPET images of c-neu oncomice at 30, 60, and 150 minutes (5-minute static image) after intravenous injection of ^{18}F-FPRGD4. (C) Decay-corrected whole-body coronal microPET images of orthotopic MDA-MB-435 tumor-bearing mouse at 30, 60, and 150 minutes after intravenous injection of ^{18}F-FPRGD4. (D) Decay-corrected whole-body coronal microPET images of DU-145 tumor-bearing mouse (5-minute static image) after intravenous injection of ^{18}F-FPRGD4. (E) Coronal microPET images of a U87MG tumor-bearing mouse at 30 and 60 minutes after coinjection of ^{18}F-FPRGD4 and a blocking dose of c(RGDyK). Arrows indicate tumors in all cases. (From Wu Z, Li ZB, Chen K, et al. MicroPET of tumor integrin $\alpha_v\beta_3$ expression using ^{18}F-labeled PEGylated tetrameric RGD peptide (^{18}F-FPRGD4). J Nucl Med 2007;48(9):1540; with permission.)

in a Wister rat model. PET imaging and autoradiography revealed focal accumulation in the infarct area started at day 3, peaked between 1 and 3 weeks, and decreased to day 3 level at 6 months after reperfusion. The time course of focal tracer uptake paralleled vascular density as measured by CD31 immunohistochemical analysis, indicating that ^{18}F-Galacto-RGD is promising for the monitoring of myocardial repair processes.[153] The results from this study encourage the application of RGD-PET imaging to monitor the angiogenesis in other noncancer diseases.

PET imaging of VEGF and its receptors

VEGF, a potent mitogen in embryonic and somatic angiogenesis, plays a pivotal role in both normal vascular tissue development and many disease processes.[154,155] The VEGF family is composed of seven members with a common VEGF homology domain: VEGF-A, -B, -C, -D, -E, -F, and placenta growth factor.[5] VEGF-A is a dimeric, disulfide-bound glycoprotein existing in at least seven homodimeric isoforms, consisting of 121, 145, 148, 165, 183, 189, or 206 amino acids. Besides the difference in molecular weight, these isoforms also differ in their biologic properties such as the ability to bind to cell-surface heparin-sulfate proteoglycans.[5]

The angiogenic actions of VEGF are mainly mediated via two endothelium-specific receptor tyrosine kinases, Flt-1 (VEGFR-1) and Flk-1/KDR (VEGFR-2).[156] Both VEGFRs are largely restricted to vascular endothelial cells and all VEGF-A isoforms bind to both VEGFR-1 and VEGFR-2. It is now generally accepted that VEGFR-1 is critical for physiologic and developmental angiogenesis and its function varies with the stages of development, the states of physiologic and pathologic conditions, and the cell types in which it is expressed.[5,155] VEGFR-2 is the major mediator of the mitogenic, angiogenic, and permeability-enhancing effects of VEGF. Over-expression of VEGF and VEGFRs has been implicated as poor prognostic markers in various clinical studies.[5] Agents that prevent VEGF-A binding to its receptors,[157] antibodies that directly block VEGFR-2[158,159] and small molecules that inhibit the kinase activity of VEGFR-2 and thereby block growth factor signaling,[65,160,161] are all currently under active development. The critical role of VEGF-A in cancer progression has been highlighted by the approval of the humanized anti-VEGF monoclonal antibody bevacizumab for first-line cancer treatment.[162] Development of VEGF- or VEGFR-targeted molecular imaging probes could serve as a new paradigm for the assessment of antiangiogenic therapeutics and for better

understanding the role and expression profile of VEGF/VEGFR in many angiogenesis-related diseases. VEGF/VEGFR has been imaged by various imaging modalities, though PET is the dominant technique for direct VEGF/VEGFR imaging.[163] In the clinical setting, the right timing can be critical for VEGFR-targeted cancer therapy and noninvasive imaging of VEGF/VEGFR can help in determining whether to start and when to start VEGFR-targeted treatment. With the development of new tracers with better targeting efficacy and desirable pharmacokinetics, clinical translation will be critical for the maximum benefit of VEGF-based imaging agents.

VEGF imaging has been investigated, especially with radiolabeled-specific antibodies.[164] VG76e, an IgG1 monoclonal antibody that binds to human VEGF, was labeled with [124]I for PET imaging of solid tumor xenografts in immune-deficient mice.[165] Whole-animal PET imaging studies revealed a high tumor-to-background contrast. Although VEGF specificity in vivo was demonstrated in this report, the poor immunoreactivity (< 35%) of the radiolabeled antibody limits the potential use of this tracer. HuMV833, the humanized version of a mouse monoclonal anti-VEGF antibody MV833, was also labeled with [124]I and the distribution and biologic effects of HuMV833 in patients in a phase I clinical trial were investigated.[166] Patients with progressive solid tumors were treated with various doses of HuMV833, and PET imaging using [124]I-HuMV833 was performed to measure the antibody distribution in and clearance from tissues. It was found that antibody distribution and clearance were quite heterogeneous not only between and within patients but also between and within individual tumors. Bevacizumab, a humanized monoclonal antibody against VEGF, has been labeled with ^{111}In to image VEGF-A expression in nude mice models or patients with colorectal liver metastases.[167] Although enhanced uptake of ^{111}In-bevacizumab in the liver metastases was observed in 9 of the 12 patients, there was no correlation between the level of ^{111}In-antibody accumulation and the level of VEGF-A expression in the tissue, as determined by in situ hybridization and ELISA.[167]

Bevacizumab has also been labeled with the PET isotope [89]Zr for noninvasive in vivo VEGF visualization and quantification. On small-animal PET images, radiolabeled bevacizumab showed higher uptake compared with radiolabeled human IgG in a human SKOV-3 ovarian tumor xenograft. Tracer uptake in other organs was seen primarily in the liver and spleen (**Fig. 3**).[164] A recent study showed that there was a significant ^{18}F-FDG kinetics correlation between k1 (the transport coefficient) and VEGF-A mRNA level determined

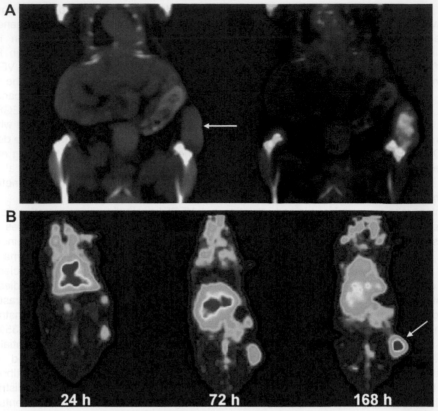

Fig. 3. (*A*) Coronal CT image and fusion of microPET and CT images (168 hours after injection) enables adequate quantitative measurement of ^{89}Zr-bevacizumab in the tumor. (*B*) Coronal planes of microPET images after injection of ^{89}Zr-bevacizumab. *Arrows* indicate SKOV-3 tumors. (*Reproduced from* Nagengast WB, de Vries EG, Hospers GA, et al. In vivo VEGF imaging with radiolabeled bevacizumab in a human ovarian tumor xenograft. J Nucl Med 2007;48(8):1316; with permission.)

by gene chip assay ($r = 0.51$), indicating the possibility to predict the gene expression of VEGF-A with the regression functions from the FDG-PET parameters.[168]

VEGF/VEGFR interactions is one of the most extensively studied angiogenesis-related signaling pathways.[163] The alternative to overcome the difficulty induced by the soluble and more dynamic nature of VEGF is to image VEGFRs, other indicators of angiogenesis that have superior accessibility. VEGF isoforms exist in nature and have very strong binding affinity and specificity to VEGFRs.[163,169] Therefore, a generic strategy is to label these VEGF isoforms with radionuclides to image VEGFR expression. VEGF$_{121}$ is a soluble, nonheparin-binding variant that exists in solution as a disulfide-linked homodimer containing the full biologic and receptor-binding activity of the larger variants.[5] VEGF$_{121}$ has been labeled with ^{64}Cu ($t_{1/2} = 12.7$ hours) for PET imaging of tumor angiogenesis and VEGFR expression.[170] DOTA-VEGF$_{121}$ exhibited nanomolar receptor-binding

affinity (comparable to VEGF$_{121}$) in vitro. MicroPET imaging revealed rapid, specific, and prominent uptake of ^{64}Cu-DOTA-VEGF$_{121}$ (10%~15%ID/g) in highly vascularized small U87MG tumor (60 mm^3) with high VEGFR-2 expression but significantly lower and sporadic uptake (~3%ID/g) in large U87MG tumor (1,200 mm^3) with low VEGFR-2 expression (**Fig. 4**). Western blotting of tumor tissue lysate, immunofluorescence staining, and blocking studies with unlabeled VEGF$_{121}$ confirmed that the tumor uptake is VEGFR-specific. This was the first report on PET imaging of VEGFR expression. This study also demonstrated the dynamic nature of VEGFR expression during tumor progression in that even for the same tumor model, VEGFR expression level can be dramatically different at different stages. Successful demonstration of the ability of ^{64}Cu-DOTA-VEGF$_{121}$ to visualize VEGFR expression in vivo should allow for clinical translation of this tracer to image tumor angiogenesis and to guide VEGFR-targeted cancer therapy.[170]

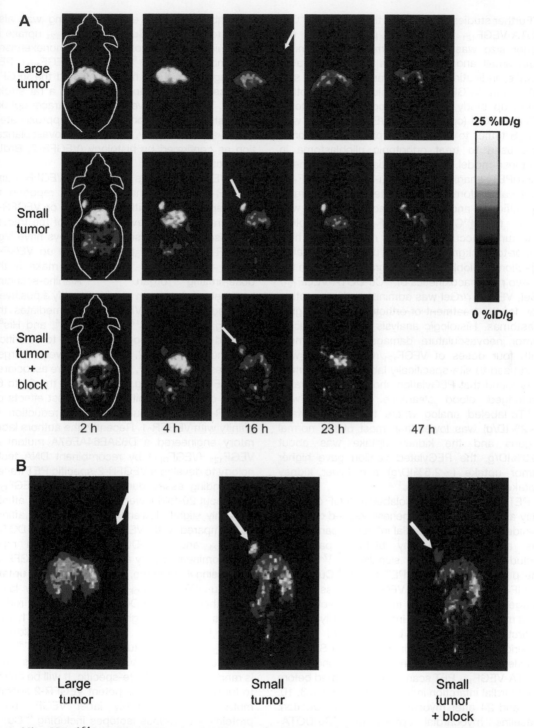

Fig. 4. MicroPET of ^{64}Cu-DOTA-VEGF$_{121}$ in U87MG tumor-bearing mice. (*A*) Serial microPET scans of large and small U87MG tumor-bearing mice injected intravenously with 5 MBq to 10 MBq of ^{64}Cu-DOTA-VEGF$_{121}$. Mice injected with ^{64}Cu-DOTA-VEGF$_{121}$ 30 minutes after injection of 100 µg VEGF$_{121}$ are also shown (denoted as "small tumor + block"). (*B*) Two-dimensional whole-body projection of the three mice shown in (*A*) at 16 hours after injection of ^{64}Cu-DOTA-VEGF$_{121}$. Tumors are indicated by arrows. (*Reproduced from* Cai W, Chen K, Mohamedali KA, et al. PET of vascular endothelial growth factor receptor expression. J Nucl Med 2006;47(12):2052; with permission.)

Further studies showed that the uptake of ^{64}Cu-DOTA-VEGF$_{121}$ in the tumor peaked when the tumor size was about 100 mm^3 to 250 mm^3. Both small and large tumors had lower tracer uptake, indicating a narrow range of tumor size with high VEGFR-2 expression.[171] In another follow-up study, a VEGFR-specific fusion toxin VEGF$_{121}$/rGel (composed of VEGF$_{121}$ linked with a G$_4$S tether to recombinant plant toxin gelonin) was used to treat orthotopic glioblastoma in a mouse model.[169] Before initiation of treatment, microPET imaging with ^{64}Cu-labeled VEGF$_{121}$/rGel was performed to evaluate the tumor targeting efficacy and the pharmacokinetics. It was found that ^{64}Cu-DOTA-VEGF$_{121}$/rGel exhibited high tumor accumulation and retention and high tumor-to-background contrast up to 48 hours after injection in glioblastoma xenografts. Based on the in vivo pharmacokinetics of ^{64}Cu-DOTA-VEGF$_{121}$/rGel, VEGF$_{121}$/rGel was administered every other day for the treatment of orthotopic U87MG glioblastomas. Histologic analysis revealed specific tumor neovasculature damage after treatment with four doses of VEGF$_{121}$/rGel.[169] ^{64}Cu was also used to site-specifically label VEGF$_{121}$ and it was found that PEGylation showed considerably prolonged blood clearance. Compared with ^{99m}Tc-labeled analog where the tumor uptake ($\sim$2%ID/g) was lower than most of the normal organs and the kidney uptake was about 120%ID/g, the PEGylated version gave higher tumor uptake ($\sim$2.5%ID/g) and lower kidney uptake at about 65%ID/g.[172]

PET imaging using radiolabeled VEGF can also play a role in other angiogenesis-related diseases besides cancer. Myocardial infarction can lead to the activation of many biologic pathways, including VEGF/VEGFR signaling.[173,174] Using the previously validated PET tracer ^{64}Cu-DOTA-VEGF$_{121}$, the kinetics of VEGFR expression was imaged for the first time in living subjects using a rat model of myocardial infarction.[175] Myocardial infarction was induced by ligation of the left anterior descending coronary artery in Sprague-Dawley rats and confirmed by ultrasound. ^{64}Cu-DOTA-VEGF$_{121}$ PET scans were performed before myocardial infarction induction, and at days 3, 10, 17, and 24 after myocardial infarction induction. Baseline myocardial uptake of ^{64}Cu-DOTA-VEGF$_{121}$ was minimal (0.3 ± 0.1%ID/g). After myocardial infarction, ^{64}Cu-DOTA-VEGF$_{121}$ myocardial uptake significantly increased (up to 1.0 ± 0.1%ID/g) and was elevated for 2 weeks, after which it returned to baseline levels. In a hindlimb ischemia model, PET imaging showed significantly higher ^{64}Cu-DOTA-VEGF$_{121}$ uptake in ischemic hindlimbs than in nonischemic

hindlimbs. Treadmill exercise training was also found to increase ^{64}Cu-DOTA-VEGF$_{121}$ uptake in ischemic hindlimbs compared with nonexercised hindlimbs.[176] With ^{64}Cu-DOTA-VEGF$_{121}$ PET imaging, the authors have evaluated the VEGFR expression kinetics noninvasively in a rat stroke model. The results revealed that the tracer uptake in the stroke border zone peaked at approximately 10 days after surgery, indicating neovascularization as confirmed by histology (VEGFR-2, BrdU, and lectin staining).[177]

All VEGF-A isoforms bind to both VEGFR-1 and VEGFR-2.[5] In the imaging studies reported to date, specificity to either VEGFR-1 or VEGFR-2 has rarely been achieved as most of the tracers are based on VEGF isoforms. Kidneys have high VEGFR-1 expression that can take up VEGF-A based tracer, which thus usually make it the dose-limiting organ.[170,178] Alanine-scanning mutagenesis has been used to identify a positively charged surface in VEGF$_{165}$ that mediates the binding to VEGFR-2.[179] Arg^{82}, Lys^{84}, and His^{86}, located in a hairpin loop, were found to be critical for binding VEGFR-2, while negatively charged residues, Asp^{63}, Glu^{64}, and Glu^{67}, were associated with VEGFR-1 binding. Mutations in the 63 to 67 region of VEGF exhibited only modest effects on VEGFR-2 binding but significant reduction in affinity with VEGFR-1. Recently, the authors laboratory engineered a D63AE64AE67A mutant of VEGF$_{121}$ (VEGF$_{DEE}$) by recombinant DNA technology to develop a VEGFR-2-specific PET tracer. Cell-binding assay demonstrated that VEGF$_{DEE}$ had about 20-fold lower VEGFR-1 binding affinity and only slightly lower VEGFR-2 binding affinity as compared with VEGF$_{121}$. Both ^{64}Cu-DOTA-VEGF$_{121}$ and ^{64}Cu-DOTA-VEGF$_{DEE}$ had rapid and prominent activity accumulation in VEGFR-2-expressing 4T1 tumors. However, the renal uptake of ^{64}Cu-DOTA-VEGF$_{DEE}$ was significantly lower than that of ^{64}Cu-DOTA-VEGF$_{121}$ as rodent kidneys expressed high levels of VEGFR-1, indicating that VEGF$_{DEE}$ is superior to wild-type VEGF$_{121}$ for imaging tumor angiogenesis.[180] The DOTA conjugation of VEGF proteins in this study is random instead of site-specific. It will be critical to further develop more potent VEGFR-2 specific mutants, site-specifically label VEGF analog proteins with various isotopes including ^{64}Cu, to improve angiogenesis imaging quality and result analysis.[175]

Imaging of matrix metalloproteinases

MMPs are a family of zinc- and calcium-dependent endopeptidases that are responsible for the enzymatic degradation of connective tissue und thus facilitate endothelial cell migration during angiogenesis.[181] Additionally, MMPs process and release bioactive molecules, such as growth factors, proteinase inhibitors, cytokines and chemokines.[182] From the more than 18 members of the MMP family, the gelatinases MMP-2 and -9 are most consistently detected in malignancies.[117] In the progression of the atherosclerotic lesions, MMP-3 and -9 have been shown to limit plaque growth and promote a stable plaque phenotype, and MMP-12 supports atherosclerotic lesion expansion and destabilization.[183] Many strategies have been developed to image MMPs level for the assessment of angiogenesis.[184,185]

The so-called "smart probes" have been developed to contain fluorescent dyes and MMP-cleavable sequences.[186,187] It has been reported a MMP-2-sensitive probe was activated by MMP-2 in vitro, producing up to an 850% increase in near-infrared fluorescent signal intensity, and MMP-2-positive tumors were easily identified as high-signal-intensity regions as early as 1 hour after intravenous injection of the MMP-2 probe.[188]

Via phage display techniques, the MMP-specific decapeptide H-Cys-Thr-Thr-His-Trp-Gly-Phe-Thr-leu-Cys-OH (CTT) was found and could be labeled with ^{125}I and [99m]Tc. However, this tracer has unfavorable characteristics for in vivo imaging because the metabolic stability of the compound is low and lipophilicity is high.[189] Another group labeled this peptide with ^{111}In after conjugating it with a highly hydrophilic and negatively charged chelator DTPA. A significant correlation was observed between the accumulation in the tumor as well as tumor-to-blood ratio of ^{111}In-DTPA-CTT and gelatinase activity. Moreover, ^{111}In-DTPA-CTT showed low levels of radioactivity in the liver and kidneys.[190] CTT peptide also has been labeled with ^{64}Cu after DOTA conjugation for PET imaging of MMP. [64]Cu DOTA CTT inhibited hMMP-2 and mMMP-9 with similar affinity to CTT. MicroPET imaging studies showed that ^{64}Cu-DOTA-CTT was taken up by MMP-2/9-positive B16F10 murine melanoma tumors, however, the low affinity for MMP-2 and MMP-9 and in vivo instability of CTT-based imaging probes need to be overcome for further applications.[191]

Another approach is to label small-molecule MMP inhibitors (MMPIs), which are typically used as antiangiogenic drugs. In general, MMPIs possess a zinc-binding group complexing the zinc ion of the active site and are classified into several groups because of their lead structures.[181] Different ^{18}F and ^{11}C labeled MMPIs have been synthesized and evaluated preclinically with mixed results.[192,193] Fluorinated MMPIs based on lead structures of the broad-spectrum inhibitors N-hydroxy-2(R)-[[(4-methoxyphenyl)sulfonyl](benzyl)-amino]-3-methyl-butanamide (CGS 25,966) and N-hydroxy-2(R)-[[(4-methoxyphenyl)sulfonyl](3-picolyl)-amino]-3-methyl-butanamide (CGS 27,023A) have been synthesized and showed high in vitro MMP inhibition potencies for MMP-2, -8, -9, and -13.[194] However, in vivo microPET study with ^{11}C-CGS 25,966 failed to demarcate MMP-positive tumors.[195] A ^{11}C-labeled MMPI (2R)-2-[[4-(6-fluorohex-1-ynyl)phenyl]sulfonylamino]-3-methylbutyric acid ^{11}C-methyl ester (^{11}C-FMAME), has also been synthesized and applied to two animal models of breast cancer, MCF-7 xenograft transfected with interleukin-1 and MDA-MB-435 xenograft in athymic mice. Again, low tumor-to-blood and tumor-to muscle ratios of these tracers do not allow visualization of the tumors in microPET studies.[192,196] However, biodistribution study with ^{18}F-labeled similar compound, (2R)-2-[4-(6-^{18}F-Fluorohex-1-ynyl)-benzenesulfonylamino]-3-methylbutyric acid (^{18}F-SAV03), showed higher tumor uptake of the tracer than normal organs.[193] Other MMPIs have also been synthesized and labeled with radionuclides including ^{111}In and [18]F.[194,197] Nevertheless, significant improvements in tumor MMP targeting and in vivo pharmacokinetics are necessary before the use of MMP-radiotracer imaging will be translated into the clinic.

Imaging of other angiogenesis-related targets

Fibronectin is a large glycoprotein, which can be found physiologically in plasma and tissues. However, the extra-domain B of fibronectin (EDB), consisting of 91 amino acids, is not present in the fibronectin molecule under normal conditions, except for the endometrium in the proliferative phase and some vessels of the ovaries. EDB is interesting as a marker of angiogenesis as it is expressed in a variety of solid tumors, as well as in ocular angiogenesis and wound healing.[198] The human antibody fragment scFv(L19) has been shown to efficiently localize on neovasculature both in animal models and in cancer patients. In a study with patients suffering from various solid tumors, 16 of 20 tumor lesions could be identified by SPECT using ^{123}I-scFv(L19). Whether the unidentified tumors were not detected because they were either in a phase of slow growth with low levels of angiogenesis, or because of the technical limitations of SPECT imaging, is not clear.[199] No reports about PET tracers targeting EDB are available up to now. Other angiogenesis-related biomarkers, such as angiopoietins/Tie receptors,[200] and CD276[201] are also potential targets for angiogenesis imaging. Angiopoietins/Tie receptors are involved in regulation of complex interactions between endothelium and surrounding cells. CD276 has been observed to be over-expressed in tumor versus normal endothelium.

SUMMARY AND PERSPECTIVE

Numerous imaging techniques are available for assessing tissue vasculature on a structural, functional, and molecular level. A wide variety of targeting ligands (small molecules, peptides, peptidomimetics, and antibodies) have been conjugated with various imaging labels for MR imaging, US, optical, SPECT, PET, and multimodality imaging of angiogenesis. All these methods have been successfully used preclinically and will hopefully aid in antiangiogenic drug evaluation in animal studies. Because of its high sensitivity and the low amounts of tracer that have to be used, PET will probably be the first to be used on a wide scale in patients in the intermediate term. In addition, toxicity issues of PET tracers are of less importance compared with MR imaging or US imaging probes as only pica molar amount will be used for imaging purpose. However, it is likely that not one single parameter, target structure, or imaging technique will be used for the assessment of angiogenesis in the future, but rather a multimodality, multiplexing imaging that will allow for evaluation of the angiogenic cascade in its full complexity to acquire comprehensive information. It is predictable that the new generation clinical PET/CT and microPET/microCT, as well as PET/MR imaging and microPET/microMR imaging currently in active development,[202–204] will likely play a major role in molecular imaging of angiogenesis for the years to come.

Although it is generally assumed that noninvasive imaging results correlate with the target expression level, such assumption has not been extensively validated. In most reports, two tumor models are studied, where one acts as a positive control and the other as a negative control. Quantitative correlation between the target expression level in vivo and the noninvasive imaging data is rare.[137,145,205,206] Such correlation is critical for future therapeutic response monitoring, as it would be ideal to be able to monitor the changes in the target expression level quantitatively, rather than qualitatively, in each individual patient. Lack of accurate quantification is one of the hindrances why only a few radiotracers including PET tracers have been used in human beings up to now, and their role in assessment of anti- or proangiogenic therapies is still unsettled.

To further improve imaging of the angiogenesis process at molecular level, it is necessary to identify new angiogenesis-related targets and corresponding specific ligands and to optimize currently available imaging probes. Thorough and full understanding of the physiologic and pathologic changes during angiogenesis will be critical for new target identification. Optimization of currently available imaging probes can be achieved in several ways. First, oligomerization (homo or hetero) the targeting ligand (typically peptide) can improve the binding affinity as well as tissue retention, likely because of the polyvalency effect.[207] Second, site-specific labeling may be advantageous than randomly labeling on lysine residues in terms of retaining the binding affinity and functional activity.[175] Third, incorporation of a linker between the targeting ligand and the label can improve the pharmacokinetic properties. Glycosylation, PEGylation, and various other linkers have been shown to improve the imaging quality. Last, development of new strategies to improve the labeling yield (most applicable to ^{18}F-based tracers) is critical for future clinical studies. To foster the continued discovery and development of angiogenesis-targeted imaging agents, cooperative efforts are needed from cellular and molecular biologists to identify and validate novel imaging targets, chemists and radiochemists to synthesize and characterize the imaging probes, and engineers and medical physicists and mathematicians to develop high-sensitivity and high-resolution imaging devices and hybrid instruments and better image reconstruction algorithms.

Noninvasive imaging of angiogenesis has clinical applications in many aspects, including lesion detection, patient stratification, new drug development and validation, treatment monitoring, and dose optimization. For example, glucosamino ^{99m}Tc-d-c(RGDfK) gamma-camera imaging has been applied to monitor the therapeutic efficacy of paclitaxel in Lewis lung carcinoma tumor-bearing mice.[208] With the development of new tracers with better targeting efficacy and desirable pharmacokinetics, clinical translation will be critical for the maximum benefit of these imaging probes. Most of the molecular imaging probes suffer from the slow translation from bench to bedside. Multiple steps in preclinical development, especially the investigational new drug-directed toxicology, significantly slowed down the process of converting a newly developed agent into a diagnostic imaging probe for clinical testing. The high specificity required for molecular imaging not only leads to higher costs of development but also smaller market potential, which may make them considered too risky by investors for commercial development. However, the situation has gradually changed over the last several years thanks to the continued development and wider availability of scanners dedicated to small-animal imaging studies, as well as the exploratory investigational new drug mechanism proposed by the FDA to allow faster first-in-human studies. Now the molecular imaging techniques can bridge the gap between preclinical and clinical research to develop candidate drugs that have the optimal target specificity, pharmacodynamics, and efficacy. It is expected that in the foreseeable future, anigogenesis imaging with PET tracers will be routinely applied in anticancer clinical trials, paving the way to personalized molecular therapy.

REFERENCES

1. Folkman J. Angiogenesis in cancer, vascular, rheumatoid and other disease. Nat Med 1995;1(1):27–31.
2. Atluri P, Woo YJ. Pro-angiogenic cytokines as cardiovascular therapeutics: assessing the potential. BioDrugs 2008;22(4):209–22.
3. Pathak AP, Gimi B, Glunde K, et al. Molecular and functional imaging of cancer: advances in MRI and MRS. Methods Enzymol 2004;386:3–60.
4. Rajagopalan S, Trachtenberg J, Mohler E, et al. Phase I study of direct administration of a replication deficient adenovirus vector containing the vascular endothelial growth factor cDNA (CI-1023) to patients with claudication. Am J Cardiol 2002;90(5):512–6.
5. Ferrara N. Vascular endothelial growth factor: basic science and clinical progress. Endocr Rev 2004;25(4):581–611.
6. Hurwitz H, Fehrenbacher L, Novotny W, et al. Bevacizumab plus irinotecan, fluorouracil, and leucovorin for metastatic colorectal cancer. N Engl J Med 2004;350(23):2335–42.
7. Kerbel RS. Antiangiogenic therapy: a universal chemosensitization strategy for cancer? Science 2006;312(5777):1171–5.
8. Faivre S, Demetri G, Sargent W, et al. Molecular basis for sunitinib efficacy and future clinical development. Nat Rev Drug Discov 2007;6(9):734–45.
9. Jaffe CC. Measures of response: RECIST, WHO, and new alternatives. J Clin Oncol 2006;24(20):3245–51.
10. Cai W, Rao J, Gambhir SS, et al. How molecular imaging is speeding up anti-angiogenic drug development. Mol Cancer Ther 2006;5(11):2624–33.
11. Choe YS, Lee KH. Targeted in vivo imaging of angiogenesis: present status and perspectives. Curr Pharm Des 2007;13(1):17–31.
12. Haubner R. Noninvasive tracer techniques to characterize angiogenesis. Handb Exp Pharmacol 2008;185(II):323–39.
13. Berthelot T, Lasne MC, Deleris G. New trends in molecular imaging of tumor angiogenesis. Anticancer Agents Med Chem 2008;8(5):497–522.
14. Auguste P, Lemiere S, Larrieu-Lahargue F, et al. Molecular mechanisms of tumor vascularization. Crit Rev Oncol Hematol 2005;54(1):53–61.
15. Carmeliet P. Mechanisms of angiogenesis and arteriogenesis. Nat Med 2000;6(4):389–95.
16. Holash J, Maisonpierre PC, Compton D, et al. Vessel cooption, regression, and growth in tumors mediated by angiopoietins and VEGF. Science 1999;284(5422):1994–8.
17. Folkman J. Tumor angiogenesis: therapeutic implications. N Engl J Med 1971;285(21):1182–6.
18. Kalluri R. Basement membranes: structure, assembly and role in tumour angiogenesis. Nat Rev Cancer 2003;3(6):422–33.
19. Bergers G, Benjamin LE. Tumorigenesis and the angiogenic switch. Nat Rev Cancer 2003;3(6):401–10.
20. Nguyen M. Angiogenic factors as tumor markers. Invest New Drugs 1997;15(1):29–37.
21. Landgren E, Schiller P, Cao Y, et al. Placenta growth factor stimulates MAP kinase and mitogenicity but not phospholipase C-gamma and migration of endothelial cells expressing Flt 1. Oncogene 1998;16(3):359–67.
22. Nor JE, Christensen J, Mooney DJ, et al. Vascular endothelial growth factor (VEGF)-mediated angiogenesis is associated with enhanced endothelial cell survival and induction of Bcl-2 expression. Am J Pathol 1999;154(2):375–84.
23. Paku S, Paweletz N. First steps of tumor-related angiogenesis. Lab Invest 1991;65(3):334–46.
24. Djonov V, Schmid M, Tschanz SA, et al. Intussusceptive angiogenesis: its role in embryonic vascular network formation. Circ Res 2000,00(3),280–92.
25. Metzger RJ, Krasnow MA. Genetic control of branching morphogenesis. Science 1999;284(5420):1635–9.
26. Pepper MS, Ferrara N, Orci L, et al. Vascular endothelial growth factor (VEGF) induces plasminogen activators and plasminogen activator inhibitor-1 in microvascular endothelial cells. Biochem Biophys Res Commun 1991;181(2):902–6.
27. Asahara T, Chen D, Takahashi T, et al. Tie2 receptor ligands, angiopoietin-1 and angiopoietin-2, modulate VEGF-induced postnatal neovascularization. Circ Res 1998;83(3):233–40.
28. Brooks PC, Clark RA, Cheresh DA. Requirement of vascular integrin $a_v b_3$ for angiogenesis. Science 1994;264(5158):569–71.
29. Friedlander M, Brooks PC, Shaffer RW, et al. Definition of two angiogenic pathways by distinct alpha v integrins. Science 1995;270(5241):1500–2.

30. Sang QX. Complex role of matrix metalloproteinases in angiogenesis. Cell Res 1998;8(3):171–7.

31. Gamble J, Meyer G, Noack L, et al. B1 integrin activation inhibits in vitro tube formation: effects on cell migration, vacuole coalescence and lumen formation. Endothelium 1999;7(1):23–34.

32. Nakao N, Miura K, Takayasu Y, et al. CT angiography in hepatocellular carcinoma. J Comput Assist Tomogr 1983;7(5):780–7.

33. Less JR, Skalak TC, Sevick EM, et al. Microvascular architecture in a mammary carcinoma: branching patterns and vessel dimensions. Cancer Res 1991;51(1):265–73.

34. Konerding MA, Miodonski AJ, Lametschwandtner A. Microvascular corrosion casting in the study of tumor vascularity: a review. Scanning Microsc 1995;9(4):1233–43.

35. Schlingemann RO, Rietveld FJ, Kwaspen F, et al. Differential expression of markers for endothelial cells, pericytes, and basal lamina in the microvasculature of tumors and granulation tissue. Am J Pathol 1991;138(6):1335–47.

36. Miettinen M, Lindenmayer AE, Chaubal A. Endothelial cell markers CD31, CD34, and BNH9 antibody to H- and Y-antigens–evaluation of their specificity and sensitivity in the diagnosis of vascular tumors and comparison with von Willebrand factor. Mod Pathol 1994;7(1):82–90.

37. Schlaeger TM, Bartunkova S, Lawitts JA, et al. Uniform vascular-endothelial-cell-specific gene expression in both embryonic and adult transgenic mice. Proc Natl Acad Sci U S A 1997;94(7):3058–63.

38. Motoike T, Loughna S, Perens E, et al. Universal GFP reporter for the study of vascular development. Genesis 2000;28(2):75–81.

39. Trotter MJ, Olive PL, Chaplin DJ. Effect of vascular marker Hoechst 33342 on tumour perfusion and cardiovascular function in the mouse. Br J Cancer 1990;62(6):903–8.

40. Hashizume H, Baluk P, Morikawa S, et al. Openings between defective endothelial cells explain tumor vessel leakiness. Am J Pathol 2000;156(4):1363–80.

41. Usami N, Iwano S, Yokoi K. Solitary fibrous tumor of the pleura: evaluation of the origin with 3D CT angiography. J Thorac Oncol 2007;2(12):1124–5.

42. McDonald DM, Choyke PL. Imaging of angiogenesis: from microscope to clinic. Nat Med 2003;9(6):713–25.

43. van Vliet M, van Dijke CF, Wielopolski PA, et al. MR angiography of tumor-related vasculature: from the clinic to the micro-environment. Radiographics 2005;25(Suppl 1):S85–97 [discussion: S97–8].

44. Boudghene FP, Gouny P, Tassart M, et al. Subungual glomus tumor: combined use of MRI and three-dimensional contrast MR angiography. J Magn Reson Imaging 1998;8(6):1326–8.

45. Foster FS, Burns PN, Simpson DH, et al. Ultrasound for the visualization and quantification of tumor microcirculation. Cancer Metastasis Rev 2000;19(1-2):131–8.

46. Jiang Y, Zhao J, White DL, et al. Micro CT and Micro MR imaging of 3D architecture of animal skeleton. J Musculoskelet Neuronal Interact 2000;1(1):45–51.

47. Tozer GM, Ameer-Beg SM, Baker J, et al. Intravital imaging of tumour vascular networks using multiphoton fluorescence microscopy. Adv Drug Deliv Rev 2005;57(1):135–52.

48. Galbraith SM. Antivascular cancer treatments: imaging biomarkers in pharmaceutical drug development. Br J Radiol 2003;76(Spec No 1):S83–6.

49. Choyke PL, Dwyer AJ, Knopp MV. Functional tumor imaging with dynamic contrast-enhanced magnetic resonance imaging. J Magn Reson Imaging 2003;17(5):509–20.

50. O'Connor JP, Jackson A, Parker GJ, et al. DCE-MRI biomarkers in the clinical evaluation of antiangiogenic and vascular disrupting agents. Br J Cancer 2007;96(2):189–95.

51. Zhang C, Jugold M, Woenne EC, et al. Specific targeting of tumor angiogenesis by RGD-conjugated ultrasmall superparamagnetic iron oxide particles using a clinical 1.5-T magnetic resonance scanner. Cancer Res 2007;67(4):1555–62.

52. Liu G, Rugo HS, Wilding G, et al. Dynamic contrast-enhanced magnetic resonance imaging as a pharmacodynamic measure of response after acute dosing of AG-013736, an oral angiogenesis inhibitor, in patients with advanced solid tumors: results from a phase I study. J Clin Oncol 2005;23(24):5464–73.

53. Thomas AL, Morgan B, Horsfield MA, et al. Phase I study of the safety, tolerability, pharmacokinetics, and pharmacodynamics of PTK787/ZK 222584 administered twice daily in patients with advanced cancer. J Clin Oncol 2005;23(18):4162–71.

54. Medved M, Karczmar G, Yang C, et al. Semiquantitative analysis of dynamic contrast enhanced MRI in cancer patients: Variability and changes in tumor tissue over time. J Magn Reson Imaging 2004;20(1):122–8.

55. Padhani AR. MRI for assessing antivascular cancer treatments. Br J Radiol 2003;76(Spec No 1):S60–80.

56. Marzola P, Degrassi A, Calderan L, et al. In vivo assessment of antiangiogenic activity of SU6668 in an experimental colon carcinoma model. Clin Cancer Res 2004;10(2):739–50.

57. Faccioli N, Marzola P, Boschi F, et al. Pathological animal models in the experimental evaluation of tumour microvasculature with magnetic resonance imaging. Radiol Med (Torino) 2007;112(3):319–28.

58. Williams DS. Quantitative perfusion imaging using arterial spin labeling. Methods Mol Med 2006;124:151–73.

59. Liu TT, Brown GG. Measurement of cerebral perfusion with arterial spin labeling: Part 1. Methods. J Int Neuropsychol Soc 2007;13(3):517–25.

60. Wolf RL, Detre JA. Clinical neuroimaging using arterial spin-labeled perfusion magnetic resonance imaging. Neurotherapeutics 2007;4(3):346–59.

61. Hsu YY, Chang CN, Jung SM, et al. Blood oxygenation level-dependent MRI of cerebral gliomas during breath holding. J Magn Reson Imaging 2004;19(2):160–7.

62. Baudelet C, Cron GO, Gallez B. Determination of the maturity and functionality of tumor vasculature by MRI: correlation between BOLD-MRI and DCE-MRI using P792 in experimental fibrosarcoma tumors. Magn Reson Med 2006;56(5):1041–9.

63. Fleischer AC, Wojcicki WE, Donnelly EF, et al. Quantified color Doppler sonography of tumor vascularity in an animal model. J Ultrasound Med 1999;18(8):547–51.

64. Forsberg F, Ro RJ, Potoczek M, et al. Assessment of angiogenesis: implications for ultrasound imaging. Ultrasonics 2004;42(1–9):325–30.

65. Drevs J, Hofmann I, Hugenschmidt H, et al. Effects of PTK787/ZK 222584, a specific inhibitor of vascular endothelial growth factor receptor tyrosine kinases, on primary tumor, metastasis, vessel density, and blood flow in a murine renal cell carcinoma model. Cancer Res 2000;60(17):4819–24.

66. Liang JD, Yang PM, Liang PC, et al. Three-dimensional power Doppler ultrasonography for demonstrating associated arteries of hepatocellular carcinoma. J Formos Med Assoc 2003;102(6): 367–74.

67. Stride E, Saffari N. Microbubble ultrasound contrast agents: a review. Proc Inst Mech Eng [H] 2003;217(6):429–47.

68. Niermann KJ, Fleischer AC, Huamani J, et al. Measuring tumor perfusion in control and treated murine tumors: correlation of microbubble contrast-enhanced sonography to dynamic contrast-enhanced magnetic resonance imaging and fluorodeoxyglucose positron emission tomography. J Ultrasound Med 2007;26(6):749–56.

69. Wilson SR, Burns PN, Muradali D, et al. Harmonic hepatic US with microbubble contrast agent: initial experience showing improved characterization of hemangioma, hepatocellular carcinoma, and metastasis. Radiology 2000;215(1):153–61.

70. Burns PN, Wilson SR, Simpson DH. Pulse inversion imaging of liver blood flow: improved method for characterizing focal masses with microbubble contrast. Invest Radiol 2000;35(1):58–71.

71. Quaia E. Microbubble ultrasound contrast agents: an update. Eur Radiol 2007;17(8):1995–2008.

72. Cornud F, Hamida K, Flam T, et al. Endorectal color Doppler sonography and endorectal MR imaging features of nonpalpable prostate cancer:

73. correlation with radical prostatectomy findings. Am J Roentgenol 2000;175(4):1161–8.

73. McCarville MB, Streck CJ, Dickson PV, et al. Angiogenesis inhibitors in a murine neuroblastoma model: quantitative assessment of intratumoral blood flow with contrast-enhanced gray-scale US. Radiology 2006;240(1):73–81.

74. Stieger SM, Bloch SH, Foreman O, et al. Ultrasound assessment of angiogenesis in a matrigel model in rats. Ultrasound Med Biol 2006;32(5):673–81.

75. Ferrara KW, Merritt CR, Burns PN, et al. Evaluation of tumor angiogenesis with US: imaging, Doppler, and contrast agents. Acad Radiol 2000;7(10): 824–39.

76. Hughes MS, Marsh JN, Zhang H, et al. Characterization of digital waveforms using thermodynamic analogs: detection of contrast-targeted tissue in vivo. IEEE Trans Ultrason Ferroelectr Freq Control 2006;53(9):1609–16.

77. Lassau N, Lamuraglia M, Chami L, et al. Gastrointestinal stromal tumors treated with imatinib: monitoring response with contrast-enhanced sonography. Am J Roentgenol 2006;187(5):1267–73.

78. Li PC, Yang MJ. Transfer function analysis of ultrasonic time-intensity measurements. Ultrasound Med Biol 2003;29(10):1493–500.

79. Lavisse S, Lejeune P, Rouffiac V, et al. Early quantitative evaluation of a tumor vasculature disruptive agent AVE8062 using dynamic contrast-enhanced ultrasonography. Invest Radiol 2008;43(2):100–11.

80. Haider MA, Milosevic M, Fyles A, et al. Assessment of the tumor microenvironment in cervix cancer using dynamic contrast enhanced CT, interstitial fluid pressure and oxygen measurements. Int J Radiat Oncol Biol Phys 2005;62(4):1100–7.

81. Bisdas S, Konstantinou GN, Lee PS, et al. Dynamic contrast-enhanced CT of head and neck tumors: perfusion measurements using a distributed-parameter tracer kinetic model. Initial results and comparison with deconvolution-based analysis. Phys Med Biol 2007;52(20):6181–96.

82. Larson DR, Zipfel WR, Williams RM, et al. Water-soluble quantum dots for multiphoton fluorescence imaging in vivo. Science 2003;300(5624):1434–6.

83. Brown EB, Campbell RB, Tsuzuki Y, et al. In vivo measurement of gene expression, angiogenesis and physiological function in tumors using multiphoton laser scanning microscopy. Nat Med 2001;7(7):864–8.

84. Montet X, Ntziachristos V, Grimm J, et al. Tomographic fluorescence mapping of tumor targets. Cancer Res 2005;65(14):6330–6.

85. Jones T. The imaging science of positron emission tomography. Eur J Nucl Med 1996;23(7):807–13.

86. Laking GR, Price PM. Positron emission tomographic imaging of angiogenesis and vascular function. Br J Radiol 2003;76(Spec No 1):S50–9.

87. Phelps ME, Hoffman EJ, Mullani NA, et al. Application of annihilation coincidence detection to transaxial reconstruction tomography. J Nucl Med 1975;16(3):210–24.

88. Phelps ME. PET: the merging of biology and imaging into molecular imaging. J Nucl Med 2000;41(4):661–81.

89. Willmann JK, van Bruggen N, Dinkelborg LM, et al. Molecular imaging in drug development. Nat Rev Drug Discov 2008;7(7):591–607.

90. Beyer T, Townsend DW, Brun T, et al. A combined PET/CT scanner for clinical oncology. J Nucl Med 2000;41(8):1369–79.

91. Kamel E, Hany TF, Burger C, et al. CT vs 68Ge attenuation correction in a combined PET/CT system: evaluation of the effect of lowering the CT tube current. Eur J Nucl Med Mol Imaging 2002; 29(3):346–50.

92. Cherry SR, Shao Y, Silverman RW, et al. MicroPET: a high resolution PET scanner for imaging small animals. IEEE Trans Nucl Sci 1997;44(3):1161–6.

93. Chatziioannou AF, Cherry SR, Shao Y, et al. Performance evaluation of microPET: a high-resolution lutetium oxyorthosilicate PET scanner for animal imaging. J Nucl Med 1999;40(7):1164–75.

94. Pichler BJ, Judenhofer MS, Pfannenberg C. Multimodal imaging approaches: PET/CT and PET/MRI. Handb Exp Pharmacol 2008;185(I):109–32.

95. Laking GR, West C, Buckley DL, et al. Imaging vascular physiology to monitor cancer treatment. Crit Rev Oncol Hematol 2006;58(2):95–113.

96. Anderson RE. Cerebral blood flow xenon-133. Neurosurg Clin N Am 1996;7(4):703–8.

97. Wilson RA, Shea MJ, De Landsheere CM, et al. Validation of quantitation of regional myocardial blood flow in vivo with 11C-labeled human albumin microspheres and positron emission tomography. Circulation 1984;70(4):717–23.

98. Dimitrakopoulou-Strauss A, Strauss LG, Burger C. Quantitative PET studies in pretreated melanoma patients: a comparison of 6-[^{18}F]fluoro-L-dopa with ^{18}F-FDG and ^{15}O-water using compartment and noncompartment analysis. J Nucl Med 2001; 42(2):248–56.

99. Acierno LJ. Adolph Fick: mathematician, physicist, physiologist. Clin Cardiol 2000;23(5):390–1.

100. Lammertsma AA, Jones T. Low oxygen extraction fraction in tumours measured with the oxygen-15 steady state technique: effect of tissue heterogeneity. Br J Radiol 1992;65(776):697–700.

101. Iida H, Takahashi A, Tamura Y, et al. Myocardial blood flow: comparison of oxygen-15-water bolus injection, slow infusion and oxygen-15-carbon dioxide slow inhalation. J Nucl Med 1995;36(1):78–85.

102. Wilson CB, Lammertsma AA, McKenzie CG, et al. Measurements of blood flow and exchanging water space in breast tumors using positron emission tomography: a rapid and noninvasive dynamic method. Cancer Res 1992;52(6):1592–7.

103. Anderson H, Price P. Clinical measurement of blood flow in tumours using positron emission tomography: a review. Nucl Med Commun 2002;23(2):131–8.

104. Tseng J, Dunnwald LK, Schubert EK, et al. 18F-FDG kinetics in locally advanced breast cancer: correlation with tumor blood flow and changes in response to neoadjuvant chemotherapy. J Nucl Med 2004;45(11):1829–37.

105. Hoffend J, Mier W, Schuhmacher J, et al. Gallium-68-DOTA-albumin as a PET blood-pool marker: experimental evaluation in vivo. Nucl Med Biol 2005;32(3):287–92.

106. Sipkins DA, Cheresh DA, Kazemi MR, et al. Detection of tumor angiogenesis in vivo by alphaVbeta3-targeted magnetic resonance imaging. Nat Med 1998;4(5):623–6.

107. Wierzbicka-Patynowski I, Niewiarowski S, Marcinkiewicz C, et al. Structural requirements of echistatin for the recognition of alpha vbeta 3 and alpha 5beta 1 Integrins. J Biol Chem 1999; 274(53):37809–14.

108. Cai W, Shin DW, Chen K, et al. Peptide-labeled near-infrared quantum dots for imaging tumor vasculature in living subjects. Nano Lett 2006; 6(4):669–76.

109. Hood JD, Cheresh DA. Role of integrins in cell invasion and migration. Nat Rev Cancer 2002;2(2):91–100.

110. Chen X. Multimodality imaging of tumor integrin alphavbeta3 expression. Mini Rev Med Chem 2006; 6(2):227–34.

111. Hynes RO. Integrins: bidirectional, allosteric signaling machines. Cell 2002;110(6):673–87.

112. Xiong JP, Stehle T, Zhang R, et al. Crystal structure of the extracellular segment of integrin a_vb_3 in complex with an Arg-Gly-Asp ligand. Science 2002;296(5565):151–5.

113. Ruoslahti E, Pierschbacher MD. New perspectives in cell adhesion: RGD and integrins. Science 1987; 238(4826):491–7.

114. Jin H, Varner J. Integrins: roles in cancer development and as treatment targets. Br J Cancer 2004; 90(3):561–5.

115. Mizejewski GJ. Role of integrins in cancer: survey of expression patterns (44435). Proc Soc Exp Biol Med 1999;222(2):124–38.

116. Cai W, Chen X. Anti-angiogenic cancer therapy based on integrin a_vb_3 antagonism. Anticancer Agents Med Chem 2006;6:407–28.

117. Brooks PC, Stromblad S, Sanders LC, et al. Localization of matrix metalloproteinase MMP-2 to the surface of invasive cells by interaction with integrin a_vb_3. Cell 1996;85(5):683–93.

118. Yang JT, Rayburn H, Hynes RO. Embryonic mesodermal defects in a_5 integrin-deficient mice. Development 1993;119(4):1093–105.

119. Goh KL, Yang JT, Hynes RO. Mesodermal defects and cranial neural crest apoptosis in a_5 integrin-null embryos. Development 1997; 124(21):4309–19.

120. Taverna D, Hynes RO. Reduced blood vessel formation and tumor growth in a_5-integrin-negative teratocarcinomas and embryoid bodies. Cancer Res 2001;61(13):5255–61.

121. Yang JT, Rayburn H, Hynes RO. Cell adhesion events mediated by a_4 integrins are essential in placental and cardiac development. Development 1995;121(2):549–60.

122. Aumailley M, Gurrath M, Muller G, et al. Arg-Gly-Asp constrained within cyclic pentapeptides. Strong and selective inhibitors of cell adhesion to vitronectin and laminin fragment P1. FEBS Lett 1991;291(1):50–4.

123. Haubner R, Finsinger D, Kessler H. Stereoisomeric peptide libraries and peptidomimetics for designing selective inhibitors of the $\alpha_v\beta_3$ integrin for a new cancer therapy. Angew Chem Int Ed Engl 1997;36:1374–89.

124. Haubner R, Wester HJ, Reuning U, et al. Radiolabeled alpha(v)beta3 integrin antagonists: a new class of tracers for tumor targeting. J Nucl Med 1999;40(6):1061–71.

125. Haubner R, Wester HJ, Weber WA, et al. Noninvasive imaging of alpha(v)beta3 integrin expression using 18F-labeled RGD-containing glycopeptide and positron emission tomography. Cancer Res 2001;61(5):1781–5.

126. Haubner R. Alphavbeta3-integrin imaging: a new approach to characterise angiogenesis? Eur J Nucl Med Mol Imaging 2006;33(Suppl 1):54–63.

127. Harris JM, Martin NE, Modi M. PEGylation: a novel process for modifying pharmacokinetics. Clin Pharmacokinet 2001;40(7):539–51.

128. Chen X, Park R, Shahinian AH, et al. Pharmacokinetics and tumor retention of 125I-labeled RGD peptide are improved by PEGylation. Nucl Med Biol 2004;31(1):11–9.

129. Noiri E, Goligorsky MS, Wang GJ, et al. Biodistribution and clearance of 99mTc-labeled Arg-Gly-Asp (RGD) peptide in rats with ischemic acute renal failure. J Am Soc Nephrol 1996;7(12):2682–8.

130. Chen X, Hou Y, Tohme M, et al. PEGylated Arg-Gly-Asp peptide: 64Cu labeling and PET imaging of brain tumor alphavbeta3 integrin expression. J Nucl Med 2004;45(10):1776–83.

131. Dijkgraaf I, Liu S, Kruijtzer JA, et al. Effects of linker variation on the in vitro and in vivo characteristics of an 111In-labeled RGD peptide. Nucl Med Biol 2007;34(1):29–35.

132. Li ZB, Chen K, Chen X. (68)Ga-labeled multimeric RGD peptides for microPET imaging of integrin alpha(v)beta (3) expression. Eur J Nucl Med Mol Imaging 2008;35(6):1100–8.

133. van Hagen PM, Breeman WA, Bernard HF, et al. Evaluation of a radiolabelled cyclic DTPA-RGD analogue for tumour imaging and radionuclide therapy. Int J Cancer 2000;90(4):186–98.

134. Bach-Gansmo T, Danielsson R, Saracco A, et al. Integrin receptor imaging of breast cancer: a proof-of-concept study to evaluate 99mTc-NC100692. J Nucl Med 2006;47(9):1434–9.

135. Haubner R, Wester HJ, Burkhart F, et al. Glycosylated RGD-containing peptides: tracer for tumor targeting and angiogenesis imaging with improved biokinetics. J Nucl Med 2001;42(2): 326–36.

136. Haubner R, Kuhnast B, Mang C, et al. [18F]Galacto-RGD: synthesis, radiolabeling, metabolic stability, and radiation dose estimates. Bioconjug Chem 2004;15(1):61–9.

137. Haubner R, Weber WA, Beer AJ, et al. Noninvasive visualization of the activated alphavbeta3 integrin in cancer patients by positron emission tomography and [18F]Galacto-RGD. PLoS Med 2005; 2(3):e70.

138. Beer AJ, Haubner R, Goebel M, et al. Biodistribution and pharmacokinetics of the alphavbeta3-selective tracer 18F-galacto-RGD in cancer patients. J Nucl Med 2005;46(8):1333–41.

139. Beer AJ, Haubner R, Wolf I, et al. PET-based human dosimetry of 18F-galacto-RGD, a new radiotracer for imaging alpha v beta3 expression. J Nucl Med 2006;47(5):763–9.

140. Beer AJ, Haubner R, Sarbia M, et al. Positron emission tomography using [18F]Galacto-RGD identifies the level of integrin alpha(v)beta3 expression in man. Clin Cancer Res 2006;12(13):3942–9.

141. Beer AJ, Grosu AL, Carlsen J, et al. [18F]galacto-RGD positron emission tomography for imaging of alphavbeta3 expression on the neovasculature in patients with squamous cell carcinoma of the head and neck. Clin Cancer Res 2007;13(22 Pt 1):6610–6.

142. Beer AJ, Lorenzen S, Metz S, et al. Comparison of integrin alphaVbeta3 expression and glucose metabolism in primary and metastatic lesions in cancer patients: a PET study using 18F-galacto-RGD and 18F-FDG. J Nucl Med 2008;49(1):22–9.

143. Boturyn D, Coll JL, Garanger E, et al. Template assembled cyclopeptides as multimeric system for integrin targeting and endocytosis. J Am Chem Soc 2004;126(18):5730–9.

144. Chen X, Tohme M, Park R, et al. Micro-PET imaging of alphavbeta3-integrin expression with 18F-labeled dimeric RGD peptide. Mol Imaging 2004; 3(2):96–104.

145. Zhang X, Xiong Z, Wu Y, et al. Quantitative PET imaging of tumor integrin alphavbeta3 expression with 18F-FRGD2. J Nucl Med 2006;47(1):113–21.

146. Chen X, Park R, Tohme M, et al. MicroPET and autoradiographic imaging of breast cancer alpha

v-integrin expression using 18F- and 64Cu-labeled RGD peptide. Bioconjug Chem 2004;15(1):41–9.

147. Chen X, Liu S, Hou Y, et al. MicroPET imaging of breast cancer alphav-integrin expression with 64Cu-labeled dimeric RGD peptides. Mol Imaging Biol 2004;6(5):350–9.

148. Wu Z, Li ZB, Chen K, et al. MicroPET of tumor integrin alphavbeta3 expression using 18F-labeled PEGylated tetrameric RGD peptide (18F-FPRGD4). J Nucl Med 2007;48(9):1536–44.

149. Li ZB, Cai W, Cao Q, et al. (64)Cu-labeled tetrameric and octameric RGD peptides for small-animal PET of tumor alpha(v)beta(3) integrin expression. J Nucl Med 2007;48(7):1162–71.

150. Thumshirn G, Hersel U, Goodman SL, et al. Multimeric cyclic RGD peptides as potential tools for tumor targeting: solid-phase peptide synthesis and chemoselective oxime ligation. Chemistry 2003;9(12):2717–25.

151. Poethko T, Schottelius M, Thumshirn G, et al. Two-step methodology for high-yield routine radiohalogenation of peptides: (18)F-labeled RGD and octreotide analogs. J Nucl Med 2004;45(5):892–902.

152. Cai W, Wu Y, Chen K, et al. In vitro and in vivo characterization of 64Cu-labeled AbegrinTM, a humanized monoclonal antibody against integrin avb3. Cancer Res 2006;66(19):9673–81.

153. Higuchi T, Bengel FM, Seidl S, et al. Assessment of alphavbeta3 integrin expression after myocardial infarction by positron emission tomography. Cardiovasc Res 2008;78(2):395–403.

154. Ferrara N. VEGF and the quest for tumour angiogenesis factors. Nat Rev Cancer 2002;2(10):795–803.

155. Broumas AR, Pollard RE, Bloch SH, et al. Contrast-enhanced computed tomography and ultrasound for the evaluation of tumor blood flow. Invest Radiol 2005;40(3):134–47.

156. Hicklin DJ, Ellis LM. Role of the vascular endothelial growth factor pathway in tumor growth and angiogenesis. J Clin Oncol 2005;23(5):1011–27.

157. Sun J, Wang DA, Jain RK, et al. Inhibiting angiogenesis and tumorigenesis by a synthetic molecule that blocks binding of both VEGF and PDGF to their receptors. Oncogene 2005;24(29):4701–9.

158. Watanabe H, Mamelak AJ, Wang B, et al. Antivascular endothelial growth factor receptor-2 (Flk-1/KDR) antibody suppresses contact hypersensitivity. Exp Dermatol 2004;13(11):671–81.

159. Prewett M, Huber J, Li Y, et al. Antivascular endothelial growth factor receptor (fetal liver kinase 1) monoclonal antibody inhibits tumor angiogenesis and growth of several mouse and human tumors. Cancer Res 1999;59(20):5209–18.

160. Ciardiello F, Caputo R, Damiano V, et al. Antitumor effects of ZD6474, a small molecule vascular endothelial growth factor receptor tyrosine kinase inhibitor, with additional activity against epidermal growth factor receptor tyrosine kinase. Clin Cancer Res 2003;9(4):1546–56.

161. Wedge SR, Ogilvie DJ, Dukes M, et al. ZD4190: an orally active inhibitor of vascular endothelial growth factor signaling with broad-spectrum antitumor efficacy. Cancer Res 2000;60(4):970–5.

162. Kennedy JE, ter Haar GR, Wu F, et al. Contrast-enhanced ultrasound assessment of tissue response to high-intensity focused ultrasound. Ultrasound Med Biol 2004;30(6):851–4.

163. Cai W, Chen X. Multimodality imaging of vascular endothelial growth factor and vascular endothelial growth factor receptor expression. Front Biosci 2007;12:4267–79.

164. Nagengast WB, de Vries EG, Hospers GA, et al. In vivo VEGF imaging with radiolabeled bevacizumab in a human ovarian tumor xenograft. J Nucl Med 2007;48(8):1313–9.

165. Collingridge DR, Carroll VA, Glaser M, et al. The development of [124I]iodinated-VG76e: a novel tracer for imaging vascular endothelial growth factor in vivo using positron emission tomography. Cancer Res 2002;62(20):5912–9.

166. Jayson GC, Zweit J, Jackson A, et al. Molecular imaging and biological evaluation of HuMV833 anti-VEGF antibody: implications for trial design of antiangiogenic antibodies. J Natl Cancer Inst 2002;94(19):1484–93.

167. Scheer MG, Stollman TH, Boerman OC, et al. Imaging liver metastases of colorectal cancer patients with radiolabelled bevacizumab: Lack of correlation with VEGF-A expression. Eur J Cancer 2008;44(13):1835–40.

168. Strauss LG, Koczan D, Klippel S, et al. Impact of angiogenesis-related gene expression on the tracer kinetics of 18F-FDG in colorectal tumors. J Nucl Med 2008;49(8):1238–44.

169. Hsu AR, Cai W, Veeravagu A, et al. Multimodality molecular imaging of glioblastoma growth inhibition with vasculature-targeting fusion toxin VEGF121/rGel. J Nucl Med 2007;48(3):445–54.

170. Cai W, Chen K, Mohamedali KA, et al. PET of vascular endothelial growth factor receptor expression. J Nucl Med 2006;47(12):2048–56.

171. Chen K, Cai W, Li ZB, et al. Quantitative PET Imaging of VEGF receptor expression. Mol Imaging Biol 2008;11(1):15–22.

172. Backer MV, Levashova Z, Patel V, et al. Molecular imaging of VEGF receptors in angiogenic vasculature with single-chain VEGF-based probes. Nat Med 2007;13(4):504–9.

173. Li J, Brown LF, Hibberd MG, et al. VEGF, flk-1, and flt-1 expression in a rat myocardial infarction model of angiogenesis. Am J Physiol 1996;270(5 Pt 2): H1803–11.

174. Soeki T, Tamura Y, Shinohara H, et al. Serial changes in serum VEGF and HGF in patients with

acute myocardial infarction. Cardiology 2000; 93(3):168–74.

175. Rodriguez-Porcel M, Cai W, Gheysens O, et al. Imaging of VEGF receptor in a rat myocardial infarction model using PET. J Nucl Med 2008; 49(4):667–73.

176. Willmann JK, Paulmurugan R, Chen K, et al. Ultrasonic imaging of tumor angiogenesis with contrast microbubbles targeted to vascular endothelial growth factor type 2 receptor [revision]. Radiology 2007;246(2):508–18.

177. Cai W, Guzman R, Hsu AR, et al. Positron emission tomography imaging of poststroke angiogenesis. Stroke 2008;40(1):270–7.

178. Simon M, Rockl W, Hornig C, et al. Receptors of vascular endothelial growth factor/vascular permeability factor (VEGF/VPF) in fetal and adult human kidney: localization and [125I]VEGF binding sites. J Am Soc Nephrol 1998;9(6):1032–44.

179. Keyt BA, Nguyen HV, Berleau LT, et al. Identification of vascular endothelial growth factor determinants for binding KDR and FLT-1 receptors. Generation of receptor-selective VEGF variants by site-directed mutagenesis. J Biol Chem 1996; 271(10):5638–46.

180. Wang H, Cai W, Chen K, et al. A new PET tracer specific for vascular endothelial growth factor receptor 2. Eur J Nucl Med Mol Imaging 2007; 34(12):2001–10.

181. Wagner S, Breyholz HJ, Faust A, et al. Molecular imaging of matrix metalloproteinases in vivo using small molecule inhibitors for SPECT and PET. Curr Med Chem 2006;13(23):2819–38.

182. Folgueras AR, Pendas AM, Sanchez LM, et al. Matrix metalloproteinases in cancer: from new functions to improved inhibition strategies. Int J Dev Biol 2004;48(5–6):411–24.

183. Johnson JL, George SJ, Newby AC, et al. Divergent effects of matrix metalloproteinases 3, 7, 9, and 12 on atherosclerotic plaque stability in mouse brachiocephalic arteries. Proc Natl Acad Sci U S A 2005;102(43):15575–80.

184. Hidalgo M, Eckhardt SG. Development of matrix metalloproteinase inhibitors in cancer therapy. J Natl Cancer Inst 2001;93(3):178–93.

185. Li WP, Anderson CJ. Imaging matrix metalloproteinase expression in tumors. Q J Nucl Med 2003; 47(3):201–8.

186. Lee S, Park K, Kim K, et al. Activatable imaging probes with amplified fluorescent signals. Chem Commun (Camb) 2008;(36):4250–60.

187. Lee S, Park K, Lee SY, et al. Dark quenched matrix metalloproteinase fluorogenic probe for imaging osteoarthritis development in vivo. Bioconjug Chem 2008;19(9):1743–7.

188. Bremer C, Bredow S, Mahmood U, et al. Optical imaging of matrix metalloproteinase-2 activity in tumors: feasibility study in a mouse model. Radiology 2001;221(2):523–9.

189. Medina OP, Kairemo K, Valtanen H, et al. Radionuclide imaging of tumor xenografts in mice using a gelatinase-targeting peptide. Anticancer Res 2005;25(1A):33–42.

190. Hanaoka H, Mukai T, Habashita S, et al. Chemical design of a radiolabeled gelatinase inhibitor peptide for the imaging of gelatinase activity in tumors. Nucl Med Biol 2007;34(5):503–10.

191. Sprague JE, Li WP, Liang K, et al. In vitro and in vivo investigation of matrix metalloproteinase expression in metastatic tumor models. Nucl Med Biol 2006;33(2):227–37.

192. Zheng QH, Fei X, Liu X, et al. Synthesis and preliminary biological evaluation of MMP inhibitor radiotracers [11C]methyl-halo-CGS 27023A analogs, new potential PET breast cancer imaging agents. Nucl Med Biol 2002;29(7):761–70.

193. Furumoto S, Takashima K, Kubota K, et al. Tumor detection using 18F-labeled matrix metalloproteinase-2 inhibitor. Nucl Med Biol 2003;30(2):119–25.

194. Wagner S, Breyholz HJ, Law MP, et al. Novel fluorinated derivatives of the broad-spectrum MMP inhibitors N-hydroxy-2(R)-[[(4-methoxyphenyl)sulfonyl](benzyl)- and (3-picolyl)-amino]-3-methylbutanamide as potential tools for the molecular imaging of activated MMPs with PET. J Med Chem 2007;50(23):5752–64.

195. Zheng QH, Fei X, Liu X, et al. Comparative studies of potential cancer biomarkers carbon-11 labeled MMP inhibitors (S)-2-(4′-[11C]methoxybiphenyl-4-sulfonylamino)-3-methylbutyric acid and N-hydroxy-(R)-2-[[(4′-[11C]methoxyphenyl)sulfonyl]benzylamino]-3-methylbut anamide. Nucl Med Biol 2004;31(1):77–85.

196. Zheng QH, Fei X, DeGrado TR, et al. Synthesis, biodistribution and micro-PET imaging of a potential cancer biomarker carbon-11 labeled MMP inhibitor (2R)-2-[[4-(6-fluorohex-1-ynyl)phenyl]sulfonylamino]-3-methylbutyric acid [11C]methyl ester. Nucl Med Biol 2003;30(7):753–60.

197. Kulasegaram R, Giersing B, Page CJ, et al. In vivo evaluation of 111In-DTPA-N-TIMP-2 in Kaposi sarcoma associated with HIV infection. Eur J Nucl Med 2001;28(6):756–61.

198. Neri D, Carnemolla B, Nissim A, et al. Targeting by affinity-matured recombinant antibody fragments of an angiogenesis associated fibronectin isoform. Nat Biotechnol 1997;15(12):1271–5.

199. Santimaria M, Moscatelli G, Viale GL, et al. Immunoscintigraphic detection of the ED-B domain of fibronectin, a marker of angiogenesis, in patients with cancer. Clin Cancer Res 2003;9(2):571–9.

200. Suri C, Jones PF, Patan S, et al. Requisite role of angiopoietin-1, a ligand for the TIE2 receptor, during embryonic angiogenesis. Cell 1996;87(7):1171–80.

201. Seaman S, Stevens J, Yang MY, et al. Genes that distinguish physiological and pathological angiogenesis. Cancer Cell 2007;11(6):539–54.

202. Shao Y, Cherry SR, Farahani K, et al. Simultaneous PET and MR imaging. Phys Med Biol 1997;42(10):1965–70.

203. Townsend DW, Beyer T. A combined PET/CT scanner: the path to true image fusion. Br J Radiol 2002;75(Spec No):S24–30.

204. Catana C, Wu Y, Judenhofer MS, et al. Simultaneous acquisition of multislice PET and MR images: initial results with a MR-compatible PET scanner. J Nucl Med 2006;47(12):1968–76.

205. Cai W, Chen K, He L, et al. Quantitative PET of EGFR expression in xenograft-bearing mice using

^{64}Cu-labeled cetuximab, a chimeric anti-EGFR monoclonal antibody. Eur J Nucl Med Mol Imaging 2007;34:850–8 [Epub].

206. Cai W, Ebrahimnejad A, Chen K, et al. Quantitative radioimmunoPET imaging of EphA2 in tumour-bearing mice. Eur J Nucl Med Mol Imaging 2007; 34(12):2024–36.

207. Li ZB, Wu Z, Chen K, et al. 18F-labeled BBN-RGD heterodimer for prostate cancer imaging. J Nucl Med 2008;49(3):453–61.

208. Jung KH, Lee KH, Paik JY, et al. Favorable biokinetic and tumor-targeting properties of 99mTc-labeled glucosamino RGD and effect of paclitaxel therapy. J Nucl Med 2006;47(12):2000–7.

PET Imaging of Hypoxia

Suzanne E. Lapi, PhD*, Thomas F. Voller, BSc, Michael J. Welch, PhD

KEYWORDS

- Positron emission tomography (PET) • Hypoxia
- ^{18}F-MISO • ^{64}Cu-ATSM • Nitroimidazole

Hypoxia in tissue is characterized as a lack of oxygen required for cells to function normally. It usually is defined as the oxygen tension at which the metabolic demand in stoma, endothelial cells, and tumor cells exceeds the supply.[1] This imbalance between oxygen and delivery causes numerous downstream effects, which have implications in various situations and disease states.

Hypoxia imaging has applications in functional recovery in ischemic events such as stroke and myocardial ischemia, but especially in tumors in which hypoxia can be predictive of treatment response and overall prognosis.

Hypoxia can occur in both heart and brain tissue following arterial occlusions and other events.[2] The heart is a very aerobic organ, consuming some 8 to 15 mL O_2/min/100 g tissue at rest, and it requires a constant supply of oxygen to maintain function and viability.[3] The heart can become exposed to ischemic conditions resulting from acute coronary events. Brief periods of ischemia (less than 20 minutes) are reversible if followed by reperfusion.[4] If the duration of oxygen deprivation becomes longer, sections of the heart may become necrotic and nonviable.[4] During a stroke, blood flow to the brain is interrupted, and if this condition persists, brain function becomes impaired, sometimes irreversibly.[5] The longer the duration of hypoxia, the larger and more diffuse the area of the brain that is affected. The high energy requirements of the brain render this organ particularly vulnerable to hypoxia.[4]

Hypoxia usually develops in tumors through a disruption in the vascular blood supply to the growing tumor mass. Tumor vessels are typically structurally and functionally abnormal compared with normal tissue, with the vasculature being characterized by vigorous proliferation, which leads to structurally immature, defective, and ineffective vessels. This results in vessels that are tortuous and leaky, which can contribute to heterogeneity in blood flow and thus varied levels of oxygenation in tumors.[6,7] Blood flow in these abnormal vessels can vary considerably, from 0.01 to 2.0 mL/g/min[7]; thus tumors can exhibit perfusion that is characteristic of a range of metabolic rates. In addition to the abnormal vasculature, fluid accumulating in the tumor matrix and the rapidly proliferating cancer cells themselves can cause high interstitial pressure that restricts and compresses the intratumor vessels, causing collapse and reducing blood supply even further.[7,8] Hypoxia also can be caused by a deterioration of diffusion geometry within the tumor (again caused by abnormal blood vessels) or disease/therapy-associated anemia, which leads to a reduced oxygen transport by the blood.[9] Thus hypoxia can result from diffusion and effusion issues and is usually the result of a combination of these problems.[1] There is evidence that tumors may consist of up to 50% to 60% hypoxic or anoxic tissue heterogeneously distributed within the tumor mass with tumor to tumor variability greater than intra-tumor variability.[9] Clinically relevant hypoxia is detected in 50% of all solid tumors irrespective of size, stage, nodal status, or other histopathological features, with local recurrences typically having a higher hypoxic fraction than that of primary tumors.[7]

Mallinckrodt Institute of Radiology, Washington University, 510 South Kingshighway Boulevard, St. Louis, MO 63110, USA
* Corresponding author.
E-mail address: lapis@mir.wustl.edu (S.E. Lapi).

PET Clin 4 (2009) 39–47
doi:10.1016/j.cpet.2009.05.009
1556-8598/09/$ – see front matter

Hypoxia is associated with restrained proliferation, differentiation, necrosis, or apoptosis, and it can lead to the development of a more aggressive cancer phenotype.[9] Hypoxia-induced proteome or genome changes may trigger mechanisms that enable cells to escape this hostile environment and hence favor unrestricted growth and mobility.[7] Lack of nutrients to the cells (caused by reduced blood supply) in combination with hypoxia also may lead to these cellular changes, thus causing progression, local growth, and metastasis.[7] This situation can manifest as a higher rate of recurrence and metastasis, and in the long term, decreased survival.

Hypoxia cells have been shown to have an increased resistance to radiotherapy. Radiotherapy is thought to rely mainly on the formation of free radicals, which cause DNA damage, a mechanism that is enhanced by the presence of oxygen. Because of this oxygen enhancement effect, hypoxia can be a key factor in tumor development and therapy because of the increased radioresistance of hypoxic cells compared with normally oxygenated cells.[10] Early on, Gray and colleagues[11] determined the radiation dose required to achieve the same biologic effect is 2.8 to 3 times higher in the absence of oxygen than in its prescence. Hypoxia is one of the major factors that negatively affects radiotherapy outcome.[1] Sustained hypoxia also can lead to alterations in the number of quiescent cells, which leads to alterations in the response to radiation and chemotherapy,[7] as these therapies are primarily effective against rapidly proliferating cells.[12]

In patients who have cervical carcinoma, tumor hypoxia is an important prognostic factor that predicts for decreased overall and disease-free survival. Moreover, hypoxic tumors are less responsive to irradiation than are normoxic tumors. A higher frequency of metastatic disease has been reported in patients who have hypoxic soft tissue sarcomas and cervical cancer.[13,14] Brizel and colleagues[14] have reported that a combination of radiotherapy and hyperthermia (to improve tumor oxygenation) in 38 patients who had nonmetastatic high-grade soft tissue sarcoma resulted in improvement of tumor oxygenation measured by polarographic oxygen electrodes and had an impact on treatment outcome. They reported that patients who had less than 90% tumor necrosis in the resected specimen experienced longer disease-free survival than those who had at least 90% necrosis. Höckel and colleagues[13] have studied 103 patients with advanced cervical cancer. In cervical cancer, the oxygen status of the tumor measured by invasive oxygen electrodes was noted to be the single most important prognostic factor. Patients who had hypoxic cervical tumors had significantly worse disease-free survival and overall survival compared with nonhypoxic tumors. The poor outcomes in patients who had hypoxic tumors was because of locoregional failure, irrespective of the mode of therapy (surgery or radiation) applied as primary treatment.[13]

Direct correlations have been made between imaging protocols and pO_2 measurements taken with an Eppendorf (Eppendorf, Westbury, NY) pO2 hypoximeter, which measures oxygen tensions using a polargraphic oxygen microelectrode. This direct real-time measurement of oxygen tension in tissues provided the first concrete evidence that intratumoral oxygen tension was indicative of survival in human cancers.[13] This method of oxygen measurement has demonstrated the clinical relevance of tumor hypoxia, although this methodology is limited by its invasiveness and is feasible only for superficial or easily accessible tumors.[15] It also can yield variable results because of sampling errors. In addition, the pO2 electrode only measures average oxygen tension and thus does not distinguish necrotic tissue from hypoxic but viable tissue, which is a disadvantage for this technique.[13]

Noninvasive imaging protocols for detecting hypoxia have been developed for magnetic resonance (MR). These techniques can be based on endogenous or exogenous contrast agents and can include electron paramagnetic resonance (EPR),[16,17] magnetic resonance spectroscopy (MRS),[18] and blood oxygen-dependent level (BOLD) imaging.[19,20] EPR relies on the injections of free radical contrast agents, which reflect the absolute oxygen tension present in the tissue.[17] Although hypoxia cannot be detected by MRS directly, physiologic conditions (uptake of binding markers) associated with the lack of oxygenation can be detected, usually by ^{19}F MRS. The patient is injected with perfluorocarbons to measure oxygen tension. This technique relies on the change in the relaxation rate of the ^{19}F being enhanced in direct proportion to the O_2 concentration;[21] however, these relaxation rates may depend on other physiologic factors present in the tissue. Magnetic resonance imaging (MRI) can be used to detect paramagnetic deoxyhemoglobin distinctly from oxyhemoglobin and thus obtains a measure of blood oxygenation.[20] This technique is known as BOLD imaging and has been used to indirectly measure oxygen levels in animal[20] and human[22] tumors. A disadvantage of this technique is the inability to separate confounding effects related to blood flow heterogeneity,[12] which is likely to be present in hypoxic tissue. Despite the development of these techniques, studies in people with MR are limited.[12]

Recently there has been development of imaging agents using positron emission tomography (PET) and single photon emission computed tomography (SPECT agents). Despite the wider availability of SPECT, many PET agents have come to the forefront of hypoxia imaging. Halogenated PET nitroimidazole imaging agents labeled with ^{18}F ($t_{1/2}$ = 110 m) and ^{124}I ($t_{1/2}$ = 110 m) have been under investigation for the last 25 years, with radiometal agents (^{64}Cu-ATSM) being developed more recently. The structures of several of these agents are shown in **Fig. 1**. With the use of these specific hypoxia tracers, PET can be used for assessing and quantifying tumor hypoxia in a noninvasive manner. This method has potential for determining the intratumor distribution of regional tumor hypoxia and thus may be used to select patients for hypoxia therapies. This article focuses on these PET imaging agents for hypoxia.

RADIOLABLED 2-NITROIMIDAZOLES AS MARKERS FOR HYPOXIA

Nitroimidazoles first were proposed as reducible hypoxia markers in 1979.[23] These compounds enter cells by passive diffusion and undergo reduction forming a reactive intermediate species. In the presence of oxygen, the molecule is reoxidized, and the nitroimidazole diffuses back out of the cell. Under hypoxic conditions, however, further reduction occurs, forming covalent bonds with intracellular macromolecules, thus trapping the compound inside the cell.[24] This mechanism is shown in **Fig. 2**. Because the rate of uptake depends strictly on the oxygen concentration in the cell, correlations can be made between tracer concentration and hypoxia conditions. There are several fluorinated and iodinated agents that have been developed based on the nitroimidazole basic structure.

[^{18}F]-fluoromisonidazole

^{18}F-labeled misonidazole (FMISO) was proposed as a radioactive derivative of the nitroimidazoles in 1984.[25,26] Over the last decade, [^{18}F]FMISO

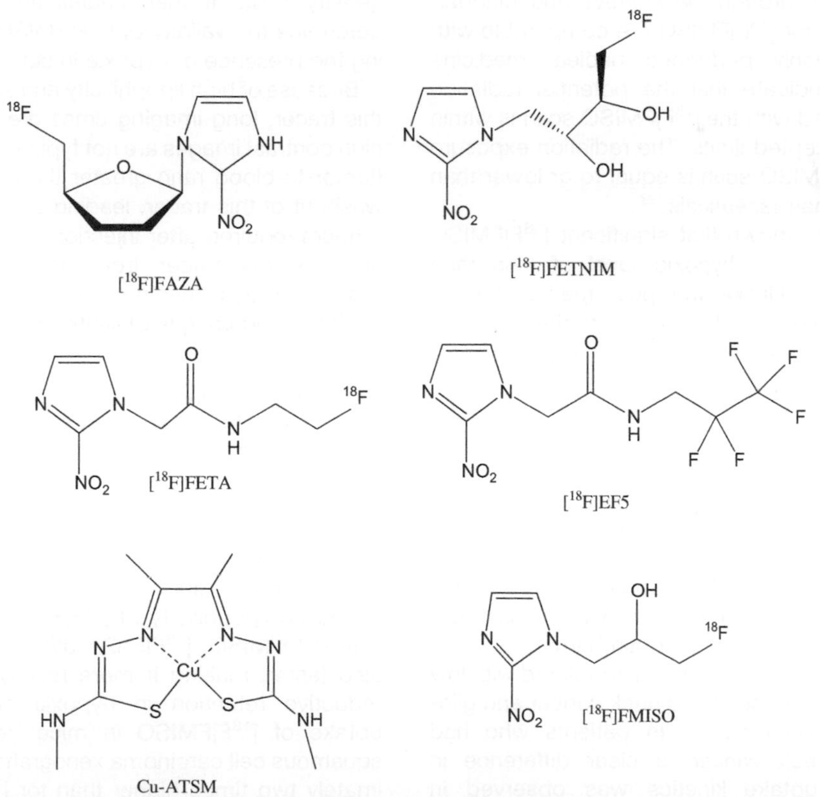

Fig. 1. Structure of hypoxia positron emission tomography imaging agents.

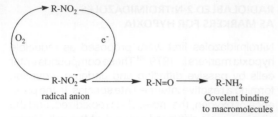

Fig. 2. Mechanism of Nitroimidazole retention in hypoxic tissue.

has been studied as a PET agent for imaging hypoxia, and [18F]FMISO is currently the most widely used PET agent for mapping regional hypoxia. It generally is considered the gold standard for PET hypoxia imaging. It has been shown to be retained in hypoxic cells in vivo and in vitro.

In patients, time activity curves of this agent have shown that FMISO in normal tissue equilibrates with plasma levels within 30 minutes but is retained selectively in hypoxic tissue for up to 2.5 hours.[27] Imaging protocols are typically 20 to 30 minutes and start from 75 to 150 minutes after injection of the radiotracer.[28] A typical threshold of tumor-to-plasma ratio of 1.4 at 2 hours after injection can be considered to be indicative of hypoxia.[27] This agent is metabolized by the liver and excreted through the kidneys and bladder. Organ doses for [18F]FMISO are comparable with other commonly performed nuclear medicine scans and indicate that the potential radiation risk associated with the [18F]FMISO scan is within generally accepted limits. The radiation exposure for the [18F]FMISO scan is equal to or lower than other radiopharmaceuticals.[29]

It has been shown that significant [18F]FMISO uptake requires a hypoxic level of less than 10 mm Hg.[27] Unlike the pO2 measurements, however, FMISO is only sensitive to the presence of hypoxia in viable cells,[28] which may be advantageous for in vivo imaging in people.

[18F]FMISO has been used in numerous oncology clinical studies including gliomas,[8] head and neck cancer,[30] and nonsmall cell lung cancer. In an early study involving patients who had malignant glioma, a feasibility study demonstrated the use of FMISO to detect hypoxia in the brain in vivo.[31] [18F]FMISO uptake also has been observed in the brain, indicating that it is freely diffusible across the blood–brain barrier.

[18F]FMISO uptake has been correlated with low prognosis in both head and neck cancer and glioblastoma multiforme.[30,32] In patients who had head and neck cancer, a clear difference in [18F]FMISO uptake kinetics was observed in patients who responded to radiation therapy

compared with nonresponders.[30] Although [18F]FMISO uptake varied widely between patients and considerably between different parts of tumors, patients who were nonresponsive to radiation therapy generally displayed higher levels of [18F]FMISO accumulation. Nonresponders also showed initially low perfusion of the tracers followed by accumulation indicating hypoxia, while responders showed high perfusion followed by rapid washout, indicating well-oxygenated, viable tumor tissue.[30] In this study, no pattern was observed in patients who had nonsmall cell lung cancer, indicating that the choice of hypoxia imaging agent should depend on tumor type. In glioblastoma multiforme patients, the volume and intensity of hypoxia as determined by [18F]FMISO scans before radiotherapy were correlated with shortened time to progression and survival.[32]

One study concluded that [18F]FMISO was not suitable for detecting tumor hypoxia in various soft tissue tumors, with no correlation found between hypoxic tumors (as determined by O2 electrode measurements) and those displaying enhanced [18F]FMISO uptake.[33] The authors of the publication with these negative [18F]FMISO findings speculated that the low uptake of FMISO in the tumors could be caused by large amounts of necrosis in the soft tissue tumors or tumor heterogeneity,[33] but further studies are warranted to determine the validity of [18F]FMISO in ascertaining the presence of hypoxia in soft tissue tumors.

Because of high lipophilicity and slow kinetics of this tracer, long imaging times are required, and high contrast images are not typical with this agent (tumor-to-blood ratio greater than 1.2). The slow washout of this tracer, leading to a delay time of 2 hours required after injection to allow for clearance of the tracer from normal background tissues, delays imaging and can result in poor statistics and images of limited quality.[34]

[18F]Fluoroazomycin Arabinoside and [124I]Iodoazomycin Arabinoside

[18F]fluoroazomycin arabinoside (FAZA) recently has been shown to have superior pharmacokinetics than [18F]FMISO, primarily because of faster clearance from normal tissues resulting in higher tumor-to-background ratios.[35] This is caused by increased lipophilicity of [18F]FAZA as compared with [18F]FMISO. [18F]FAZA diffusion into cells is also faster, making it more readily available for reductive retention in hypoxia cells.[36] Tumor uptake of [18F]FMISO in mice bearing human squamous cell carcinoma xenografts was approximately two times higher than for [18F]FAZA, but tumor-to-blood ratios was significantly higher for

[^{18}F]FAZA than [^{18}F]FMISO because of slower clearance of [^{18}F]FMISO. In people, imaging with [^{18}F]FAZA appears feasible in patients who have head and neck cancer.[15] Image quality in these patients in a preliminary clinical study was determined to be adequate for clinical use. Tumor uptake was heterogeneous within individual tumors and between individuals, suggesting large intertumor and intratumor variability.[15] The authors from this study concluded that imaging at approximately 2 hours after radiotracer injection seemed to be a reasonable choice for [^{18}F[FAZA] tumor imaging, as early time points largely depended on perfusion of the radiotracer into the tumor. The arbitrary hypoxia threshold chosen (tumor-to-muscle ratio of 1.5) in this study was slightly higher than with [^{18}F]FMISO (between 1.2 and 1.4), again possibly indicating superior kinetics.[15] More studies are required, however, to fully ascertain the benefits of imaging with [^{18}F]FAZA as opposed to [^{18}F]FMISO.

The iodinated analog [^{124}I]IAZA also has been prepared, but imaging at later time points, which were not possible with the fluorinated versions, resulted in no advantage. Significant thyroid uptake also was reported in this study, indicating possible deiodination of the [^{124}I]IAZA.[35]

[^{124}I]-iodoazomycin Galactopyranoside

[^{124}I]-iodoazomycin galactopyranoside (IAZG) was developed as a longer-lived nitroimidazole PET radiotracer to obtain images at extended time points. Theoretically, in this manner, images could be obtained after washout of the unbound tracer, thus yielding images with better contrast. [^{124}I]IAZG uptake was shown to be consistent with independent measures of hypoxia in rat liver tumors.[37] In a comparison study between [^{18}F]FMISO and [^{124}I]IAZG in rats bearing liver and peritoneal metastasis, both tracers were shown to accumulate in hypoxic tumor tissue. The two tracers also demonstrated similar tumor-to-background ratios, although the optimal imaging time differed (3 hours for [^{18}F]FMISO and 6 hours for [^{124}I]IAZG).[38] The [^{18}F]FMISO agent, however, yielded higher quality scans as the absolute concentration of the tracer was higher in the tumor; thus higher counting statistics were obtained. The difference in kinetic behavior between these two molecules may be attributed to the difference in lipophilicity of these two tracers. The authors suggest that deiodination of the [^{124}I]IAZG compound also may be responsible for the varied biodistribution, but as thyroid uptake in the animals in this study was not reported, it is difficult to determine.[38] A similar PET imaging

agent—[^{124}I]-iodoazomycin galactoside—in another study by the same group, was shown to have high tumor-to-whole body ratios in both hypoxic fibrosarcoma and breast cancer models.[39] Comparisons with [^{18}F]FMISO showed optimal imaging at later time points (24 hours after injection versus 3 hours after injection for [^{18}F]FMISO), and higher tumor-to-normal tissue ratios were obtained. Higher absolute values of tracer accumulation also obtained with [^{124}I]-iodoazomycin galactoside (17% as compared with 5% to 10% for [^{18}F]FMISO).[39] Considerable deiodination was observed in vivo with this tracer, as observed by the amount of radioactivity present in the thyroid in the animals. These data reinforce the notion that hypoxia agent selection may need to be tumor-specific.

[^{18}F]1-(2-fluoro-1-[hydroxymethyl]ethoxy)methyl-2-nitroimidazole

[^{18}F]1-(2-fluoro-1-[hydroxymethyl]ethoxy)methyl-2-nitroimidazole (FRP170) was developed recently as a new 2-nitroimidazole analog with a hydrophilic side chain in attempts to increase the target to background ratios obtained with [^{18}F]FMISO. Radiofluorination of this compound yields [^{18}F]FRP170, which would be expected to yield superior images are earlier time points than [^{18}F]FMISO.[40] A recent study in four healthy male volunteers and three lung cancer patients who underwent dynamic scanning after injection of [^{18}F]FRP170 revealed rapid elimination though the kidneys and liver, with early uptake in lung cancer lesions.[40] Tumor uptake was observed on all lung cancer subjects, with contrast increasing over time. The authors concluded that [^{18}F]FRP170 was almost equivalent to [^{18}F]FMISO, although no match protocols were performed.[40]

The same group also evaluated [^{18}F]FRP170 in myocardial tissue in an animal model.[41] Visualization of ischemic but viable myocardial tissue was accomplished ex vivo, with confirmation of the location of the damaged areas by histology. Further studies would be necessary to confirm the use of [^{18}F]FRP170 for imaging hypoxic cardiac tissue.

[^{18}F]2-(2-nitro-^{1}H-imidazol-1-yl)-N-(2,2,3,3-pentafluoropropyl)-acetimide

[^{18}F]2-(2-nitro-^{1}H-imidazol-1-yl)-N-(2,2,3,3- pentafluoropropyl)-acetimide (EF5) first was developed as a biopsy-based staining agents. A positron emitting version of this compound recently was developed as an imaging agent of hypoxia. The enhanced lipophicity of this drug substantially increases its biologic half-life and signal from hypoxia-dependent metabolism.[42] EF5 also is reported to be the most stable of the 2-nitroimidazoles studies to date.

In a recent human trial with patients who had newly diagnosed head and neck squamous cell carcinoma (HNSCC), the time course of [^{18}F]EF5 was studied to determine the feasibility of this tracer as a hypoxia imaging agent.[43] The initial distribution of [^{18}F]EF5 was found to be dominated by blood flow, whereas binding and uptake at later time points were found to be hypoxia-specific. A tumor-to-muscle ratio of 1.5 was determined to be an appropriate threshold for the presence of clinically significant hypoxia. Additionally, increased [^{18}F]EF5 uptake was found to be predictive of higher grade tumor and of shorter time to metastasis in patients who had soft tissue sarcomas.[44] This also was reported in patients who had brain tumors.[45] The authors concluded that [^{18}F]EF5 could be used to identify patients at high risk for metastases.

One possible drawback to EF5 is that its labeling chemistry is more complex than that for the other ^{18}F-labeled agents, thus possibly leading to reduced availability of this radiotracer.[46]

COPPER-BASED RADIOPHARMACEUTICALS FOR IMAGING HYPOXIA
[[60,61,62,64]Cu]copper(II)-diacetyl-bis(N[4]-methylthiosemicarbazone)

Dithiosemicarbazones were discovered to possess antitumor properties in the 1960s. This led to the development of this class of ligands as radiopharmaceuticals because of the simplicity of the chemistry and the availability of copper positron- emitting isotopes.[47] [[60,61,62,64]Cu]copper(II)-diacetyl-bis(N[4]-methylthiosemicarbazone) (Cu-ATSM) is a neutral lipophilic molecule that is highly membrane-permeable and undergoes reduction and becomes trapped in the cell. This complex has been synthesized with a multitude of copper isotopes with varying half-lives, including [60]Cu ($t_{1/2}$ = 23.7 minutes), [61]Cu ($t_{1/2}$ = 3.35 hours), [62]Cu ($t_{1/2}$ = 9.74 minutes), and [64]Cu ($t_{1/2}$ = 12.7 hours).[47] [60]Cu, [61]Cu, and ^{64}Cu can be produced by proton bombardment of solid targets using a medical cyclotron, while [62]Cu is available from a generator similar to that used for [99m]Tc.[47]

[64]Cu-ATSM was developed as an alternative to [^{18}F]FMISO. [^{64}Cu] ($t_{1/2}$ = 12.7 hours, β^+ = 17.4%) can be produced in high specific activity in reliable quantities, and the longer half-life allows for distribution to centers without a cyclotron over longer distances than possible with [18]F. This isotope also decays by β^- and therefore can have potential as both a diagnostic and therapeutic agent.[48]

The radiopharmaceutical [62]Cu-ATSM initially was reported an agent for delineating hypoxic myocardial tissue in an isolated rat heart model.[49] The reduction of Cu(II) to Cu(I), which is the retention mechanism by which the copper is trapped in hypoxic tissue, was measured by electron spin resonance using nonradioactive Cu-ASTM, and this study determined that the Cu-ATSM was reduced in hypoxic but not in normal mitochondria. Rapid washout of this tracer from other tissues, as well as favorable blood pool clearance, may allow for screening for patients who have myocardial hypoxia with this agent. Retention of the radiopharmaceutical was increased under hypoxic conditions, and in this heart model, the [62]Cu-ATSM retention was correlated inversely with ^{201}Tl, a known blood flow marker.[49] Additional studies in several canine models determined quantitative and selective Cu-ATSM radiotracer uptake in hypoxic myocardium.[50] This study was performed to determine the oxygen-deprived myocardial state in both hypoxia and ischemia. The authors concluded that Cu-ATSM was an effective tracer for global hypoxia, which was also useful in situations such as myocardial infarction, where flow may be limited. This study additionally demonstrated that Cu-ATSM was not retained in necrotic tissue; thus this tracer could differentiate between hypoxic, viable tissue and nonfunctional, dead, myocardial tissue.[50] In addition, these scans were performed only 20 minutes after tracer injection, thus showing differences between hypoxic and normal tissue can be obtained rapidly.[50] In a preliminary human study, [62]Cu-ASTM PET imaging was performed in seven patients who had coronary heart disease. Increased uptake was observed in one patient with unstable angina.[51]

Yuan and colleagues[52] evaluated ^{64}Cu-ATSM as a hypoxia agent by comparing autoradiography distributions of the radiotracers in animal studies with nonradioactive EF5, a validated hypoxia marker drug. This group studied the uptake and immunohistochemistry in mammary adenocarcinomas, fibrosarcomas, and gliomas. Although they determined that high tumor-to-muscle ratios could be observed for the adenocarcinomas and gliomas, this was not the case for the fibrosarcomas.[52] This shows that although Cu-ATSM may be a valid hypoxia agent for some tumor types, this cannot be extrapolated to all tumors, and hence this may not be a universal hypoxia marker.

The first report of Cu-ASTM in a human study was with [62]Cu-ATSM in 2000. This study was

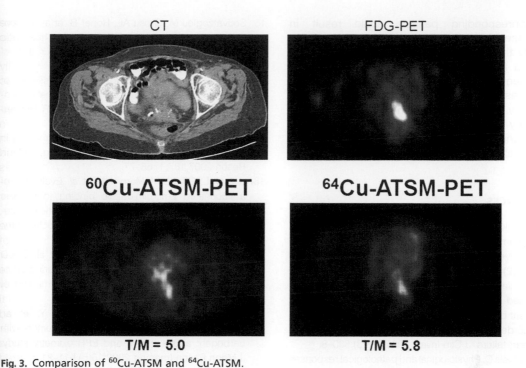

CT

FDG-PET

^{60}Cu-ATSM-PET

^{64}Cu-ATSM-PET

T/M = 5.0

T/M = 5.8

Fig. 3. Comparison of ^{60}Cu-ATSM and ^{64}Cu-ATSM.

conducted in normal subjects and patients who had lung cancer.[53] Intense uptake of the ^{62}Cu-ATSM was observed in all lung cancer patients, reaching a plateau within a few minutes after injections. The mean tumor-to-background ratio of ^{62}Cu-ATSM was 3.00, with a maximum of 9.33.[53] The radiotracer cleared rapidly from the blood and lungs of all normal subjects. In addition to this, a negative correlation was observed in three out of four patients between flow and flow-normalized ^{62}Cu-ATSM uptake, indicating that ^{62}Cu-ATSM uptake might be increased by low flow.

Cu-ATSM also has been evaluated in patients with rectal[54] and cervical cancer.[55] These were correlative studies designed to determine if uptake of ^{60}Cu-ATSM was predictive of a response to therapy. In patients who had rectal cancer, a pilot study indicated that ^{60}Cu-ATSM uptake may be predictive of survival but that further studies were needed to confirm this.[54] In a small study in cervical cancer patients, the interpatient ^{60}Cu-ATSM uptake was variable and found to correlate strongly with response to therapy and overall survival.[55] A tumor-to-muscle ratio of 3.5 was determined to be an accurate cutoff for distinguishing patients who did and did not develop disease recurrence after radiation therapy. In addition, this study determined that the prognostic information obtained from ^{60}Cu-ATSM could not be derived from Fluorodeoxyglucose (FDG-PET). Further studies comparing ^{60}Cu-ATSM with

^{64}Cu-ATSM in patients who had cancer of the uterine cervix found that patterns of these radiopharmaceuticals were similar, and image quality of the ^{64}Cu-ATSM was superior to the ^{60}Cu-ATSM.[56] Representative images from this study are shown in **Fig. 3**. The use of this longer-lived analog in this crossover study demonstrated the utility of ^{64}Cu-ATSM, which would allow for production and shipping of this radiopharmaceutical to supply large multicenter trials.

Overall, this agent shows rapid delineation of tumor hypoxia and higher tumor-to- background ratios (>>2.0), thus showing advantages over Fluoromisonidazole ([^{18}F]FMISO).[47] A current large-scale clinical trial with this radiopharmaceutical may shed more light on the advantages of Cu-ATSM.

SUMMARY

A recent review concluded "PET imaging with specific hypoxia tracers is becoming a must in radiation therapy planning."[10] With the developments of new therapies in phase 3 clinical trials to overcome hypoxia in tumors, the testing of predictive assays that can identify patient populations that can benefit from these treatments is necessary.[57] In addition, it has been suggested that dynamic hypoxia measurements during oxygen-modifying treatments could aid in the determination of responding and nonresponding patients.[1] Reduction of unnecessary treatments in nonresponding patients could result in decreased adverse effects and the opportunity to modify the patient treatment regime. Assays are needed for predicting patient outcome, and as treatment selection tools and for evaluating treatment response. These techniques may be used to apply hypoxia-directed interventions such as intensity modulation radiation therapy (IMRT) and chemotherapy with hypoxia selective drugs such as tirapazamine.[12]

REFERENCES

1. Ljungkvist AS, Bussink J, Kaanders JH, et al. Dynamics of tumor hypoxia measured with bioreductive hypoxic cell markers. Radiat Res 2007; 167(2):127–45.
2. Mathias CJ, Welch MJ, Kilbourn MR, et al. Radiolabeled hypoxic cell sensitizers: tracers for assessment of ischemia. Life Sci 1987;41(2):199–206.
3. Giordano FJ. Oxygen, oxidative stress, hypoxia, and heart failure. J Clin Invest 2005;115(3):500–8.
4. Michiels C. Physiological and pathological responses to hypoxia. Am J Pathol 2004;164(6):1875–82.
5. Won SJ, Kim DY, Gwag BJ. Cellular and molecular pathways of ischemic neuronal death. J Biochem Mol Biol 2002;35(1):67–86.
6. Jain RK. Normalization of tumor vasculature: an emerging concept in antiangiogenic therapy. Science 2005;307(5706):58–62.
7. Vaupel P. Tumor microenvironmental physiology and its implications for radiation oncology. Semin Radiat Oncol 2004;14(3):198–206.
8. Padera TP, Stoll BR, Tooredman JB, et al. Cancer cells compress intratumour vessels. Nature 2004; 427(6976):695.
9. Vaupel P, Mayer A. Hypoxia in cancer: significance and impact on clinical outcome. Cancer Metastasis Rev 2007;26(2):225–39.
10. Lucignani G. PET imaging with hypoxia tracers: a must in radiation therapy. Eur J Nucl Med Mol Imaging 2008;35(4):838–42.
11. Gray LH, Conger AD, Ebert M, et al. The concentration of oxygen dissolved in tissues at the time of irradiation as a factor in radiotherapy. Br J Radiol 1953; 26(312):638–48.
12. Foo SS, Abbott DF, Lawrentschuk N, et al. Functional imaging of intratumoral hypoxia. Mol Imaging Biol 2004;6(5):291–305.
13. Hockel M, Knoop C, Schlenger K, et al. Intratumoral pO_2 predicts survival in advanced cancer of the uterine cervix. Radiother Oncol 1993;26(1):45–50.
14. Brizel DM, Scully SP, Harrelson JM, et al. Tumor oxygenation predicts for the likelihood of distant metastases in human soft tissue sarcoma. Cancer Res 1996;56(5):941–3.
15. Souvatzoglou M, Grosu AL, Koper B, et al. Tumour hypoxia imaging with [18F]FAZA PET in head and neck cancer patients: a pilot study. Eur J Nucl Med Mol Imaging 2007;34(10):1566–75.
16. Gallez B, Baudelet C, Jordan BF. Assessment of tumor oxygenation by electron paramagnetic resonance: principles and applications. NMR Biomed 2004;17(5):240–62.
17. Pan X, Xia D, Halpern H. Targeted-ROI imaging in electron paramagnetic resonance imaging. J Magn Reson 2007;187(1):66–77.
18. Kwock L, Gill M, McMurry HL, et al. Evaluation of a fluorinated 2-nitroimidazole binding to hypoxic cells in tumor-bearing rats by 19F magnetic resonance spectroscopy and immunohistochemistry. Radiat Res 1992;129(1):71–8.
19. Landuyt W, Hermans R, Bosmans H, et al. BOLD contrast fMRI of whole rodent tumour during air or carbogen breathing using echoplanar imaging at 1.5 T. Eur Radiol 2001;11(11):2332–40.
20. Dunn JF, O'Hara JA, Zaim-Wadghiri Y, et al. Changes in oxygenation of intracranial tumors with carbogen: a BOLD MRI and EPR oximetry study. J Magn Reson Imaging 2002;16(5):511–21.
21. Clark LC Jr, Ackerman JL, Thomas SR, et al. Perfluorinated organic liquids and emulsions as biocompatible NMR imaging agents for 19F and dissolved oxygen. Adv Exp Med Biol 1984;180:835–45.
22. Griffiths JR, Taylor NJ, Howe FA, et al. The response of human tumors to carbogen breathing, monitored by gradient-recalled echo magnetic resonance imaging. Int J Radiat Oncol Biol Phys 1997;39(3): 697–701.
23. Chapman JD, Franko AJ, Sharplin J. A marker for hypoxic cells in tumors with potential clinical applicability. Br J Cancer 1981;43(4):546–50.
24. Whitmore GF, Varghese AJ. The biological properties of reduced nitroheterocyclics and possible underlying biochemical mechanisms. Biochem Pharmacol 1986;35(1):97–103.
25. Rajendran JG, Schwartz DL, O'Sullivan J, et al. Tumor hypoxia imaging with [F-18] fluoromisonidazole positron emission tomography in head and neck cancer. Clin Cancer Res 2006;12(18):5435–41.
26. Gronroos T, Eskola I, Lehtio K, et al. Pharmacokinetics of [F-18]FETNIM: a potential hypoxia marker for PET. J Nucl Med 2001;42(9):1397–404.
27. Lee ST, Scott AM. Hypoxia positron emission tomography imaging with [F-18]-fluoromisonidazole. Semin Nucl Med 2007;37(6):451–61.
28. Padhani A. PET imaging of tumour hypoxia. Cancer Imaging 2006;6:S117–21.
29. Krohn KA, Link JM, Mason RP. Molecular imaging of hypoxia. J Nucl Med 2008;49:129s–48s.
30. Eschmann SM, Paulsen F, Reimold M, et al. Prognostic impact of hypoxia imaging with [F-18]-misonidazole PET in nonsmall cell lung cancer and head

and neck cancer before radiotherapy. J Nucl Med 2005;46(2):253–60.

31. Valk PE, Mathis CA, Prados MD, et al. Hypoxia in human gliomas—demonstration by PET with fluorine-18-fluoromisonidazole. J Nucl Med 1992; 33(12):2133–7.

32. Spence AM, Muzi M, Swanson KR, et al. Regional hypoxia in glioblastoma multiforme quantified with [18F]-fluoromisonidazole positron emission tomography before radiotherapy: correlation with time to progression and survival. Clin Cancer Res 2008; 14(9):2623–30.

33. Bentzen L, Keiding S, Nordsmark M, et al. Tumour oxygenation assessed by [F-18]-fluoromisonidazole PET and polarographic needle electrodes in human soft tissue tumours. Radiother Oncol 2003;67(3): 339–44.

34. Nunn A, Linder K, Strauss HW. Nitroimidazoles and imaging hypoxia. Eur J Nucl Med 1995;22(3):265–80.

35. Reischl G, Dorow DS, Cullinane C, et al. Imaging of tumor hypoxia with [I-124] IAZA in comparison with [F-18] FMISO and [F-18]FAZA—first small animal PET results. J Pharm Pharm Sci 2007;10(2):203–11.

36. Kumar P, Stypinski D, Xia H, et al. Fluoroazomycin arabinoside (FAZA): synthesis, H-2 and H-3-labelling and preliminary biological evaluation of a novel 2-nitroimidazole marker of tissue hypoxia. J Labelled Comp Radiopharm 1999;42(1):3–16.

37. Riedl CC, Brader P, Zanzonico PB, et al. Imaging hypoxia in orthotopic rat liver tumors with iodine 124-labeled iodoazomycin galactopyranoside PET. Radiology 2008;248(2):561–70.

38. Riedl CC, Brader P, Zanzonico P, et al. Tumor hypoxia imaging in orthotopic liver tumors and peritoneal metastasis: a comparative study featuring dynamic F-18-MISO and I-124-IAZG PET in the same study cohort. Eur J Nucl Med Mol Imaging 2008;35(1):39–46.

39. Zanzonico P, O'Donoghue J, Chapman JD, et al. Iodine-124-labeled iodo-azomycin-galactoside imaging of tumor hypoxia in mice with serial microPET scanning. Eur J Nucl Med Mol Imaging 2004; 31(1):117–28.

40. Kaneta T, Takai Y, Iwata R, et al. Initial evaluation of dynamic human imaging using F-18-FRP170 as a new PET tracer for imaging hypoxia. Ann Nucl Med 2007;21(2):101–7.

41. Kaneta T, Takai Y, Kagaya Y, et al. Imaging of ischemic but viable myocardium using a new F-18-labeled 2-nitroimidazole analog, F-18-FRP170. J Nucl Med 2002;43(1):109–16.

42. Koch CJ, Hahn SM, Rockwell K, et al. Pharmacokinetics of EF5 [2-(2-nitro-1-H-imidazol-1-yl)-N-(2,2,3,3,3-pentafluoropropyl) acetamide] in human patients: implications for hypoxia measurements in vivo by 2-nitrolmidazoles. Cancer Chemother Pharmacol 2001;48(3):177–87.

43. Komar G, Seppanen M, Eskola O, et al. F-18-EF5: a New PET tracer for imaging hypoxia in head and neck cancer. J Nucl Med 2008;49(12):1944–51.

44. Evans SM, Fraker D, Hahn SM, et al. EF5 binding and clinical outcome in human soft tissue sarcomas. Int J Radiat Oncol Biol Phys 2006;64(3):922–7.

45. Evans SM, Judy KD, Dunphy I, et al. Comparative measurements of hypoxia in human brain tumors using needle electrodes and EF5 binding. Cancer Res 2004;64(5):1886–92.

46. Dolbier WR, Li AR, Koch CJ, et al. [F-18]-EF5, a marker for PET detection of hypoxia: synthesis of precursor and a new fluorination procedure. Appl Radiat Isot 2001;54(1):73–80.

47. Vavere AL, Lewis JS. Cu-ATSM: a radiopharmaceutical for the PET imaging of hypoxia. Dalton Trans 2007;43:4893–902.

48. Blower PJ, Lewis JS, Zweit J. Copper radionuclides and radiopharmaceuticals in nuclear medicine. Nucl Med Biol 1996;23(8):957–80.

49. Fujibayashi Y, Taniuchi H, Yonekura Y, et al. Copper-62-ATSM: a new hypoxia imaging agent with high membrane permeability and low redox potential. J Nucl Med 1997;38(7):1155–60.

50. Lewis JS, Herrero P, Sharp TL, et al. Delineation of hypoxia in canine myocardium using PET and copper(II)-diacetyl-bis(N-4-methylthiosemicarbazone). J Nucl Med 2002;43(11):1557–69.

51. Takahashi N, Fujibayashi Y, Yonekura Y, et al. Copper-62 ATSM as a hypoxic tissue tracer in myocardial ischemia. Ann Nucl Med 2001;15(3):293–6.

52. Yuan H, Schroeder T, Bowsher JE, et al. Intertumoral differences in hypoxia selectivity of the PET imaging agent 64Cu(II)-diacetyl-bis(N4-methylthiosemicarbazone). J Nucl Med 2006;47(6):989–98.

53. Takahashi N, Fujibayashi Y, Yonekura Y, et al. Evaluation of 62Cu labeled diacetyl-bis(N4-methylthiosemicarbazone) as a hypoxic tissue tracer in patients with lung cancer. Ann Nucl Med 2000;14(5):323–8.

54. Dietz DW, Dehdashti F, Grigsby PW, et al. Tumor hypoxia detected by positron emission tomography with 60Cu-ATSM as a predictor of response and survival in patients undergoing neoadjuvant chemoradiotherapy for rectal carcinoma: a pilot study. Dis Colon Rectum 2008;51(11):1641–8.

55. Dehdashti F, Grigsby PW, Mintun MA, et al. Assessing tumor hypoxia in cervical cancer by positron emission tomography with 60Cu-ATSM: relationship to therapeutic response—a preliminary report. Int J Radiat Oncol Biol Phys 2003;55(5):1233–8.

56. Lewis JS, Laforest R, Dehdashti F, et al. An imaging comparison of 64Cu-ATSM and 60Cu-ATSM in cancer of the uterine cervix. J Nucl Med 2008; 49(7):1177–82.

57. Kaanders JH, Bussink J, van der Kogel AJ. Clinical studies of hypoxia modification in radiotherapy. Semin Radiat Oncol 2004;14(3):233–40.

Copper-64 Radiopharmaceuticals for Oncologic Imaging

Jason P. Holland, DPhil[a], Riccardo Ferdani, PhD[b],
Carolyn J. Anderson, PhD[b], Jason S. Lewis, PhD[a,*]

KEYWORDS

- Copper 64 • Radiopharmaceuticals
- Peptides • Antibodies • PET

Over the last century, advances in imaging technology have revolutionized clinical practice and the importance of medical imaging is apparent. More recently, the use of nuclear medicine, which includes aspects of diagnostic imaging and radiotherapy, has become one of the primary tools available to clinicians and research scientists in the fight against cancer.[1] In combination with the use of radiolabeled pharmaceuticals, single photon computerized tomography (SPECT), and positron emission tomography (PET) provide detailed information about the physiology of, for example, a solid tumor. This information is complementary with the more familiar anatomic imaging techniques, which include conventional radiography (X rays), CT scans, MR imaging, and ultrasound. The principal advantage of nuclear imaging lies in its ability to identify the location of cancerous or otherwise diseased tissue, and simultaneously allows conclusions to be made about its physiologic state. The complementarity between anatomic CT or MRI imaging and the functional detail available from SPECT and PET have driven new developments in hybrid imaging modalities. For example, simultaneous PET/CT images are routinely used in oncology. In an elegant study, Quon and colleagues[2] obtained three-dimensional images by using hybrid PET/CT in combination with the well-established metabolic marker, [18F]-2-fluoro-2-deoxyglucose,

[18F]-FDG, as a presurgical tool to identify the location of cancer lesions in the lungs of a patient at John Hopkins University Hospital (Baltimore, USA). Although images recorded by using [18F]-FDG and other 18F radiolabeled compounds account for the majority of PET scans, there is currently significant interest in the development of new PET radiopharmaceuticals based on the coordination of metallic radionuclides including ^{68}Ga, ^{89}Zr, and ^{64}Cu.[3–7]

Copper has a range of radionuclides with varying decay characteristics which offer the potential for use in imaging and radiotherapy.[6] The production, decay, and relevant chelation chemistry of copper has been the subject of several excellent reviews.[6,8–10] This review article will focus on the use of ^{64}Cu as a radionuclide with the potential to be used for PET imaging applications. Copper-64 has a radioactive half-life of 12.7 hours and decays to either ^{64}Ni by positron emission (β^+ = 17.9%, E_{max} = 660 keV, $E_{average}$ = 288 keV) or electron capture (EC = 43.1%, E = 1675 and 1346 keV), or ^{64}Zn by β-decay (β^- = 39.0%, E = 190.2 keV) as shown in **Fig. 1**.[10] These decay modes mean that ^{64}Cu has the potential to be used in diagnostic PET imaging and radiotherapeutic applications. Resolution measurements using the "Derenzo" phantom indicate that PET images acquired using ^{64}Cu are comparable in quality to those obtained

---

[a] Department of Radiology, Memorial Sloan-Kettering Cancer Center, 1275 York Avenue, New York, NY 10065, USA
[b] Mallinckrodt Institute of Radiology, Washington University School of Medicine, 510 South Kingshighway Boulevard, Campus Box 8225, St. Louis, MO 63110, USA
* Corresponding author.
E-mail address: lewisj2@mskcc.org (J.S. Lewis).

PET Clin 4 (2009) 49–67
doi:10.1016/j.cpet.2009.04.013

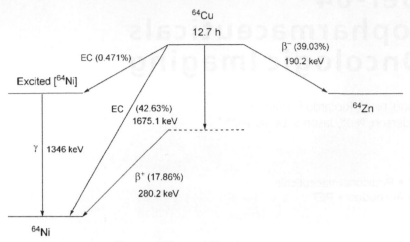

Fig. 1. The pathways for the decay of ^{64}Cu into ^{64}Ni and ^{64}Zn.

using ^{18}F as the nuclide.[11] The longer half-life allows ^{64}Cu to be produced at regional or national cyclotron facilities and distributed to local nuclear medicine departments with minimal loss in activity. In addition, the longer half-life is compatible with the timescales required for optimal biodistribution of monoclonal antibodies (mAbs) and oligopeptides for use in radioimmunotherapy (RIT). This article will describe the synthesis and evaluation of a variety of ^{64}Cu radiolabeled complexes, oligopeptides, and mAb conjugates which have been, or are close to being, translated to the clinic.

The most common production method for ^{64}Cu uses the ^{64}Ni$(p,n)^{64}$Cu reaction,[12–16] which involves the irradiation of enriched ^{64}Ni which has been electroplated on a gold[12–14,17,18] or rhodium platform.[19] McCarthy and colleagues[12] have described the efficient production of high specific-activity ^{64}Cu by using a small biomedical cyclotron and a ^{64}Ni enriched (>95%) target. The ^{64}Ni$(p,n)^{64}$Cu transmutation reaction is high yielding (2.3–5.0 mCi h^{-1}) and after purification by using an ion exchange column, high specific activity samples of [^{64}Cu]-CuCl$_2$(aq) were obtained (95–310 mCi µg^{-1}). Obata and colleagues,[14] reported yields of 0.6 to greater than 3.0 mCi/µAh, averaging 1.983 mCi/µAh with a radionuclidic purity of over 99% using a 12 MeV cyclotron. Using a tangential target on the National Institutes of Health CS-30 cyclotron, Szajek and colleagues[18] reported yields of 10.5 ± 3 mCi/µAh, when bombarded with a 12.5 MeV proton beam, which was comparable to the theoretical yield, and in over 3 hours produced greater than 1 Ci of radioactivity. The use of ^{64}Cu has increased dramatically in the past decade[20] and its production has now been reported by academic sources in the United States,[12,18] Europe,[15,19] and Japan.[14]

TUMOR HYPOXIA AND $^{60/62/64}$Cu-ATSM

It is well-established that hypoxia is an important determinant of the overall response of the tumor to conventional therapy. The presence of hypoxia can result in an increase in tumor aggressiveness, failure of local control, and activation of transcription factors that support cell survival and migration.[21–27] The ability to locate and quantify the extent of hypoxia (Fig. 2) within solid tumors by using noninvasive nuclear imaging would facilitate early diagnosis and help clinicians select the most appropriate treatment for each individual patient.[22,28]

In 1997, Fujibayashi and colleagues discovered that the neutral, lipophilic copper(II) complex of the N$_2$S$_2$ tetradentate ligand, diacetyl-2,3-bis(N^4-methyl-3-thiosemicarbazone), commonly referred to as Cu-ATSM, showed hypoxia-selective uptake in ex vivo ischemic, perfused, isolated rat-heart models (Fig. 3).[29,30] Copper-ATSM was later shown to be hypoxia-selective in vitro (Fig. 4) and for tumor hypoxia in vivo.[29,31–46] Recent experimental and computational work provided the first experimental evidence directly probing the reduction, reoxidation, and pH-mediated ligand dissociation reactions of Cu-ATSM and their relationship to hypoxia selectivity.[41] Several questions remain, particularly pertaining to the processes involved in cellular uptake, but the current revised mechanism indicates that hypoxia selectivity of Cu-ATSM (Fig. 5) arises because of a delicate balance of equilibria in which the rates of reduction (most likely enzyme-mediated), reoxidation, and protonation are fast relative to the rate of pH-mediated ligand dissociation.

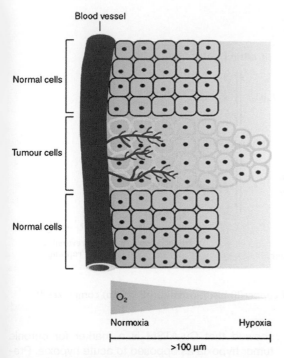

Fig. 2. The decrease in oxygen tension with increasing distance from the blood supply.

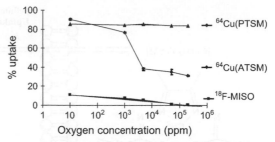

Fig. 4. Percentage uptake of ^{64}Cu-ATSM, ^{18}F-Fluoromisonidazole ([^{18}F]-FMISO) and pyruvaldehyde-bis(4-n-methyl-3-thiosemicarbazonato)copper(II) (^{64}Cu-PTSM) in EMT6 cells at varying oxygen concentrations. (*From* Lewis JS, McCarthy DW, McCarthy TJ, et al. Evaluation of ^{64}Cu-ATSM in vitro and in vivo in a hypoxic tumor model. J Nucl Med 1999;40:177–83; with permission.)[34]

PATIENT STUDIES WITH $^{60/62/64}$Cu-ATSM

Takahashi and colleagues[47] reported the first human studies of the uptake of Cu-ATSM in 10 subjects: four normal subjects and six with lung cancer. In this study the short-lived ^{62}Zn/^{62}Cu generator-produced radionuclide, ^{62}Cu ($t_{1/2}$ = 0.16 h, β^+ = 98%, EC = 2%), was used; however, the biodistribution will be unaffected by the change in radionuclide. Preliminary results suggested that ^{62}Cu-ATSM was cleared rapidly from the blood with only a small fraction being accumulated in normal lung tissue (0.43 ± 0.09 uptake ratio; divided by the arterial input function). In contrast,

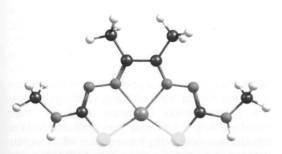

Fig. 3. Chemical structure of Cu-ATSM. Copper = silver, sulfur = yellow, nitrogen = blue, carbon = gray and hydrogen = white.

high tumor uptake was observed (3.00 ± 1.50 uptake ratio) in all subjects with lung cancer. Further human studies followed in which the efficacy of using ^{62}Cu-ATSM for identifying myocardial ischemia was measured in seven subjects with coronary artery disease.[48] [^{18}F]-FDG uptake was also measured. Four subjects displayed clinically unstable angina and showed abnormal [^{18}F]-FDG uptake. In these subjects, ^{62}Cu-ATSM uptake was higher, and the main conclusion was that Cu-ATSM showed promise as a PET tracer for imaging hypoxia in acute ischemia.

Dehdashti and colleagues reported the first correlative studies comparing the uptake of ^{60}Cu-ATSM ($t_{1/2}$ = 0.16 h, β^+ = 98%, EC = 2%)[6,17] with response to conventional therapies in patients with non-small cell lung cancer (NSCLC),[49] and cervical cancer.[50] In the NSCLC study, response to therapy was evaluated using ^{60}Cu-ATSM tumor to muscle (T:M) uptake ratios. Imaging with [^{18}F]-FDG was also conducted as part of routine clinical evaluation. Of the 14 subjects studied, eight responded to radiotherapy (five showed a complete response with three partial responders) and six showed no response. The mean ^{60}Cu-ATSM T:M ratio of nonresponders (3.4 ± 0.8) was found to be much larger than uptake observed in responders (1.5 ± 0.4) [P = 0.002]. However, no significant differences were observed in the standardized uptake values (SUV) between the tumors of responders (3.5 ± 1.0) and nonresponders (2.8 ± 1.1) [P = 0.2]. The threshold T:M value of 3.0 was identified as an reliable cutoff value for distinguishing responders from nonresponders. In contrast to the results with ^{60}Cu-ATSM, no significant differences were observed in either the mean T:M ratios or SUV for the uptake of [^{18}F]-FDG in

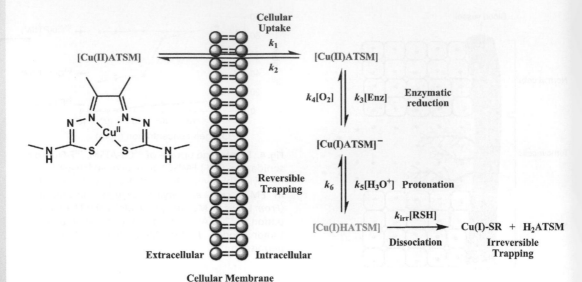

Fig. 5. The proposed mechanism of hypoxia-selectivity of copper(II) bis(thiosemicarbazonato) complexes.[41]

responders (12.7 ± 10.4) and nonresponders (10.9 ± 4.1) [P = 0.7]. In addition, no statistically significant correlation between [60]Cu-ATSM and [^{18}F]-FDG uptake was observed.

Clinical studies have also assessed the ability of [60]Cu-ATSM to predict response to neoadjuvant chemoradiotherapy in patients with rectal carcinoma.[51] A total of 19 subjects were enrolled in the study, and the data from 17 was analyzed. After chemoradiotherapy, which consisted of 45 Gy administered in 25 fractions to the pelvis and combined with continuous intravenous infusion of 5-fluorouracil (225 mg/m^2.day), 14 subjects had a reduction in tumor size and 13 were down staged. As with the studies on patients with NSCLC, the median T:M ratio for uptake of Cu-ATSM of 2.6 was found to discriminate responders from nonresponders. T:M values greater than 2.6 indicate the presence of hypoxia in the tumors and correlate with poor prognosis for progression-free patient survival.

Since the first PET study demonstrating the ability of [60]Cu-ATSM to act as an indicator of response to radiotherapy in patients with cervical cancer,[50] several additional studies have been conducted.[52–54] These reports include the first clinical comparison between the imaging characteristics of [60]Cu-ATSM and ^{64}Cu-ATSM (and [^{18}F]-FDG) in cancers of the uterine cervix conducted after Cu-ATSM was approved for study as an Investigational New Drug (IND 62,675) **(Fig. 6)**.[54] The study concluded that tumor uptake of Cu-ATSM as measured in images recorded between 1 to 9 days was reproducible, irrespective of the radionuclide used. This important result

showed that Cu-ATSM is a marker for chronic tumor hypoxia as opposed to acute hypoxia. Pre-therapy imaging has also confirmed previous results indicating that PET imaging of Cu-ATSM provides clinically relevant information about tumor oxygenation and is predictive of the likelihood of disease-free survival post-treatment in patients with cervical cancer.[53]

Before radiolabeled Cu-ATSM could be used for routine clinical analysis, accurate dosimetry measurements were required. In 2005, Laforest and colleagues[55] used the Medical Internal Radionuclide Dose approach to provided estimates of human absorbed doses from [60/61/62/64]Cu-ATSM by extrapolating data acquired from biodistribution data in rat models. Calculated organ doses for [61]Cu, [62]Cu and ^{64}Cu were extrapolated from the results obtained for [60]Cu-ATSM dosimetry. For ^{64}Cu-ATSM, the liver was identified as the dose limiting organ with an average radiation dose of 1.443 rad/mCi. Whole body doses were predicted to be 0.096 rad/mCi and the effective dose was 0.133 rad/mCi. In the animal model, measurable activity was identified in the gastrointestinal tract, suggesting that this is the primary excretion pathway for Cu-ATSM. However, humans have slower metabolism than rodents, which may account for the fact that no activity was observed in the bladder or gastrointestinal tract of human patients. Therefore, gastrointestinal residence times for ^{64}Cu-ATSM are likely to be higher than predicted and the actual doses received by these organs will be slightly elevated. Human doses using ^{64}Cu-ATSM have also been estimated from biodistribution data in nontumor bearing hamsters.[33]

A   **B**

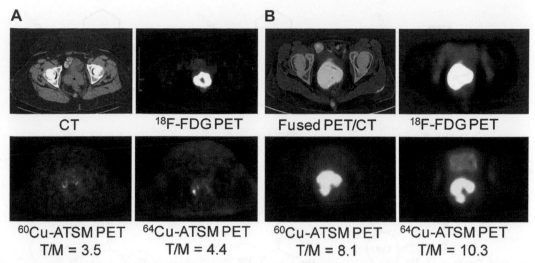

CT   [18F]-FDG PET   Fused PET/CT   [18F]-FDG PET

60Cu-ATSM PET   64Cu-ATSM PET   60Cu-ATSM PET   64Cu-ATSM PET
T/M = 3.5   T/M = 4.4   T/M = 8.1   T/M = 10.3

Fig. 6. Transaxial PET/CT images showing the CT image (top left), [18F]-FDG image, 60Cu-ATSM and 64Cu-ATSM images recorded between 30 to 60 minutes in two subjects with known cervical cancers. (*A*) Images recorded for a patient who responded to conventional radiotherapy and (*B*) images from a nonresponder. (*From* Lewis JS, Laforest R, Dehdashti F, et al. An imaging comparison of 64Cu-ATSM and 60Cu-ATSM in cancer of the uterine cervix. J Nucl Med 2008;49:1177–82; with permission.)[54]

64Cu-ATSM AS A RADIOTHERAPEUTIC AGENT

Due to the electron capture and β-decay pathways, 64Cu-ATSM has also been characterized as a potential radiotherapeutic agent.[33,56] Hamsters bearing either 7-day or 15-day old human GW39 colon cancer tumors were treated with 10 mCi of 64Cu-ATSM. After treatment, animals with 7-day old tumors showed a 6-fold increase in survival (135 days) in 50% of the population compared with controls (20 days, [*P* = 0.002]). In animals with 15-day old tumors, greater than 6 mCi caused a statistically significant increase in survival time compared with controls (*P* = 0.001). Administration of the proligand, H2ATSM, or the nonradioactive Cu-ATSM showed no difference in survival compared with controls. Again, high liver uptake was observed with a calculated human dose of 0.693 ± 0.037 rad/mCi ± SD. In hamsters, higher uptake in both the upper and lower large intestine walls was observed with extrapolated human doses of 1.201 ± 0.383 and 1.430 ± 0.186 rad/mCi, respectively.

64Cu-LABELED SOMATOSTATIN ANALOGS FOR TARGETING NEUROENDOCRINE TUMORS

Somatostatin is a 14-amino-acid peptide that is involved in the regulation of several hormones (growth factor, insulin, glucagon, prolactin, and so forth) in organs, such as the gastrointestinal tract, the exocrine and endocrine tissue of the pancreas, the hypothalamus, the pituitary gland, and the central nervous system. The inhibitory effect of somatostatin is mediated by somatostatin receptors (SSTr) which are surface proteins that belong to the G-protein coupled receptor family. There are at least five known SSTr subtypes (SSTr1-SSTr5),[57] and because they have been found to be abundant on the surface of several human tumors,[57–61] (SSTr2 in particular)[62,63] the use of somatostatin analogs to target these biomarkers for diagnostic and therapeutic purposes has been investigated for many years.[64–69] Somatostatin analogs are used instead of somatostatin itself because the latter has a very short half-life in circulation, due to rapid metabolism by ubiquitous peptidase enzymes.[70] Two of these analogs, octreotide (Sandostatin)[71–74] and lanreotide (Somatuline)[73,75,76] are already used clinically, and further derivatives with potentially higher SSTr affinity and improved activity are under investigation.[77,78]

Somatostatin analogs have been linked to bifunctional chelators which are able to complex 64Cu, and the resulting compounds have been studied as potential radiotracers for PET imaging of SSTr-positive tumors (**Fig. 7**). Anderson and colleagues[79] conjugated octreotide (OC) to 1,4,8,1-tetraazacyclotetradecane-1,4,8,1-tetraacetic acid (TETA) and labeled the resulting compound with 64Cu. This compound (64Cu-TETA-OC) showed high affinity for SSTr,[80] and in some subjects it delineated SSTr-positive lesions that were not observed with commonly used imaging agents.[81,82] Other somatostatin analogs were also conjugated to

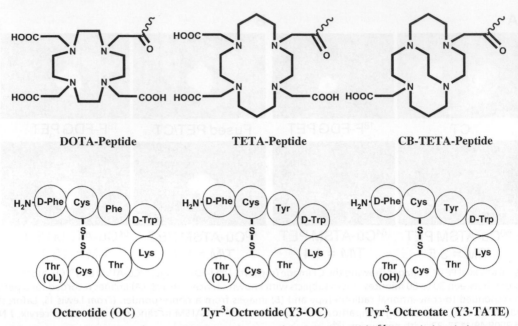

Fig. 7. Amino acid sequences of somatostatin analogs used in imaging with ^{64}Cu and the chelators used to complex [64]Cu.

TETA, and the ^{64}Cu-labeled compound ^{64}Cu-TETA-Tyr3-Octreotate (^{64}Cu-TETA-Y3-TATE) was found to have the highest receptor targeting/affinity and good clearance properties.[83–86]

Evidence that compounds, such as ^{64}Cu-TETA-OC, dissociate to give free Cu^{2+} ions in vivo[81,87,88] stimulated the search for new chelates with higher kinetic stability for conjugation to somatostatin derivatives. The Cu^{2+} complex of the 1,4-bis(carboxymethyl)-1,4,8,11-tetraazabicyclo[6.6.2]hexadecane proligand (CB-TE2A)[89] was found to have higher thermodynamic and kinetic stability than the ^{64}Cu complex of TETA in vivo.[90] Metabolism studies in normal rat liver revealed that ^{64}Cu-CB-TE2A resulted in significantly lower values of protein-associated ^{64}Cu than ^{64}Cu-TETA [13 ± 6% versus 75 ± 9% at 4 h],[90] and as a consequence the corresponding octreotate (^{64}Cu-CB-TE2A-Y3-TATE) conjugate demonstrated improved tumor uptake and blood and liver clearance compared with ^{64}Cu-TETA-OC.[91,92]

[64]Cu-LABELED INTEGRIN-TARGETING PEPTIDES

Integrins are transmembrane proteins that regulate cell-cell and cell-matrix interactions. They are dimers that consist of two non-covalently bound subunits (α and β) that have an extracellular domain arranged in a characteristic way that imparts different adhesion properties to the cell.[93–95] Integrin proteins have been found to play important roles in angiogenesis and vasculogenesis and tumor

metastasis. In addition, cell adhesion mediated by integrin-protein interactions, directly impacts cell migration, survival and proliferation.[96] So far, 24 different integrins have been identified, constituted by combinations of 18 α and 8 β subunits. Alpha-v beta-3 ($\alpha_v\beta_3$) is one of the most widely studied integrin since it is up-regulated in endothelial cells involved in active angiogenesis but not in quiescent endothelial cells,[96] making it an ideal biomarker for angiogenesis and tumor imaging.[97] Tumors where $\alpha_v\beta_3$ is found to be highly expressed include glioblastomas, breast and prostate tumors, malignant melanomas, and ovarian carcinomas.[98–101] The $\alpha_v\beta_3$ integrin binds to extracellular proteins through a specific binding pocket that recognizes the three amino acid sequence arginine-glycine-aspartic acid (Arg-Gly-Asp or RGD).[102–106] This discovery has lead to the design of many RGD-based imaging agents[97,107–115] and several investigations involving the ^{64}Cu radiolabeled complexes have been reported (Fig. 8).

Chen and colleagues[116] conjugated 1,4,7,10-tetraazacyclododecane-1,4,7,10-tetraacetic acid (DOTA) to c(RGDyK) and labeled it with ^{64}Cu for cancer imaging studies but found only moderate uptake in U87MG human glioma tumors (1.44 ± 0.09% ID/g at 4 hours post-injection) with high liver and kidney retention (2.84 ± 0.17 and 1.98 ± 0.06% ID/g at 4 hours post-injection, respectively). To improve tumor uptake and in vivo kinetics, they substituted the monomeric RGD derivative for dimeric compounds (E[c(RGDyK)$_2$ and

E[c(RGDfK)$_2$] and observed improved tumor targeting. However, kidney uptake remained too high for the compounds to be considered for further clinical studies.[117] In an attempt to modulate the kidney retention, polyethylene glycol (PEG) groups were added to the monomeric RGD peptide derivative and it was observed that ^{64}Cu-DOTA-c(RGDyK)-PEG had very similar uptake in brain tumors compared with ^{64}Cu-DOTA-c(RGDyK), but a much lower liver uptake and a faster clearance from blood and kidneys.[118] In a lung cancer study, the PEG-ylated dimeric RGD derivative ^{64}Cu-DOTA-E[c(RGDyK)$_2$-PEG was found to be an excellent PET imaging agent despite a lower binding affinity. The superior image quality was a direct result of minimal activity accumulation in normal heart and lung tissue which allowed for ideal imaging of the primary lung tumor.[119] By using tetrameric[120] and octameric[121] RGD derivatives, binding affinity and tumor uptake in glioblastoma cells improved; however, liver and kidney uptake also increased. In a recent article, the same group

reported a DOTA-conjugated RGD derivative (RGD4C) linked to tumor necrosis factor-α (TNFα). Once radiolabeled with ^{64}Cu this compound was taken up by several α$_v$β$_3$-positive tumors, because of integrin and TNFα receptor recognition. The antitumor activity observed was improved compared with that of TNFα alone, since its toxicity was localized to integrin-positive cells only.[122]

Sprague and colleagues conjugated c(RGDyK) to a different chelator, CB-TE2A, and found that the corresponding ^{64}Cu complex was taken up specifically by osteoclasts,[123] which are up regulated in osteolytic lesions and bone metastases.[124] These investigations open the possibility of other applications for imaging α$_v$β$_3$ in diseases such as osteoarthritis or osteoporosis, and imaging osteolytic bone metastases.

McQuade and colleagues conjugated DOTA to bitistatin, a small protein which is part of the disintegrin family and contains an RGD motif (or an analogous sequence) at the apex of one of its loops. The ^{64}Cu-labeled bitistatin showed specific

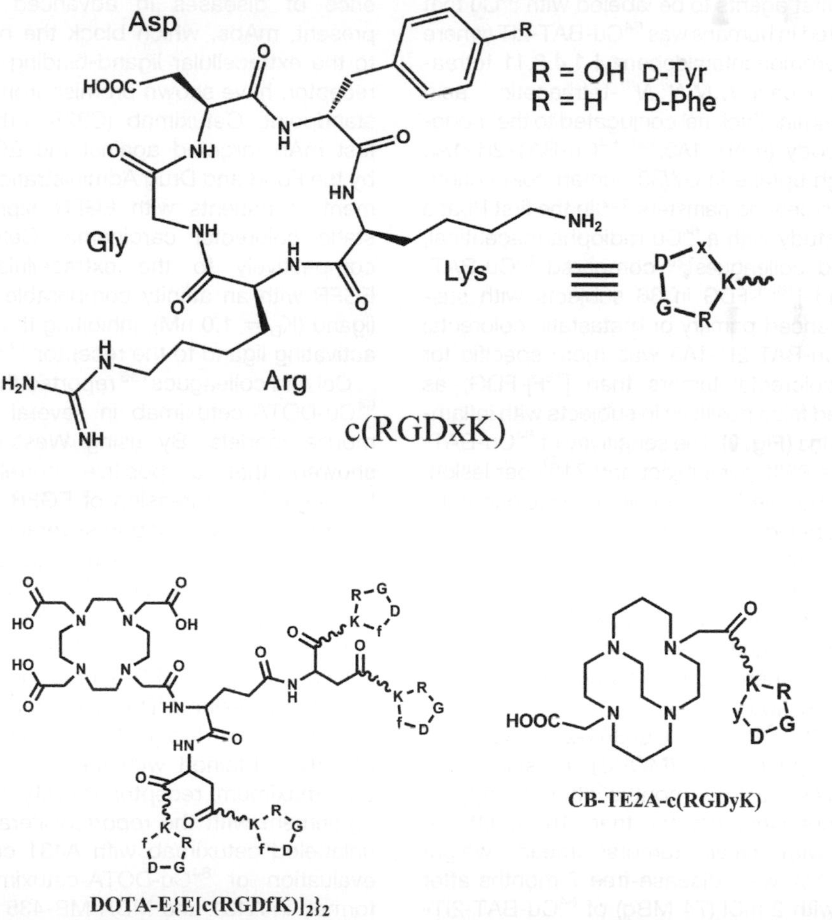

Fig. 8. Structures of c(RGDxK) peptides used in imaging of α$_v$β$_3$ expression in tumor angiogenesis and osteoclasts. x = D-Tyr or D-Phe.

uptake in mammary carcinoma tumors. However, maximum tumor uptake required around 6 hours and remained 8-fold lower than the ^{125}I-bitistatin derivative. In an attempt to improve tumor uptake and biodistribution kinetics, a spacer was introduced between DOTA and the targeting peptide; however, higher tumor uptake was accompanied by higher uptake in nontarget organs.[125]

In a recent patent, Cochran and colleagues[126] reported the conjugation of DOTA to a library of many miniproteins derived from knotting proteins whose 25 to 40 amino acid sequences have been enriched by an RGD loop. After screening for initial integrin binding ability, some of the chelators were labeled with ^{64}Cu. Biodistribution and small-animal PET imaging studies showed good specific uptake in U87MG tumors (glioblastoma). However, kidney uptake was consistently higher than tumor uptake over a 25-hour period.[126]

^{64}Cu-LABELED MONOCLONAL ANTIBODY 1A3 FOR TARGETING COLORECTAL CANCER

One of the first agents to be labeled with ^{64}Cu that was evaluated in humans was ^{64}Cu-BAT-2IT (where BAT = 6-bromoacetamidobenzyl-1,4,8,11-tetraazacyclotetradecane-N,N',N'',N'''-tetraacetic acid and 2IT = 2-iminothiolane) conjugated to the monoclonal antibody (mAb) 1A3.[127] ^{64}Cu-BAT-2IT-1A3 showed high uptake in GW39 human colon carcinoma tumor-bearing hamsters.[127] In the first Phase I/II clinical study with a ^{64}Cu radiopharmaceutical, Philpott and colleagues[128] compared ^{64}Cu-BAT-2IT-1A3 and [^{18}F]-FDG in 36 subjects with suspected advanced primary or metastatic colorectal cancer. ^{64}Cu-BAT-2IT-1A3 was more specific for detecting colorectal tumors than [^{18}F]-FDG, as FDG showed false positives in subjects with inflammatory lesions (**Fig. 9**). The sensitivity of ^{64}Cu-BAT-2IT-1A3 was 86% per subject and 71% per lesion, which was improved over radioimmunoscintigraphy with ^{111}In-labeled mAb 1A3 (76% per subject and 63% per lesion).[128,129]

^{64}Cu-BAT-2IT-1A3 was also evaluated for radioimmunotherapy in the GW39 tumor-bearing hamster model and was compared with ^{67}Cu-BAT-2IT-1A3, where ^{67}Cu is a therapeutic radionuclide ($t_{1/2}$ = 67 hours; 100% β^{-}).[130] Hamsters were injected with ^{64}Cu-, ^{67}Cu-BAT-2IT-1A3, Cu-labeled nonspecific IgG (MOPC), or saline and were sacrificed 6 to 7 months after therapy or when tumors were greater than 10 g. Of the hamsters with small tumors (mean weight 0.43 g), 87.5% were disease-free 7 months after treatment with 2 mCi (74 MBq) of ^{64}Cu-BAT-2IT-1A3 or 0.4 mCi (14.8 MBq) of ^{67}Cu- BAT-2IT-1A3. These therapeutic responses were obtained at low radiation absorbed doses, with the mean tumor doses for ^{64}Cu- and ^{67}Cu-BAT-2IT-1A3 being 586 and 1269 rad, respectively. The maximum tolerated dose of ^{64}Cu-BAT-2IT-1A3 was later determined to be 150 mCi/kg, and at this dose 62.5% of hamsters with larger GW39 tumors ($\sim$600 mg) were still alive 4 months post-treatment.[131] This study demonstrated the therapeutic capabilities of ^{64}Cu.

^{64}Cu-LABELED ANTIBODIES FOR TARGETING EPIDERMAL GROWTH FACTOR

The epidermal growth factor (EGF) family of membrane receptors (EGFR) is one of the most relevant targets in the tyrosine kinase family. EGFR expression is increased in many human tumors, such as breast cancer, squamous-cell carcinoma of the head and neck, and prostate cancer.[132] Activation of EGFR contributes to several tumorigenic mechanisms, and in many tumors, EGFR expression may act as a prognostic indicator, predicting patient survival or the presence of diseases in advanced stages.[132] At present, mAbs, which block the binding of EGF to the extracellular ligand-binding domain of the receptor, have shown promise from a therapeutic standpoint. Cetuximab (C225, Erbitux) was the first mAb targeted against the EGFR approved by the Food and Drug Administration for the treatment of patients with EGFR-expressing, metastatic colorectal carcinoma. Cetuximab binds competitively to the extracellular domain of EGFR with an affinity comparable to the natural ligand (K_D = 1.0 nM), inhibiting the binding of the activating ligand to the receptor.[133,134]

Cai and colleagues[135] reported the evaluation of ^{64}Cu-DOTA-cetuximab in several tumor-bearing mouse models. By using Western blots, they showed that a positive correlation existed between the expression of EGFR and uptake of ^{64}Cu-DOTA-cetuximab in several different EGFR-expressing tumor-bearing mouse models. At Washington University, ^{64}Cu-DOTA-cetuximab was synthesized for the small-animal PET imaging of EGFR expression.[136] For the cell binding affinity evaluation, high EGFR-expressing A431 and low EGFR-expressing MDA-MB-435 cells were used. An equilibrium dissociation constant (K_D) of 0.28 nM was obtained with the A431 cells. The K_D and maximum receptor density (B_{max}) were in agreement with the reported literature values of unlabeled cetuximab with A431 cells.[136] In vivo evaluation of ^{64}Cu-DOTA-cetuximab was performed in A431 and MDA-MB-435 tumor-bearing mice. Biodistribution and small-animal PET data showed a higher uptake in the EGFR positive

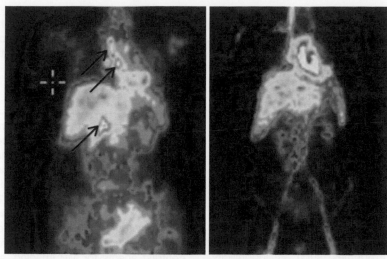

Fig. 9. Anterior volume-rendered reprojection PET images obtained after injection of FDG (*left*) and ^{64}Cu-BAT-2IT-1A3 (*right*) in a woman postresection of Dukes' C rectal cancer 1 year before enlarged mediastinal and periportal lymph nodes were observed. The lymph notes were strongly positive on FDG-PET (*left panel, see arrows*), but were completely negative with ^{64}Cu-BAT-2IT-1A3 (*right panel*). Subsequent analysis of the lymph nodes demonstrated sarcoidosis. (*Data from* Philpott GW, Schwarz SW, Anderson CJ, et al. RadioimmunoPET: detection of colorectal carcinoma with positron-emitting copper-64-labeled monoclonal antibody. J Nucl Med 1995;36(10): 1818–24.)[128]

A431 tumor than in the EGFR negative MDA-MB-435 tumor. Metabolism experiments were also performed to determine the extent of ^{64}Cu transchelation to blood, liver, and tumor proteins in A431 tumor-bearing mice. The results showed minimal metabolism of ^{64}Cu-DOTA-cetuximab in the blood out to 24 hours post-injection. Liver metabolism studies demonstrated that transchelation of ^{64}Cu to three proteins occurred. By using size-exclusion chromatography, two of these proteins were identified as superoxide dismutase and metallothionein. The third metabolite was believed to be a protein aggregate.

Over expression of EGFR has been found in over 70% of carcinomas of the cervix. The potential of [61]Cu-DOTA-cetuximab to measure EGFR concentration was evaluated by PET imaging in cervical-cancer tumors.[137] In this study, ^{64}Cu-DOTA-cetuximab was used to correlate EGFR densities on the surface of five different cervical cancer lines with the EGFR messenger RNA (mRNA) expression. Based on the cellular data, small-animal PET imaging was performed on tumor-bearing mice using the highest EGFR-expressing cervical cancer cell line, CaSki. For the in vitro analysis, five cervical-cancer cell lines were selected after a screen of 23 human cervical-cancer lines based on their level of EGFR gene expression by gene expression microarray analysis. The five cell lines had different ranges of EGFR expression with the following order: CaSki (high), ME-180 and DcTc2 4510 (mid-range),

HeLa (low), and C-33A (negative). The cell-surface EGFR expression was evaluated by conducting saturation binding assays at 4 °C, and the results paralleled the levels of EGFR expression determined by microarray analysis. In vivo biodistribution and small-animal PET studies with ^{64}Cu-DOTA-cetuximab in CaSki tumor-bearing nude mice showed high tumor uptake at 24 hours after injection (13.2% ID/g), with significant retention of radioactivity in blood and liver (**Fig. 10**). Overall, this study demonstrated that ^{64}Cu-DOTA-cetuximab is a useful marker of EGFR expression levels, and a potential PET agent for determining patient-specific therapies and therapeutic monitoring.

[64]Cu RADIOPHARMACEUTICALS IN THE PIPELINE
Thiosemicarbazonato Complexes

The neutral, lipophilic, radiolabeled copper complex of the proligand pyruvaldehyde-bis(4-N-methyl-3-thiosemicarbazone), [62/64]Cu-PTSM, has been investigated as a potential PET tracer for imaging blood perfusion,[38] and also for treating tumor growth (^{64}Cu-PTSM) at wound sites following laparoscopic surgery (**Fig. 11**).[138] In 1993, Fujibayashi and colleagues[139] also studied the [62]Cu-PTSM complex as a potential brain-imaging agent. Unlike Cu-ATSM, which is more difficult to reduce because of the additional methyl substituent on the ligand backbone (one-electron reduction potential of $E_{1/2} = -0.646$ V versus the saturated calomel reference electrode, SCE), Cu-PTSM is readily reduced ($E_{1/2}$(SCE) = -0.565 V) in normoxic and hypoxic cells.[41] Reduction followed by facile protonation,[40] leads to intracellular release of the copper ion, which leads to potential use of labile copper bis(thiosemicarbazonato) complexes, such as Cu-PTSM in the treatment of Alzheimer's Disease.[140–142]

Recently, a synthetic methodology for rapid and facile functionalization and ^{64}Cu radiolabeling of bis(thiosemicarbazonato) complexes was presented.[143] The new bifunctional chelate, H₂ATSM/A, has a reactive hydrazinic amine group, which has been successfully conjugated to a range of biologically active molecules including saccharides, amino acids, alkyl, and aromatic substituents, including derivatized 4-nitroimidazoles (see **Fig. 11**).[143,144] Properties, such as lipophilicity, reduction potentials, and pK_a, can be controlled by functionalization. In vitro and in vivo PET imaging in BALB/c mice bearing EMT6 tumors demonstrated that these new functionalized complexes remain hypoxia selective and have improved biodistribution and clearance characteristics.

In addition to bis(thiosemicarbazonato) complexes, mono-thiosemicarbazonato complexes of copper have also been investigated because of their potential use as PET imaging and therapeutic agents targeting topoisomerase-IIα (Topo-IIα).[145] Topo-IIα is a 170 kDa protein which decatenates supercoiled DNA during replication by generating transient double-strand DNA breaks while retaining genetic integrity. The mechanism by which copper mono-thiosemicarbazonato complexes, such as the copper(II) complexes of EPH144 and EPH270 (see

Fig. 11), inhibit the action of Topo-IIα is uncertain. However, it has been postulated that binding and stabilization of the intermediate Topo-IIα-DNA cleavable complex may prevent replication and induce cell apoptosis.

[64]Cu-labeled Nanoparticles

Nanotechnology is an applied science that creates and studies molecules or aggregates that have an overall size in the 1 to 1000 nm range (<1 μm). In the last few years nanodevices and nanoparticles have been used in biomedical studies investigating new and improved diagnosis and therapy agents. Oncology is one of the disciplines that has benefited the most from nanotechnology. Several nanoparticles are used in diagnostic assays for cancer, as contrast agents for MR imaging, as drug delivery agents, as tumor visualization agents during surgery, and even as therapeutic agents.[146–148] Several types of nanoparticle platforms have been evaluated for imaging applications, including iron oxide nanoparticles,[149–154] gold nanoparticles,[155–160] liposomes,[161–163] emulsions,[164–166] dendrimers,[167–172] and nanotubes (**Fig. 12**).[173–175] Nanoparticles conjugated with bifunctional chelators and targeting ligands are particularly useful for PET imaging purposes because their higher surface area per volume allows a higher number of targeting residues and radionuclides per particle, which in turn translates into higher affinity and higher specific activity, respectively.[176]

Cai and colleagues[177] conjugated c(RGDyK) and DOTA to quantum dots (QD) obtaining a 20 nm nanoparticle having approximately 28 DOTA

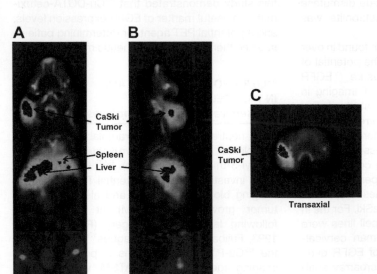

CaSki Tumor

Spleen
Liver

CaSki Tumor

Transaxial

Coronal   Sagittal

Fig. 10. Small-animal PET imaging of ^{64}Cu-DOTA-cetuximab in CaSki tumor-bearing SCID mice at 24 hours after injection: coronal (*A*), sagittal (*B*), and transaxial (*C*) views. (*From* Eiblmaier M, Meyer LA, Watson MA, et al. Correlating EGFR expression with receptor-binding properties and internalization of ^{64}Cu-DOTA-cetuximab in 5 cervical cancer cell lines. J Nucl Med 2008;49(9):1472–9; with permission.)[137]

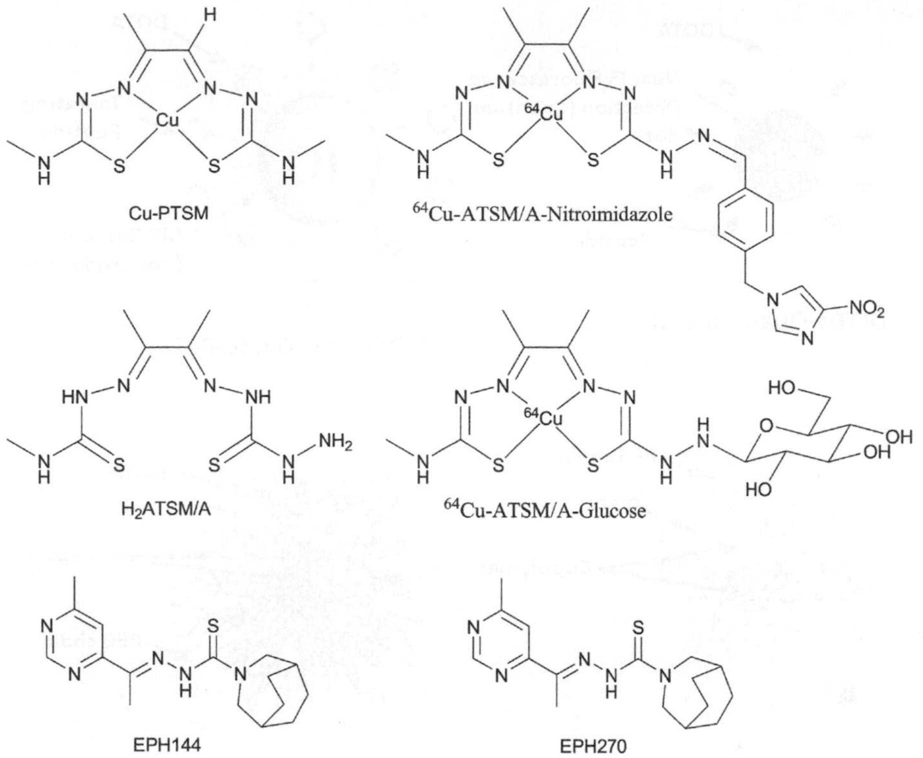

Fig. 11. Chemical structures of several promising pipeline tracers based on the chelation of ^{64}Cu and other copper radionuclides.

and 90 RGD residues on its surface. They observed selective targeting of the vasculature of $\alpha_v\beta_3$ positive tumors, such as U87MG human glioblastoma with minimal extravasation, which would be necessary for high tumor uptake. This selective targeting led to a lower than expected tumor uptake, with most of the ^{64}Cu-DOTA-QD-RGD being taken up by liver, spleen, and bone marrow. The authors concluded that smaller particles would probably have improved tumor-targeting properties because of easier extravasation and lower reticulo-endothelial system uptake.[177] Lee and colleagues[178] reported 5 nm iron oxide nanoparticles coated with polyaspartic acid functionalized with an estimated 35 RGD peptides and 30 DOTA macrocycles per particle. PET studies gave high contrast images of the tumor; however, liver uptake was still high. This behavior may be explained by the fact that while the core diameter of the particles was 5 nm, their hydrodynamic size was much larger (45 nm) so the same problems observed with the QD nanoparticles persisted.[178]

Pressly and colleagues[179] prepared well-defined amphiphilic copolymers with a predetermined number of reactive functionalities, PEG chains of variable length and low polydispersity. Upon collapsing in water, these polymers formed three-dimensional, three-layered nanoparticles with a hydrophobic inner core surrounded by a hydrophilic shell where the functional groups are located, and finally a PEG outer shell. The thickness of each layer, the number of reactive sites, and the dimension of the particle are determined by the composition of the initial linear polymer. When DOTA molecules were conjugated to these nanoparticles, ^{64}Cu labeling was achieved and biodistribution studies were conducted. Not surprisingly, particles with longer PEG chain lengths had longer circulation in blood and lower liver uptake.[179,180]

Rossin and colleagues conjugated fluorescein isothiocyanate-labeled polystyrene latex beads (100 nm diameter) with DOTA and an anti-intracellular adhesion molecule antibody for use as an imaging agent for the lung. High lung uptake of the ^{64}Cu-labeled particle was observed; however, it was accompanied by high liver uptake and partial copper transchelation.[181]

Sun and colleagues prepared shell-crosslinked nanoparticles (SCK) by crosslinking to different degrees micelles formed by amphiphilic block copolymers. When TETA was incorporated onto the final SCK the yield was low and the labeling

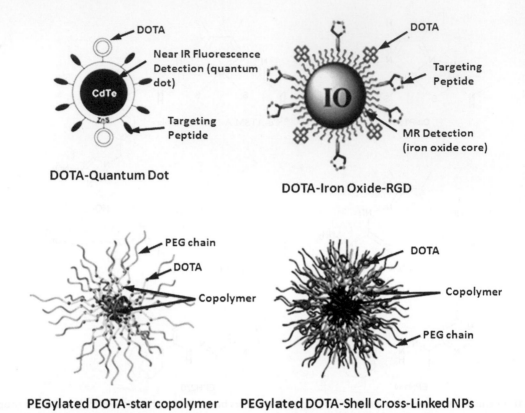

Fig. 12. Structures of nanoparticles used in imaging include DOTA-conjugated quantum dots,[177] DOTA- and RGD peptide-conjugated iron oxide nanoparticles,[178] pegylated DOTA start copolymers,[180] and pegylated DOTA-shell cross-lined nanoparticles.[183]

efficiency was unsatisfactory.[182] This problem was solved by preincorporating the copper chelator (DOTA in this case) into the copolymer before the nanoparticles were formed.[183] Tuning of the pharmacokinetics of these particles was performed by introducing different numbers and different lengths of PEG chains.[183] The extent of crosslinking and the dimensions of the linker between nanoparticle and copper chelator were found to have a dramatic impact on the specific activity of the radiolabeled particle.[184]

Bartlett and colleagues synthesized nanoparticles based on cyclodextrin polycations and DOTA-siRNA. Their study revealed that targeted (transferrin) and nontargeted particles had similar biodistribution and tumor localization; however, only the targeted ones were internalized by the tumor.[185]

Nahrendorf and colleagues[186] reported a dextranated and diethylenetriaminepentaacetic-functionalized iron oxide nanoparticle (20 nm diameter) that was labeled with ^{64}Cu and successfully used to image macrophages in inflammatory atherosclerosis.

SUMMARY

Copper-64-based radiopharmaceuticals are being explored as agents for the delineation of disease in humans. By exploitation of the chemistry of Cu(II) and the decay characteristics of ^{64}Cu, agents based on small molecules, peptides, and larger biomolecules, such as antibodies, are in development for clinical translation. Those agents already translated for use in humans have shown a high degree of success in their respective applications. A diverse array of highly specific molecular ^{64}Cu-radiopharmaceutical imaging probes will inevitably lead to improved patient-specific treatments and therefore overall survival.

REFERENCES

1. Rudin M, Weissleder R. Molecular imaging in drug discovery and development. Nat Rev Drug Discov 2003;2(2):123–31.

2. Quon A, Napel S, Beaulieu CF, et al. "Flying through" and "flying around" a PET/CT scan: Pilot study and development of 3D integrated ^{18}F-FDG

PET/CT for virtual bronchoscopy and colonoscopy. J Nucl Med 2006;47(7):1081–7.

3. Anderson CJ, Welch MJ. Radiometal-Labeled Agents (Non-Technetium) for Diagnostic Imaging. Chem Rev 1999;99(9):2219–34.

4. Blower P. Towards molecular imaging and treatment of disease with radionuclides: the role of inorganic chemistry. Dalton Trans 2006;(14):1705–11.

5. Blower PJ. Small coordination complexes as radiopharmaceuticals for cancer targeting. Trans Met Chem 1998;23:109–12.

6. Blower PJ, Lewis JS, Zweit J. Copper radionuclides and radiopharmaceuticals in nuclear medicine. Nucl Med Biol 1996;23(8):957–80.

7. Reichert DE, Lewis J, Anderson CJ. Metal complexes as diagnostic tools. Coord Chem Rev 1999;184:3–66.

8. Anderson CJ, Green MA, Fujibayashi Y. Chemistry of copper radionuclides and radiopharmaceutical products. In: Welch MJ, Redvanly CS, editors. Handbook of Radiopharmaceuticals. J. Wiley, Inc. 2003. p. 401–22.

9. Novak-Hofer I, Schubiger PA. Copper-67 as a therapeutic nuclide for radioimmunotherapy. Eur J Nucl Med Mol Imaging 2002;29(6):821–30.

10. Smith SV. Molecular imaging with copper-64. J Inorg Biochem 2004;98(11):1874–901.

11. Lewis JS, Herrero P, Sharp TL, et al. Delineation of hypoxia in canine myocardium using PET and copper(II)-diacetyl-bis(N(4)-methylthiosemicarbazone). J Nucl Med 2002;43(11):1557–69.

12. McCarthy DW, Shefer RE, Klinkowstein RE, et al. Efficient production of high specific activity ^{64}Cu using a biomedical cyclotron. Nucl Med Biol 1997;24(1):35–43.

13. Szelecsényi F, Blessing G, Qaim SM. Excitation functions of proton induced nuclear reaction on enriched ^{61}Ni and ^{64}Ni: possibility of production of no-carrier added ^{61}Cu and ^{64}Cu at a small cyclotron. Appl Radiat Isot 1993;44(3):575–80.

14. Obata A, Kawamatsu S, McCarthy DW, et al. Production of therapeutic quantities of ^{64}Cu using a 12 MeV cyclotron. Nucl Med Biol 2003;30: 535–9.

15. Hou X, Jacobsen U, Jorgensen JC. Separation of no-carrier added ^{64}Cu from a proton irradiated enriched nickel target. Appl Radiat Isot 2002;57(6): 773–7.

16. Zweit J, Smith AM, Downey S, et al. Excitation functions for deuteron induced reactions in natural nickel: production of no-carrier added ^{64}Cu from enriched ^{64}Ni target for positron emission tomography. Appl Radiat Isot 1991;42:193–7.

17. McCarthy DW, Bass LA, Cutler PD, et al. High purity production and potential applications of copper-60 and copper-61. Nucl Med Biol 1999; 26:351–8.

18. Szajek LP, Meyer W, Plascjak P, et al. Semi-remote production of [^{64}Cu]CuCl$_2$ and preparation of high specific activity [^{64}Cu]Cu-ATSM for PET studies. Radiochim Acta 2005;93:239–44.

19. Zeisler SK, Pavan RA, Orzechowski J, et al. Production of ^{64}Cu on the Sherbrooke TR-PET cyclotron. J Radioanal Nucl Chem 2003;257(1):175–7.

20. Lewis JS, Welch MJ, Tang L. Workshop on the Production, application and clinical translation of 'non-standard' PET nuclides: a meeting report. Q J Nucl Med Mol Imaging 2008;52:101–6.

21. Brown JM. The hypoxic cell: a target for selective cancer therapy-Eighteenth Bruce F. Cain Memorial Award Lecture. Cancer Res 1999;59: 5863–70.

22. Tatum JL, Kelloff GJ, Gillies RJ, et al. Hypoxia: importance in tumor biology, noninvasive measurement by imaging, and value of its measurement in the management of cancer therapy. Int J Radiat Biol 2006;82:699–757.

23. Graeber TG, Osmanian C, Jacks T, et al. Hypoxia-mediated selection of cells with diminished apoptotic potential in solid tumors. Nature 1996; 379:88–91.

24. Höckel M, Schlenger K, Aral B, et al. Association between tumor hypoxia and malignant progression in advanced cancer of the uterine cervix. Cancer Res 1996;56:4509–15.

25. Shweiki D, Itin A, Soffer D, et al. Vascular endothelial growth factor induced by hypoxia may mediate hypoxia-initiated angiogenesis. Nature 1992;359: 843–5.

26. Gray LH, Conger AD, Ebert M, et al. The concentration of oxygen dissolved in tissues at the time of irradiation as a factor in radiotherapy. Br J Radiol 1953;26:638–48.

27. Gatenby RA, Smallbone K, Maini PK, et al. Cellular adaptations to hypoxia and acidosis during somatic evolution of breast cancer. Br J Cancer 2007;97(5):646–53.

28. Carroll VA, Ashcroft M. Targeting the molecular basis for tumor hypoxia. Expert Rev Mol Med 2005;7(6):1–16.

29. Fujibayashi Y, Taniuchi H, Yonekura Y, et al. Copper-62-ATSM: a new hypoxia imaging agent with high membrane permeability and low redox potential. J Nucl Med 1997;38(7):1155–60.

30. Fujibayashi Y, Cutler CS, Anderson CJ, et al. Comparative studies of Cu-64-ATSM and C-11-Acetate in an acute myocardial infarction model: ex vivo imaging of hypoxia in rats. Nucl Med Biol 1999;26:117.

31. Dearling JLJ, Lewis JS, McCarthy DW, et al. Redox-active metal complexes for imaging hypoxic tissues: structure-activity relationships in copper(II) bis(thiosemicarbazone) complexes. Chem Commun 1998;(22):2531–2.

32. Dearling JLJ, Lewis JS, Mullen GED, et al. Copper bis(thiosemicarbazone) complexes as hypoxia imaging agents: structure-activity relationships. J Biol Inorg Chem 2002;7(3):249–59.

33. Lewis JS, Laforest R, Buettner TL, et al. Copper-64-diacetyl-bis(N[4]-methylthiosemicarbazone): an agent for radiotherapy. Proc Natl Acad Sci U S A 2001;98(3):1206–11.

34. Lewis JS, McCarthy DW, McCarthy TJ, et al. Evaluation of ^{64}Cu-ATSM in vitro and in vivo in a hypoxic tumor model. J Nucl Med 1999;40(1):177–83.

35. Lewis JS, Sharp TL, Laforest R, et al. Tumor uptake of copper-diacetyl-bis(N[4]-methylthiosemicarbazone): effect of changes in tissue oxygenation. J Nucl Med 2001;42(4):655–61.

36. Maurer RI, Blower PJ, Dilworth JR, et al. Studies on the Mechanism of Hypoxic Selectivity in Copper Bis(Thiosemicarbazone) Radiopharmaceuticals. J Med Chem 2002;45(7):1420–31.

37. Vavere AL, Lewis JS. Cu-ATSM: a radiopharmaceutical for the PET imaging of hypoxia. Dalton Trans 2007;(43):4893–902.

38. Wong TZ, Lacy JL, Petry NA, et al. PET of hypoxia and perfusion with [62]Cu-ATSM and [62]Cu-PTSM using a [62]Zn/[62]Cu generator. AJR Am J Roentgenol 2008;190(2):427–32.

39. Wood KA, Wong WL, Saunders MI. [^{64}Cu]diacetyl-bis(N[4]-methyl-thiosemicarbazone) - a radiotracer for tumor hypoxia. Nucl Med Biol 2008;35(4):393–400.

40. Holland JP, Green JC, Dilworth JR. Probing the mechanism of hypoxia selectivity of copper bis(thiosemicarbazonato) complexes: DFT calculation of redox potentials and absolute acidities in solution. Dalton Trans 2006;(6):783–94.

41. Holland JP, Barnard PJ, Collison D, et al. Spectroelectrochemical and computational studies on the mechanism of hypoxia selectivity of copper radiopharmaceuticals. Chemistry A Euro J 2008;14(19):5890–907.

42. Burgman P, O'Donoghue JA, Lewis JS, et al. Cell line-dependent differences in uptake and retention of the hypoxia-selective nuclear imaging agent Cu-ATSM. Nucl Med Biol 2005;32(6):623–30.

43. O'Donoghue JA, Zanzonico P, Pugachev A, et al. Assessment of regional tumor hypoxia using ^{18}F-fluoromisonidazole and [64]Cu(II)-diacetyl-bis(N[4]-methylthiosemicarbazone) positron emission tomography: Comparative study featuring microPET imaging, P2 probe measurement, autoradiography, and fluorescent microscopy in the R3327-AT and FaDu rat tumor models. Int J Radiat Oncol Biol Phys 2005;61(5):1493–502.

44. Dence CS, Ponde DE, Welch MJ, et al. Autoradiographic and small-animal PET comparisons between ^{18}F-FMISO, ^{18}F-FDG, ^{18}F-FLT and the hypoxic selective ^{64}Cu-ATSM in a rodent model of cancer. Nucl Med Biol 2008;35(6):713–20.

45. Yuan H, Schroeder T, Bowsher JE, et al. Intertumoral differences in hypoxia selectivity of the PET imaging agent [64]Cu(II)-diacetyl-Bis(N4-methylthiosemicarbazone). J Nucl Med 2006;47(6):989–98.

46. Tanaka T, Furukawa T, Fujieda S, et al. Double-tracer autoradiography with Cu-ATSM/FDG and immunohistochemical interpretation in four different mouse implanted tumor models. Nucl Med Biol 2006;33(6):743–50.

47. Takahashi N, Fujibayashi Y, Yonekura Y, et al. Evaluation of [62]Cu labeled diacetyl-bis(N[4]-methylthiosemicarbazone) as a hypoxic tissue tracer in patients with lung cancer. Ann Nucl Med 2000;14(5):323–8.

48. Takahashi N, Fujibayashi Y, Yonekura Y, et al. Copper-62 ATSM as a hypoxic tissue tracer in myocardial ischemia. Ann Nucl Med 2001;15(3):293–6.

49. Dehdashti F, Mintun MA, Lewis JS, et al. In vivo assessment of tumor hypoxia in lung cancer with [60]Cu-ATSM. Eur J Nucl Med Mol Imaging 2003;30(6):844–50.

50. Dehdashti F, Grigsby PW, Mintun MA, et al. Assessing tumor hypoxia in cervical cancer by positron emission tomography with [60]Cu-ATSM: relationship to therapeutic response-a preliminary report. Int J Radiat Oncol Biol Phys 2003;55(5):1233–8.

51. Dietz DW, Dehdashti F, Grigsby PW, et al. Tumor Hypoxia Detected by Positron Emission Tomography with [60]Cu-ATSM as a predictor of response and survival in patients undergoing Neoadjuvant Chemoradiotherapy for Rectal Carcinoma: a pilot study. Dis Colon Rectum 2008;51:1641–8.

52. Grigsby PW, Malyapa RS, Higashikubo R, et al. Comparison of molecular markers of hypoxia and imaging with [60]Cu-ATSM in cancer of the uterine cervix. Mol Imaging Biol 2007;9(5):278–83.

53. Dehdashti F, Grigsby PW, Lewis JS, et al. Assessing tumor hypoxia in cervical cancer by PET with [60]Cu-labeled diacetyl-bis (N[4]-methylthiosemicarbazone). J Nucl Med 2008;49(2):201–5.

54. Lewis JS, Laforest R, Dehdashti F, et al. An imaging comparison of ^{64}Cu-ATSM and [60]Cu-ATSM in cancer of the uterine cervix. J Nucl Med 2008;49(7):1177–82.

55. Laforest R, Dehdashti F, Lewis JS, et al. Dosimetry of [60/61/62/64]Cu-ATSM: a hypoxia imaging agent for PET. Eur J Nucl Med Mol Imaging 2005;32(7):764–70.

56. Obata A, Kasamatsu S, Lewis JS, et al. Basic characterization of ^{64}Cu-ATSM as a radiotherapy agent. Nucl Med Biol 2005;32(1):21–8.

57. Hoyer D, Lubbert H, Bruns C. Molecular pharmacology of Somatostatin receptors. Naunyn Schmiedebergs Arch Pharmacol 1994;350(5):441–53.

58. Reubi JC. In-vitro identification of vasoactive-intestinal-peptide receptors in human tumors - implications for tumor imaging. J Nucl Med 1995;36(10):1846–53.

59. Reubi JC, Kvols L, Krenning E, et al. Distribution of Somatostatin receptors in normal and tumor-tissue. Metab Clin Exp 1990;39(9):78–81.

60. Reubi JC, Schaer JC, Laissue JA, et al. Somatostatin receptors and their subtypes in human tumors and in peritumoral vessels. Metab Clin Exp 1996;45(8):39–41.

61. Reubi JC, Waser B, Schaer JC, et al. Somatostatin receptor sst1-sst5 expression in normal and neoplastic human tissues using receptor autoradiography with subtype-selective ligands. Eur J Nucl Med 2001;28(7):836–46.

62. Hofland LJ, Lamberts SWJ, van Hagen PM, et al. Crucial role for somatostatin receptor subtype 2 in determining the uptake of [In-111-DTPA-D-Phe(1)] octreotide in somatostatin receptor-positive organs. J Nucl Med 2003;44(8):1315–21.

63. Papotti M, Bongiovanni M, Volante M, et al. Expression of somatostatin receptor types 1-5 in 81 cases of gastrointestinal and pancreatic endocrine tumors - a correlative immunohistochemical and reverse-transcriptase polymerase chain reaction analysis. Virchows Arch 2002;440(5):461–75.

64. Harrison Louis B, Chadha M, Hill Richard J, et al. Impact of tumor hypoxia and anemia on radiation therapy outcomes. Oncologist 2002;7(6): 492–508.

65. Heppeler A, Froidevaux S, Eberle AN, et al. Receptor targeting for tumor localisation and therapy with radiopeptides. Curr Med Chem 2000;7(9):971–94.

66. Li WP, Meyer LA, Anderson CJ. Radiopharmaceuticals for positron emission tomography imaging of somatostatin receptor positive tumors. Contrast Agents Iii: Radiopharmaceuticals. Diagnostics to Therapeutics. SpringerBerlin/Heidelberg; 2005. Vol. 252. p. 179–92.

67. Weiner RE, Thakur ML. Radiolabeled peptides in diagnosis and therapy. Semin Nucl Med 2001; 31(4):296–311.

68. Weiner RE, Thakur ML. Radiolabeled peptides in the diagnosis and therapy of oncological diseases. Appl Radiat Isot 2002;57(5):749–63.

69. Weiner RE, Thakur ML. Radiolabeled peptides in oncology - role in diagnosis and treatment. BioDrugs 2005;19(3):145–63.

70. Patel YC, Wheatley T. In vivo and in vitro plasma disappearance and metabolism of somatostatin-28 and somatostatin-14 in the rat. Endocrinology 1983;112:220–5.

71. Bauer W, Briner U, Doepfner W, et al. SMS 201-995: a very potent and selective octapeptide analogue of somatostatin with prolonged action. Life Sci 1982;31(11):1133–40.

72. Bevan JS. Clinical review: The antitumoral effects of somatostatin analog therapy in acromegaly. J Clin Endocrinol Metab 2005;90(3):1856–63.

73. de Herder WW, Hofland LJ, van der Lely AJ, et al. Somatostatin receptors in gastroenteropancreatic neuroendocrine tumours. Endocr Relat Cancer 2003;10(4):451–8.

74. Lamberts SWJ. A Guide to the Clinical Use of the Somatostatin Analog Sms 201-995 (Sandostatin). Acta Endocrinol 1987;116:54–66.

75. Eriksson B, Janson ET, Bax NDS, et al. The use of new somatostatin analogues, lanreotide and octastatin, in neuroendocrine gastro-intestinal tumours. Digestion 1996;57:77–80.

76. Murray RD, Melmed S. A critical analysis of clinically available somatostatin analog formulations for therapy of acromegaly. J Clin Endocrinol Metab 2008;93(8):2957–68.

77. Ginj M, Zhang HW, Eisenwiener KP, et al. New pansomatostatin ligands and their chelated versions: affinity profile, agonist activity, internalization, and tumor targeting. Clin Cancer Res 2008;14(7): 2019–27.

78. Lewis I, Bauer W, Albert R, et al. A novel somatostatin mimic with broad somatotropin release inhibiting factor receptor binding and superior therapeutic potential. J Med Chem 2003;46(12):2334–44.

79. Anderson CJ, Pajeau TS, Edwards WB, et al. In-vitro and in-vivo evaluation of copper-64-octreotide conjugates. J Nucl Med 1995;36(12):2315–25.

80. Parry JJ, Eiblmaier M, Andrews R, et al. Characterization of somatostatin receptor subtype 2 expression in stably transfected A-427 human cancer cells. Mol Imaging 2007;6(1):56–67.

81. Anderson CJ, Dehdashti F, Cutler PD, et al. Cu-64-TETA-Octreotide as a PET imaging agent for patients with neuroendocrine tumors. J Nucl Med 2001;42(2):213–21.

82. Gulec SA, Baum R. Radio-guided surgery in neuroendocrine tumors. J Surg Oncol 2007;96(4):309–15.

83. Anderson CJ, Jones LA, Bass LA, et al. Radiotherapy, toxicity and dosimetry of copper-64-TETA-octreotide in tumor-bearing rats. J Nucl Med 1998;39(11):1944–51.

84. Lewis JS, Lewis MR, Cutler PD, et al. Radiotherapy and dosimetry of ^{64}Cu-TETA-Tyr^3-octreotate in a somatostatin receptor-positive, tumor-bearing rat model. Clin Cancer Res 1999;5(11):3608–16.

85. Lewis JS, Lewis MR, Srinivasan A, et al. Changes in target tissue uptake over a multiple dose radiotherapy regimen with copper-64-TETA-Y3-octreotate [abstract]. J Nucl Med 1999;40(5):224.

86. Lewis JS, Lewis MR, Srinivasan A, et al. Comparison of four ^{64}Cu-labeled Somatostatin analogs in vitro and in a tumor-bearing rat model: evaluation of new derivatives for positron emission tomography imaging and targeted radiotherapy. J Med Chem 1999;42(8):1341–7.

87. Bass LA, Wang M, Welch MJ, et al. In vivo transchelation of copper-64 from TETA-octreotide to

superoxide dismutase in rat liver. Bioconjug Chem 2000;11(4):527–32.

88. Wang M, Caruano AL, Lewis MR, et al. Subcellular localization of radiolabeled somatostatin analogues: Implications for targeted radiotherapy of cancer. Cancer Res 2003;63(20):6864–9.

89. Sun X, Wuest M, Weisman GR, et al. Radiolabeling and in vivo behavior of copper-64-labeled cross-bridged cyclam ligands. J Med Chem 2002;45(2):469–77.

90. Boswell CA, Sun XK, Niu WJ, et al. Comparative in vivo stability of copper-64-labeled cross-bridged and conventional tetraazamacrocyclic complexes. J Med Chem 2004;47(6):1465–74.

91. Eiblmaier M, Andrews R, Laforest R, et al. Nuclear uptake and dosimetry of ^{64}Cu-labeled chelator-somatostatin conjugates in an SSTr2-transfected human tumor cell line. J Nucl Med 2007;48(8):1390–6.

92. Sprague JE, Peng Y, Sun X, et al. Preparation and biological evaluation of copper-64-labeled Tyr3-octreotate using a cross-bridged macrocyclic chelator. Clin Cancer Res 2004;10(24):8674–82.

93. Hynes RO. Integrins - Versatility, Modulation, and Signaling in Cell-Adhesion. Cell 1992;69(1):11–25.

94. Luscinskas FW, Lawler J. Integrins as Dynamic Regulators of Vascular Function. FASEB J 1994;8(12):929–38.

95. Ruoslahti E. RGD and other recognition sequences for integrins. Annu Rev Cell Dev Biol 1996;12:697–715.

96. Hood JD, Cheresh DA. Role of integrins in cell invasion and migration. Nat Rev Cancer 2002;2(2):91–100.

97. Beer AJ, Schwaiger M. Imaging of integrin avß3 expression. Cancer Metastasis Rev 2008;27:631–44.

98. Albelda SM, Mette SA, Elder DE, et al. Integrin distribution in malignant-melanoma - association of the Beta-3-subunit with tumor progression. Cancer Res 1990;50(20):6757–64.

99. Bello L, Francolini M, Marthyn P, et al. alpha v beta 3 and alpha v beta 5 integrin expression in glioma periphery. Neurosurgery 2001;49(2):380–9.

100. Brooks PC, Stromblad S, Klemke R, et al. Anti-integrin alpha-v-beta-3 blocks human breast-cancer growth and Angiogenesis in human skin. J Clin Invest 1995;96(4):1815–22.

101. Jin H, Varner J. Integrins: roles in cancer development and as treatment targets. Br J Cancer 2004;90(3):561–5.

102. Cai WB, Chen K, Mohamedali KA, et al. PET of vascular endothelial growth factor receptor expression. J Nucl Med 2006;47(12):2048–56.

103. Horton MA. The alpha v beta 3 integrin "vitronectin receptor". Int J Biochem Cell Biol 1997;29(5):721–5.

104. Ruoslahti E. The RGD story: a personal account. Matrix Biol 2003;22(6):459–65.

105. Xiong JP, Stehle T, Diefenbach B, et al. Crystal structure of the extracellular segment of integrin alpha V beta 3. Science 2001;294(5541):339–45.

106. Xiong JP, Stehle T, Zhang RG, et al. Crystal structure of the extracellular segment of integrin alpha V beta 3 in complex with an Arg-Gly-Asp ligand. Science 2002;296(5565):151–5.

107. De Jong M, VanHagen PM, Breeman WA, et al. Evaluation of radiolabeled cyclic DTPARGD analog for tumor imaging and radionuclide therapy [abstract]. J Nucl Med 2000;41(5):232.

108. Janssen M, Buijs W, Boerman O, et al. Y-86 and In-111 labeled alpha(V beta 3) binding peptides: a comparative dosimetric study in dogs. J Nucl Med 2001;42(5):241.

109. Janssen M, Oyen WJG, Massuger LFAG, et al. Comparison of a monomeric and dimeric radiolabeled RGD-peptide for tumor targeting. Cancer Biother Radiopharm 2002;17(6):641–6.

110. Janssen ML, Oyen WJ, Dijkgraaf I, et al. Tumor targeting with radiolabeled alpha(v)beta(3) integrin binding peptides in a nude mouse model. Cancer Res 2002;62(21):6146–51.

111. Liu S, Cheung E, Ziegler MC, et al. Y-90 and Lu-177 labeling of a DOTA-conjugated vitronectin receptor antagonist useful for tumor therapy. Bioconjug Chem 2001;12(4):559–68.

112. Liu S, Edwards DS, Ziegler MC, et al. Tc-99m-Labeling of a hydrazinonicotinamide-conjugated vitronectin receptor antagonist useful for imaging tumors. Bioconjug Chem 2001;12(4):624–9.

113. Su Z, Liu GZ, Gupta S, et al. In vitro and in vivo evaluation of a technetium-99m-labeled cyclic RGD peptide as a specific marker of alpha(V) beta(3) integrin for tumor imaging. Bioconjug Chem 2002;13(3):561–70.

114. van Hagen PM, Breeman WAP, Bernard HF, et al. Evaluation of a radiolabelled cyclic DTPA-RGD analogue for tumour imaging and radionuclide therapy. Int J Cancer 2000;90(4):186–98.

115. van Hagen PM, De Jong M, Breeman WA, et al. In-111-labeled RGD analog for tumor imaging [abstract]. J Nucl Med 2000;41(5):286.

116. Chen XY, Park R, Tohme M, et al. MicroPET and autoradiographic imaging of breast cancer alpha(v)-integrin expression using F-18- and Cu-64-labeled RGD peptide. Bioconjug Chem 2004;15(1):41–9.

117. Chen XY, Liu S, Hou YP, et al. MicroPET imaging of breast cancer alpha(v)-integrin expression with Cu-64-labeled dimeric RGD peptides. Mol Imaging Biol 2004;6(5):350–9.

118. Chen XY, Hou YP, Tohme M, et al. Pegylated Arg-Gly-Asp peptide: Cu-64 labeling and PET imaging of brain tumor alpha(v)beta(3)-integrin expression. J Nucl Med 2004;45(10):1776–83.

119. Chen XY, Sievers E, Hou YP, et al. Integrin al-pha(V)beta(3)-targeted imaging of lung cancer. Neoplasia 2005;7(3):271–9.

120. Wu Y, Zhang XZ, Xiong ZM, et al. microPET imaging of glioma integrin alpha(v)beta(3) expression using Cu-64-labeled tetrameric RGD peptide. J Nucl Med 2005;46(10):1707–18.

121. Li ZB, Cai WB, Cao QZ, et al. ^{64}Cu-Labeled tetra-meric and octameric RGD peptides for small-animal PET of tumor alpha(v)beta(3) integrin expression. J Nucl Med 2007;48(7):1162–71.

122. Wang H, Chen K, Cai WB, et al. Integrin-targeted imaging and therapy with RGD4C-TNF fusion protein. Mol Cancer Ther 2008;7(5):1044–53.

123. Sprague JE, Kitaura H, Zou W, et al. Noninvasive imaging of osteoclasts in parathyroid hormone-induced osteolysis using a ^{64}Cu-labeled RGD peptide. J Nucl Med 2007;48(2):311–8.

124. Nakamura I, Duong LT, Rodan SB, et al. Involve-ment of alpha(v)beta(3) integrins in osteoclast function. J Bone Miner Metab 2007;25(6):337–44.

125. McQuade P, Knight LC, Welch MJ. Evaluation of Cu-64- and I-125-radiolabeled bitistatin as poten-tial agents for targeting alpha(v)beta(3) integrins in tumor angiogenesis. Bioconjug Chem 2004; 15(5):988–96.

126. Cochran JR, Kimura R, Levin AM, et al. Engineered integrin binding peptides [patent application]. PCT Int Appl WO. 2008045252. 2008.

127. Anderson CJ, Connett JM, Schwarz SW, et al. Copper-64-labeled antibodies for PET imaging. J Nucl Med 1992;33(9):1685–91.

128. Philpott GW, Schwarz SW, Anderson CJ, et al. RadioimmunoPET: detection of colorectal carci-noma with positron-emitting copper-64-labeled monoclonal antibody. J Nucl Med 1995;36(10): 1818–24.

129. Philpott GW, Siegel BA, Schwarz SW, et al. Immu-noscintigraphy with a new indium-111-labeled monoclonal antibody (MAb 1A3) in patients with colorectal cancer. Dis Colon Rectum 1994;37(8): 782–92.

130. Connett JM, Anderson CJ, Guo LW, et al. Radioim-munotherapy with a 64Cu-labeled monoclonal anti-body: a comparison with 67Cu. Proc Natl Acad Sci U S A 1996;93(13):6814–8.

131. Connett JM, Buettner TL, Anderson CJ. Maximum tolerated dose and large tumor radioimmunother-apy studies of 64Cu-labeled monoclonal antibody 1A3 in a colon cancer model. Clin Cancer Res 1999;5(10 Suppl):3207s–12s.

132. Laskin JJ, Sandler AB. Epidermal growth factor receptors: a promising target in solid tumors. Cancer Treat Rev 2004;30:1–17.

133. Fan Z, Masui H, Altas I, et al. Blockage of epidermal growth factor receptor function by biva-lent and monovalent fragments of C225

anti-epidermal growth factor receptor monoclonal antibodies. Cancer Res 1993;53:4322–8.

134. Mendelsohn J. Epidermal growth factor receptor inhibition by a monocolonal antobody as anti-cancer therapy. Clin Cancer Res 1997;3:2703–7.

135. Cai W, Chen K, He L, et al. Quantitative PET of EGFR expression in xenograft-bearing mice using (64)Cu-labeled cetuximab, a chimeric anti-EGFR monoclonal antibody. Eur J Nucl Med Mol Imaging 2007;34(6):850–8.

136. Li WP, Meyer LA, Capretto DA, et al. Receptor-binding, biodistribution, and metabolism studies of ^{64}Cu-DOTA-Cetuximab, a PET-imaging agent for epidermal growth-factor receptor-positive tumors. Cancer Biother Radiopharm 2008;23(2):158–71.

137. Eiblmaier M, Meyer LA, Watson MA, et al. Corre-lating EGFR expression with receptor-binding properties and internalization of ^{64}Cu-DOTA-cetux-imab in 5 cervical cancer cell lines. J Nucl Med 2008;49(9):1472–9.

138. Lewis JS, Connett JM, Garbow JR, et al. Copper-64-pyruvaldehyde-bis(N^4-methylthiosemicarba-zone) for the prevention of tumor growth at wound sites following laparoscopic surgery: monitoring therapy response with microPET and magnetic resonance imaging. Cancer Res 2002;62(2):445–9.

139. Fujibayashi Y, Wada K, Taniuchi H, et al. Mitochon-dria-selective reduction of ^{62}Cu-pyruvaldehyde bis(N^4-methylthiosemicarbazone) (^{62}Cu-PTSM) in the murine brain; a novel radiopharmaceutical for brain positron emission tomography (PET) imaging. Biol Pharm Bull 1993;16(2):146–9.

140. Donnelly PS, Caragounis A, Du T, et al. Selective intracellular release of Copper and Zinc Ions from Bis(thiosemicarbazonato) complexes reduces levels of Alzheimer disease Amyloid-beta peptide. J Biol Chem 2008;283(8):4568–77.

141. Donnelly PS, Wedd AG, Alzheimer's disease and the chemistry of copper. Aust J Chem 2007;74(7): 18–20.

142. Donnelly PS, Xiao Z, Wedd AG. Copper and Alz-heimer's disease. Curr Opin Chem Biol 2007; 11(2):128–33.

143. Holland JP, Aigbirhio FI, Betts HM, et al. Function-alized Bis(thiosemicarbazonato) Complexes of Zinc and Copper: synthetic platforms toward site-specific radiopharmaceuticals. Inorg Chem 2007; 46(2):465–85.

144. Bonnitcha PD, Vavere AL, Lewis JS, et al. In vitro and in vivo evaluation of bifunctional bisthiosemi-carbazone ^{64}Cu-complexes for the positron emis-sion tomography imaging of hypoxia. J Med Chem 2008;51(10):2985–91.

145. Wei L, Easmon J, Nagi RK, et al. ^{64}Cu-azabicy-clo[3.2.2]nonane thiosemicarbazone complexes: radiopharmaceuticals for PET of topoisomerase II

expression in tumors. J Nucl Med 2006;47(12): 2034–41.

146. Banerjee HN, Verma M. Use of nanotechnology for the development of novel cancer biomarkers. Expert Rev Mol Diagn 2006;6(5):679–83.

147. Banerjee HN, Verma M. Application of nanotechnology in cancer. Technol Cancer Res Treat 2008; 7(2):149–54.

148. Jain KK. Recent advances in nanooncology. Tech Cancer Res Treat 2008;7(1):1–13.

149. Lanza GM, Winter PM, Caruthers SD, et al. Magnetic resonance molecular imaging with nanoparticles. J Nucl Cardiol 2004;11(6):733–43.

150. Neumaier CE, Baio G, Ferrini S, et al. MR and iron magnetic nanoparticles. Imaging opportunities in preclinical and translational research. Tumori 2008;94(2):226–33.

151. Sosnovik DE, Nahrendorf M, Weissleder R. Magnetic nanoparticles for MR imaging: agents, techniques and cardiovascular applications. Not Found In Database 2008;103(2):122–30.

152. Sun C, Fang C, Stephen Z, et al. Tumor-targeted drug delivery and MRI contrast enhancement by chlorotoxin-conjugated iron oxide nanoparticles. Nanomed 2008;3(4):495–505.

153. Sun C, Lee JSH, Zhang MQ. Magnetic nanoparticles in MR imaging and drug delivery. Adv Drug Deliv Rev 2008;60(11):1252–65.

154. Waters EA, Wickline SA. Contrast agents for MRI. Basic Res Cardiol 2008;103(2):114–21.

155. Absil E, Tessier G, Fournier D, et al. Full field imaging and spectroscopy of individual gold nanoparticles. Eur Phys J Appl Phys 2008;43(2): 155–8.

156. Hirsch LR, Gobin AM, Lowery AR, et al. Metal nanoshells. Ann Biomed Eng 2006;34(1):15–22.

157. Kho KW, Kah JCY, Lee CGL, et al. Applications of gold nanoparticles in the early detection of cancer. J Mech Med Biol 2007;7(1):19–35.

158. Kogan MJ, Olmedo I, Hosta L, et al. Peptides and metallic nanoparticles for biomedical applications. Nanomedicine 2007;2(3):287–306.

159. Liong M, Lu J, Kovochich M, et al. Multifunctional inorganic nanoparticles for imaging, targeting, and drug delivery. ACS Nano 2008; 2(5):889–96.

160. Loo C, Lin A, Hirsch L, et al. Nanoshell-enabled photonics-based imaging and therapy of cancer. Tech Cancer Res Treat 2004;3(1):33–40.

161. Mulder WJM, Strijkers GJ, Habets JW, et al. MR molecular imaging and fluorescence microscopy for identification of activated tumor endothelium using a bimodal lipidic nanoparticle. FASEB J 2005;19(12):2008–10.

162. Saito R, Krauze MT, Bringas JR, et al. Gadolinium-loaded liposomes allow for real-time magnetic resonance imaging of convection-enhanced

delivery in the primate brain. Exp Neurol 2005; 196(2):381–9.

163. Al-Jamal WT, Kostarelos K. Liposome-nanoparticle hybrids for multimodal diagnostic and therapeutic applications. Nanomed 2007;2(1):85–98.

164. Caruthers SD, Wickline SA, Lanza GM. Nanotechnological applications in medicine. Curr Opin Biotechnol 2007;18(1):26–30.

165. Marsh JN, Partlow KC, Abendschein DR, et al. Molecular imaging with targeted perfluorocarbon nanoparticles: Quantification of the concentration dependence of contrast enhancement for binding to sparse cellular epitopes. Ultrasound Med Biol 2007;33(6):950–8.

166. Winter PM, Cai K, Caruthers SD, et al. Emerging nanomedicine opportunities with perfluorocarbon nanoparticles. Expert Rev Med Devices 2007;4(2):137–45.

167. Bielinska A, Eichman JD, Lee I, et al. Imaging {Au-0-PAMAM} gold-dendrimer nanocomposites in cells. J Nanoparticle Res 2002;4(5):395–403.

168. Gillies ER, Dy E, Frechet JMJ, et al. Biological evaluation of polyester dendrimer: poly(ethylene oxide) "Bow-Tie" hybrids with tunable molecular weight and architecture. Mol Pharmacol 2005;2(2):129–38.

169. Goodson T, Varnavski O, Wang Y. Optical properties and applications of dendrimer-metal nanocomposites. Int Rev Phys Chem 2004;23(1):109–50.

170. Khan MK, Nigavekar SS, Minc LD, et al. In vivo biodistribution of dendrimers and dendrimer nanocomposites - Implications for cancer imaging and therapy. Tech Cancer Res Treat 2005;4(6):603–13.

171. Kobayashi H, Kawamoto S, Jo SK, et al. Macromolecular MRI contrast agents with small dendrimers: Pharmacokinetic differences between sizes and cores. Bioconjug Chem 2003;14(2):388–94.

172. Kobayashi H, Kawamoto S, Konishi J, et al. Macromolecular MRI contrast agents with small dendrimer cores for functional kidney imaging. Radiology 2002;225:237.

173. Choi JH, Nguyen FT, Barone PW, et al. Multimodal biomedical imaging with asymmetric single-walled carbon nanotube/iron oxide nanoparticle complexes. Nano Lett 2007;7(4):861–7.

174. Keren S, Zavaleta C, Cheng Z, et al. Noninvasive molecular imaging of small living subjects using Raman spectroscopy. Proc Natl Acad Sci U S A 2008;105(15):5844–9.

175. Yu X, Munge B, Patel V, et al. Carbon nanotube amplification strategies for highly sensitive immunodetection of cancer biomarkers. J Am Chem Soc 2006;128(34):11199–205.

176. Shokeen M, Fettig NM, Rossin R. Synthesis, in vitro and in vivo evaluation of radiolabeled nanoparticles. Q J Nucl Med Mol Imaging 2008;52(3):267–77.

177. Cai W, Chen K, Li ZB, et al. Dual-function probe for PET and near-infrared fluorescence imaging of tumor vasculature. J Nucl Med 2007;48(11):1862–70.

178. Lee HY, Li Z, Chen K, et al. PET/MRI dual-modality tumor imaging using arginine-glycine-aspartic (RGD) - Conjugated radiolabeled iron oxide nanoparticles. J Nucl Med 2008;49(8):1371–9.

179. Pressly ED, Rossin R, Hagooly A, et al. Structural effects on the biodistribution and positron emission tomography (PET) imaging of well-defined Cu-64-labeled nanoparticles comprised of amphiphilic block graft copolymers. Biomacromolecules 2007; 8(10):3126–34.

180. Fukukawa KI, Rossin R, Hagooly A, et al. Synthesis and characterization of core-shell star copolymers for in vivo PET imaging applications. Biomacromolecules 2008;9(4):1329–39.

181. Rossin R, Muro S, Welch MJ, et al. In vivo imaging of Cu-64-labeled polymer nanoparticles targeted to the lung endothelium. J Nucl Med 2008;49(1): 103–11.

182. Sun XK, Rossin R, Turner JL, et al. An assessment of the effects of shell cross-linked nanoparticle size, core composition, and surface PEGylation on in vivo biodistribution. Biomacromolecules 2005;6(5):2541–54.

183. Sun G, Hagooly A, Xu J, et al. Facile, efficient approach to accomplish tunable chemistries and variable biodistributions for shell cross-linked nanoparticles. Biomacromolecules 2008;9(7): 1997–2006.

184. Xu JQ, Sun GR, Rossin R, et al. Labeling of polymer nanostructures for medical imaging: Importance of cross-linking extent, spacer length, and charge density. Macromolecules 2007;40(9): 2971–3.

185. Bartlett DW, Su H, Hildebrandt IJ, et al. Impact of tumor-specific targeting on the biodistribution and efficacy of siRNA nanoparticles measured by multimodality in vivo imaging. Proc Natl Acad Sci U S A 2007;104(39):15549–54.

186. Nahrendorf M, Zhang HW, Hembrador S, et al. Nanoparticle PET-CT imaging of macrophages in inflammatory atherosclerosis. Circulation 2008; 117(3):379–87.

PET Radiotracers of the Cardiovascular System

Robert J. Gropler, MD

KEYWORDS
- Positron emission tomography • Heart • Radiotracers
- Blood flow • Metabolism

Positron emission tomography (PET) is an established and powerful tool capable of providing in-depth measurements of cardiovascular physiology, pathophysiology, and cell biology with an accuracy that is not achievable with other methods. Examples include quantification of myocardial perfusion, oxygen consumption, various aspects of substrate metabolism and neuronal function. Moreover, recent technical advances are now permitting assessments of specific cellular and subcellular processes, such as alterations in gene expression and its consequences. As a result, the value of PET in cardiovascular investigation to identify specific pathologic mechanisms, to develop novel diagnostic approaches, or to facilitate the development and evaluation of the efficacy of new therapeutic advances is unequivocal. Moreover, clinical cardiac PET is becoming an integral component of the management paradigm for patients who have ischemic heart disease. Fundamental to the success of PET is the availability of radiotracers that faithfully track key biologic processes relevant to cardiovascular disease.

Table 1 lists PET radiotracers commonly used to evaluate the cardiovascular system. The following discussion highlights their contributions to cardiovascular investigation as well as applications pertaining to the clinical management of patients who have heart disease.

RADIOTRACERS OF MYOCARDIAL PERFUSION

Radiotracers used to assess regional myocardial blood flow (MBF) by PET fall into two broad categories: extractable tracers and diffusible tracers.

Each of these categories of tracers has relative advantages and disadvantages.

Extractable Tracers

Radiolabeled extractable tracers are partially extracted and retained by the myocardium while in transit through the capillary bed. With extractable tracers, blood activity is cleared rapidly, resulting in high quality images. However, because they are dependent on metabolic processes, extraction is inversely and nonlinearly related to myocardial blood flow. Discussed here are the positron-emitting tracers that have been most extensively studied.

Rubidum-82 chloride
Rubidium-82 chloride is a monovalent cation with several attractive qualities. First, it is produced by a generator from strontium-82, obviating the need for an on-site cyclotron and thus making it more widely available. Second, it has a short physical half-life of 76 seconds, allowing for multiple injections of tracer in rapid sequence. The extraction fraction of ^{82}Rb is inversely proportional to MBF in a nonlinear fashion, and extraction plateaus at 2 to 3 $mL \cdot g^{-1} \cdot min^{-1}$. Although this phenomenon is not significant for most clinical applications, it does inhibit the accurate quantification of blood flow.[1,2] Further complicating the process of quantification is the rapid decay of the radiotracer, which diminishes the quality of the time activity curves. Despite these limitations, quantitative values for MBF have been obtained with this radiotracer.

This work was supported by NIH grants PO1-HL13851 and RO1-HL69100.
Division of Radiological Sciences, Edward Mallinckrodt Institute of Radiology, Washington University School of Medicine, 510 S. Kingshighway, St. Louis, MO 63110, USA
E-mail address: groplerr@mir.wustl.edu

PET Clin 4 (2009) 69–87
doi:10.1016/j.cpet.2009.06.001
1556-8598/09/$ – see front matter © 2009 Elsevier Inc. All rights reserved.

Table 1
Positron-emitting compounds currently used with PET for cardiac studies

Radionuclide	Half-Life	Compound[a]	Present Use
Cyclotron-produced			
^{15}O	2.04 min	H_2O	Blood flow
		CO	Blood volume
		O_2	Oxygen consumption
^{13}N	9.9 min	NH_3	Blood flow
^{11}C	20.4 min	Acetate	Oxygen consumption
		Epinephrine	Sympathetic function
		Palmitate	Fatty acid metabolism
		Phenylephrine	Neuronal metabolism
		Glucose	Glucose metabolism
		HED	Norepinephrine distribution
		Lactate	Lactate metabolism
		MQNB	Muscarinic receptors
		CGP12177	Adrenergic receptors
		CGP12388	Adrenergic receptors
^{18}F	110 min	Deoxyglucose	Glucose metabolism
		Dopamine	Dopamine stores
		FTHA	Fatty acid metabolism
		FTP	Fatty acid metabolism
		FIAU	Probe for reporter gene
		FHBG	Probe for reporter gene
		FESP	Probe for reporter gene
Generator-produced			
^{82}Rb	1.25 min	RbCl	Blood flow

[a] ATSM, diacetyl-bis N[4]-methylthiosemicarbazone; FESP, 3-(2′-F-18-fluoroethyl)-spiperone; FHBG, 9-(4-fluoro-3-hydroxy-methylbutyl) guanine; FIAU, 5-iodo-2′-fluoro-2′deoxy-1-β-D-arabinofuranosyluracil; FTHA, fluoro-6-thio-heptodecanoic acid; FTP, 4-thia-hexadecanoic acid; HED, hydroxyephedrine; MQNB, methylquinuclidinyl benzilate.

Nitrogen-13 ammonia

Nitrogen-13 ammonia has been used extensively for the assessment of MBF with PET. Ammonia appears to enter the myocardium through a carrier-mediated mechanism and has a high extraction fraction in the myocardium and long tissue retention (tissue biologic half-life of 80–400 min).[3] As such, there is excellent tissue-to-blood–pool contrast, resulting in high-quality images. As is the case with ^{82}Rb, the extraction of ^{13}N ammonia is nonlinear and inversely related to MBF. Extraction plateaus at flow rates greater than 3 $mL \cdot gm^{-1} \cdot min^{-1}$.[4] In addition to measurements of relative MBF, accurate quantitative measurements of MBF are possible using appropriate mathematical models.[5,6]

C-11 acetate

^{11}C-acetate is a radiotracer that has been used extensively for the noninvasive assessment of myocardial oxygen consumption (MVO$_2$) with PET. However, ^{11}C-acetate also has a high first-pass extraction fraction ($\sim 50\%$ under resting conditions); thus, its initial distribution is related to blood flow.[7] These characteristics of ^{11}C-acetate kinetics allow for the assessment of MBF in both relative and absolute terms.[7,8] Like other extractable tracers, however, it is dependent on flow-dependent extraction fraction, circulating blood metabolites, and the need for kinetic modeling. Furthermore, its long half-life (20 minutes) does not allow for a sequence of studies to be performed in rapid succession.

F-18 labeled radiotracers

Recently, a new PET perfusion tracer, ^{18}F-BMS747158-02 has been developed. This agent is an analog of the insecticide pyridaben, an inhibitor of mitochondrial complex I (MC-1), a known nicotinamide adenine dinucleotide ubiquinone oxidoreductase.[9] The compound is nontoxic in its current configuration, and exhibits the favorable imaging characteristics of a high degree of cardiomyocyte uptake that occurs rapidly, and a very slow clearance. These characteristics translate into high-quality myocardial images in vivo

(**Fig. 1**). Moreover, the net myocardial extraction of ^{18}F-BMS747158-02 is proportional to blood flow over a wide range of flow rates (1.7 to 5.1 mL/g/min). The "roll-off" at increasing flow rates is less pronounced compared with either ^{99m}Tc-sestamibi or ^{201}Tl, suggesting that the myocardial distribution of ^{18}F-BMS747158-02 may more accurately track blood flow at higher flow rates. The regional myocardial distribution of ^{18}F-BMS747158-02 correlates with both regional blood flow and infarct size.[10] Moreover, it appears that with appropriate kinetic modeling methods, quantification of MBF in mL/g/min will be possible.[11] The agent is currently in Phase 2 clinical evaluation. Issues still to be resolved include the type of imaging scheme to be implemented, demonstration of the accuracy of the radiotracer under conditions where MC-1 function may be impaired, such as normal aging and ischemia/reperfusion, and minimizing radiation exposure to the staff performing the stress studies.

Diffusible Tracers

Unlike extractable tracers, the uptake and clearance of diffusible tracers are based solely on MBF and not on metabolism. Their kinetics are less complex and do not suffer from flow-related decreases in tissue extraction. Flow quantification can be performed using a modification of a one-compartment model developed by Kety[12,13] to determine blood–tissue exchange with an inert gas. Because diffusible tracers also circulate in the blood, a correction for activity in the blood pool must be performed to generate images of relative perfusion. However, such a correction is not necessary for quantitative measurements of perfusion.

Oxygen-15 water

Oxygen-15 water is the only diffusible tracer currently in common use. It has a short physical half-life that permits rapid sequential evaluations

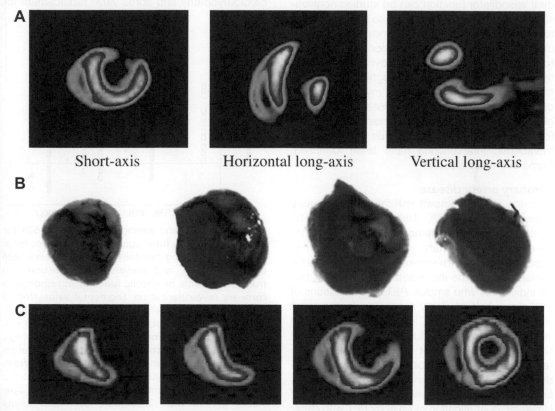

A

Short-axis   Horizontal long-axis   Vertical long-axis

B

C

Fig. 1. Representative cardiac images in rat model of left coronary ligation. (*A*) PET short- and long-axis images with BMS-747158-02 at 5 to 15 minutes after injection. (*B*) Ex vivo histologic images of heart short-axis slices from apex to base stained with blue dye. Blue areas indicate well-perfused zones, and non-blue areas indicate no-flow zones. (*C*) In vivo cardiac PET short axis images from apex to base. The dark areas in the left ventricular wall of PET images with BMS-747158-02 (*C*) match closely with the no-flow zones identified by blue stain ex vivo (*B*). (*From* Yu M, Guaraldi MT, Mistry M, et al. BMS-747158-02: a novel PET myocardial perfusion imaging agent. J Nucl Cardiol 2007;14(6):789–98; with permission.)

of MBF with only modest radiation exposure to the patient. It can be administered either intravenously or ^{15}O-carbon dioxide, which is converted to ^{15}O-water in the lungs by carbonic anhydrase, resulting in a constant intravenous infusion of ^{15}O-water.[14] For the purposes of generating images of relative perfusion, correction for blood-pool activity can be accomplished either by a separate administration of ^{15}O-carbon monoxide to label erythrocytes or from a scan early (20 sec) after the administration of the ^{15}O-water before a significant amount of tracer reaches the myocardium. Measurements of MBF by ^{15}O-water are accurate over a wide range of flow rates and the short physical half-life facilitates serial assessments.[15–18]

Research Contributions

PET assessment of MBF under conditions of stress provides a noninvasive method of assessing coronary vasodilator function. Vasodilator function comprises both endothelial-dependent and independent pathways. Endothelial-dependent vasodilator function can be studied noninvasively by assessing MBF response to cold pressor testing. In contrast, endothelial-independent vasodilation can be measured in response to vasodilators such as adenosine and dipyridamole. Using these techniques, numerous insights into the relationship between impairment in myocardial vasodilator function and cardiac disease have been gleaned. Moreover, the mechanisms responsible for the salutary effects of various cardiovascular therapeutic interventions have been identified. Some examples include:

Coronary artery disease

Smoking is a well-known risk factor for coronary artery disease (CAD). Using PET and ^{13}N-ammonia, it has been demonstrated that endothelial-dependent coronary vasodilator function is impaired in long-term smokers, providing a partial explanation for the increased cardiovascular risk for individuals who smoke. PET determinations of MBF have helped clarify the pathophysiology of hibernating myocardium, ie, reversible resting left ventricular dysfunction due to CAD. Originally, it had been proposed that myocardial hibernation represented an attempt to balance oxygen demand with a reduction in myocardial oxygen supply due to chronic hypoperfusion.[19,20] However, quantification of MBF by PET with either ^{15}O-water or ^{13}N-ammonia have shown that in a majority of cases, resting MBF in hibernating myocardium is not different from flow values in either remote tissue in the same patient or in normal healthy volunteers. Indeed, resting MBF values are markedly variable, ranging from normal

levels to frank hypoperfusion (**Fig. 2**).[21] PET measurements of MBF have demonstrated improvements in coronary endothelial function after cholesterol-lowering therapy[22] and with endurance exercise training, providing mechanistic insights as to the known beneficial effects of these interventions in patients who have CAD.[23]

Left ventricular hypertrophy

Left ventricular hypertrophy may be due to a variety of causes, most commonly essential hypertension, and others such as hypertrophic cardiomyopathy and aortic valve stenosis. Individuals who have left ventricular hypertrophy often have signs and symptoms of myocardial ischemia even in the absence of epicardial coronary obstruction.[24] A generalized abnormality in the coronary microcirculation is a likely cause; indeed, numerous studies with PET have demonstrated a reduction in vasodilator function.[24,25] Moreover, therapies designed to treat the underlying cause of the hypertrophy, such as surgical septal myomectomy in hypertrophic cardiomyopathy and aortic valve replacement for

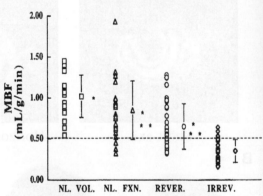

Fig. 2. Individual and average values (and i SD) for myocardial blood flow volume (□) in myocardial segments exhibiting normal function (△), reversible dysfunction (○), and irreversible dysfunction (◇) from assessments of systolic function in response to coronary revascularization. Segmental values for 19 normal subjects are also shown (average = 1.02 ± 0.26 mL/mg/min). Dotted line at 0.50 mL/gm/min, two standard deviations below mean for controls, was used as a cut-off to define abnormally low values in subjects. The range of flow in reversibly dysfunctional segments is wide. Twenty segments exhibited values within the normal range; 12 exhibited flow values greater than 2 standard deviations below mean for controls. *$P<.0001$ compared with irreversibly dysfunctional segments; **$P<.0004$ compared with normal subjects. (*From* Conversano A, Walsh JF, Geltman EM, et al. Delineation of myocardial stunning and hibernation by positron emission tomography in advanced coronary artery disease. Am Heart J 1996;131:440–50; with permission.)

aortic valve stenosis, in myocardial vasodilator function show improvement by PET.[26,27]

Assessment of patients who have cardiac allografts

Long-term survival following cardiac transplantation is frequently limited by the development of progressive vasculopathy of the intramural and epicardial coronary arteries of the allograft. The etiology of this process is unclear. Diminution in the vasodilator response to intravenous dipyridamole in recipients of cardiac transplants has been demonstrated by PET.[28,29] However, the decrease in vasodilator reserve is primarily attributable to an elevation in resting flow (most likely caused by the high prevalence of hypertension in these patients due to cyclosporine) and not to a decrease in peak hyperemic flow.[28-30]

Clinical Applications

Management of patients who have CAD

Myocardial perfusion imaging with single-photon emission computed tomography (SPECT) and either ^{201}Tl or the ^{99m}Tc-labeled tracers sestamibi or tetrofosmin is the most common method used for the detection of CAD. The ability of SPECT rest/stress myocardial perfusion imaging to accurately diagnosis CAD and to risk-stratify patients is well established; as such, SPECT perfusion imaging plays a central role in the management of patients who have CAD. However, SPECT suffers from numerous limitations, including (1) photon attenuation resulting in false-positive perfusion defects, (2) liver uptake during pharmacologic stress resulting in additional false-positive findings from back-projection errors, and (3) inability to obtain simultaneous functional information during stress imaging. PET provides many solutions to these problems, including accurate attenuation correction, high-contrast resolution and spatial resolution, and the use of radiotracers such as ^{82}Rb that are excreted by the kidneys. Furthermore, because imaging is performed at peak stress, the simultaneous measurement of myocardial perfusion and left ventricular function can be performed.[31] The use of short-lived radiopharmaceuticals allows for shorter imaging times; a rest/stress ^{13}N-ammonia study can be completed in about 60 to 75 minutes, whereas an ^{82}Rb study requires about 30 to 45 minutes. However, because of the need to begin imaging nearly simultaneously with tracer administration and the low tolerance for patient motion, exercise imaging is generally not feasible.

PET myocardial perfusion imaging has been shown to accurately identify patients who have flow-limiting CAD with reported sensitivity and specificity between ~85%–90% **(Fig. 3)**.[32,33] Moreover, PET myocardial perfusion imaging appears more accurate than SPECT in this regard, primarily because of improved specificity due to accurate attenuation correction.[34] Because of its better image quality, the confidence on image interpretation is higher with PET compared with SPECT. Analogous with SPECT, the extent and severity of perfusion abnormalities measured by PET with ^{82}Rb also provide important prognostic information.[35,36]

RADIOTRACERS OF METABOLISM

The positron-emitting radionuclides of oxygen (^{15}O), carbon (^{11}C), and nitrogen (^{13}N), as well as fluorine (^{18}F) substituting for hydrogen, can be incorporated into a wide variety of substrates or substrate analogs that participate in diverse biochemical pathways without altering the biochemical properties of the substrate of interest. Combining the knowledge of the metabolic pathways of interest with kinetic models that describe the fate of the tracer in tissue permit the assessment of the tracer kinetics as they relate to the metabolic process of interest. Metabolic processes that are typically measured with PET are:

Myocardial Oxygen Consumption

^{15}O-oxygen

Because oxygen is the final electron acceptor in all pathways of aerobic myocardial metabolism, PET with ^{15}O-oxygen has also been used to measure MVO$_2$. This method permits the measurement of myocardial oxygen extraction and measures MVO$_2$ directly. Due to the short half-life of this tracer, ^{15}O-oxygen is readily applicable in studies requiring repetitive assessments. However, the method requires the administration of multiple radiotracers (to account for MBF and blood volume) and fairly complex compartmental modeling to obtain the measurements.[37-39]

^{11}C-acetate

PET using ^{11}C-acetate is the preferred method of measuring MVO$_2$ noninvasively. Acetate is a two-carbon chain free fatty acid that is rapidly converted to acetyl–CoA in the myocyte. The primary metabolic fate of acetyl-CoA is metabolism through the tricarboxylic acid cycle. Because of the tight coupling of the tricarboxylic acid cycle and oxidative phosphorylation, the myocardial turnover of ^{11}C-acetate reflects overall flux in the tricarboxylic acid cycle and, thus, overall oxidative metabolism or MVO$_2$. Calculation of MVO$_2$ can be achieved either by exponential curve fitting or compartmental modeling.[8,40-43]

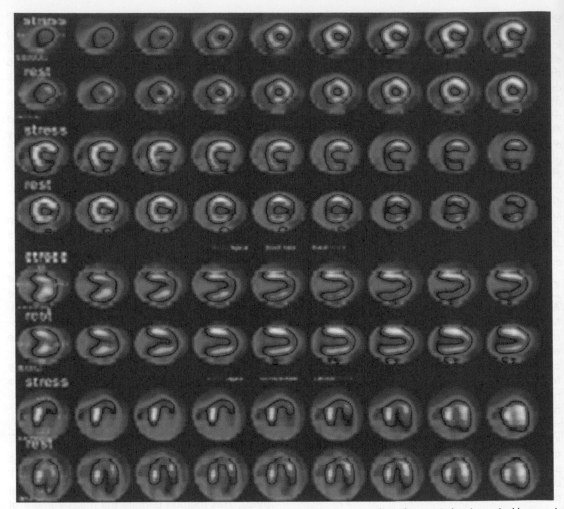

Fig. 3. Dipyridamole-stress and rest rubidium-82 PET-CT images in corresponding short-axis (*top*), vertical long-axis (*middle*), and horizontal long-axis (*bottom*) slices. Stress images are grouped on the top and rest images are grouped on the bottom. The images are abnormal and consistent with a moderately large area of severe ischemia in the lateral and inferolateral walls (left circumflex territory), and a small area of mild ischemia involving the apex (distal left anterior descending territory). (*From* Sampson UK, Dorbala S, Limaye A, et al. Diagnostic accuracy of rubidium-82 myocardial perfusion imaging with hybrid positron emission tomography/computed tomography in the detection of coronary artery disease. J Am Coll Cardiol 2007;49(10):1052–8; with permission.)

Carbohydrate Metabolism

18F-fluorodeoxyglucose

Most studies of myocardial glucose metabolism use 18F-fluorodeoxyglucose (FDG). This radiotracer competes with glucose for facilitated transport into the sarcolemma, then for hexokinase-mediated phosphorylation with trapping of the resultant F-FDG-6-phosphate. Myocardial uptake of FDG is thought to reflect overall anaerobic and aerobic myocardial glycolytic flux.[44–47] Myocardial glucose use can be assessed either in relative or absolute terms (ie, in $nmol \cdot g^{-1} \cdot min^{-1}$). For quantification, a mathematical correction for the kinetic differences between FDG and glucose, called the "lumped constant," must be used calculate rates

of glucose. However, this value may vary depending upon the prevailing plasma substrate and hormonal conditions, decreasing the accuracy of the measurement.[46,48–50] Other disadvantages of FDG include the limited metabolic fate of FDG in tissue, precluding determination of the metabolic fate (ie, glycogen formation versus glycolysis) of the extracted tracer and glucose, and limitations on the performance of serial measurements of myocardial glucose use because of the relatively long physical half-life of 18F.

Carbon-11 glucose

More recently, quantification of myocardial glucose use has been performed with PET using glucose radiolabeled in the 1-carbon position with [11]C (^{11}C-glucose). Because ^{11}C-glucose is chemically identical to unlabeled glucose, it has the same metabolic fate as glucose, thus obviating the lumped constant correction. Measurements of myocardial glucose use based on compartmental modeling of tracer kinetics are more accurate with ^{11}C-glucose than with FDG (**Fig. 4**).[51,52] Moreover, PET with ^{11}C-glucose permits the estimation of glycogen synthesis, glycolysis, and glucose oxidation.[53] Disadvantages of this method include (1) compartmental modeling that is more demanding with ^{11}C-glucose than it is with FDG, (2) the need to correct the arterial input function for the production of [11]CO$_2$ and ^{11}C-lactate, (3) a fairly complex synthesis of the tracer, and (4) short physical half-life of ^{11}C requires an on-site cyclotron.

[11]C-lactate

Recently, a multicompartmental modeling approach was developed for the assessment of myocardial lactate metabolism using PET and L-3 [^{11}C] lactic acid. Under a wide variety of conditions, PET-derived extraction of lactate correlated well with lactate oxidation measured by arterial and coronary sinus sampling.[54] This model, when combined with either FDG or ^{11}C-glucose, permits a more comprehensive measurement of myocardial carbohydrate metabolism.

Fatty Acid Metabolism

[11]C-palmitate

The major advantage of ^{11}C-palmitate is that its myocardial kinetics are identical to labeled palmitate. With appropriate mathematical modeling techniques, its use permits the assessment of various aspects of myocardial fatty acid metabolism such as uptake, oxidation, and storage.[55-58] However, this approach does suffer from several disadvantages, including reduced image quality and specificity, a more complex analysis, the need for an on-site cyclotron, and radiopharmaceutical production capability.

Fatty acid analogs

Most of the PET tracers in this category have been designed to reflect myocardial β-oxidation. 14-(R,S)-^{18}F-fluoro-6-thiaheptadecanoic acid (FTHA) was one of the first radiotracers developed using this approach. Myocardial uptake and retention tracked with changes in substrate delivery, blood flow, and workload in animal models.[59,60] As a consequence, PET with FTHA was used to evaluate the effects of various diseases, such as CAD and cardiomyopathy, on myocardial fatty acid metabolism.[61,62] However, FTHA uptake and retention has been shown to be insensitive to the inhibition of β-oxidation by hypoxia.[63] Subsequently, 16-^{18}F-fluoro-4-thiapalmitate (FTP) was developed. This modification retains the metabolic trapping function of the tracer, which is proportional to fatty acid oxidation under normal oxygenation and hypoxic conditions.[63,64] However, the accuracy of measurements of fatty acid uptake and oxidation are unclear because of the need for a lumped constant (like FDG) that may vary with the prevailing conditions. Currently, FTP is undergoing commercialization, entering early phase-1 evaluation. Recently, a new F-18–labeled fatty acid radiotracer, trans-9(RS)-^{18}F-fluoro-3,4(RS,RS)methyleneheptadecanoic acid (FCPHA), has been developed.[65] Results of initial studies showed high uptake of FCPHA into rat myocardium that remained constant for 60 minutes with low blood activity. However, the impact of alterations in plasma substrates, work load, and blood flow on myocardial kinetics is unknown. This radiotracer is undergoing commercialization and has completed phase-1 evaluation.

Overview of Myocardial Metabolism

The heart is an omnivore capable of switching between one substrate to another for energy production. This flexibility in substrate preference is fundamental to cardiac health. It permits the heart to respond to numerous stimuli, including substrate availability, the hormonal environment, the level of tissue perfusion, and the level of workload by the heart.[66,67] The control of substrate switching can either represent an acute or chronic adaptation in response to either short or prolonged alterations in the physiologic environment. Examples of acute or short-term adaptations include inhibitory effects of fatty acid oxidation on glucose oxidation and, conversely, the oxidation of fatty acids by glucose oxidation as well as the increasing oxidation of glycogen, lactate, and glucose in response to increasing workload. In contrast, chronic metabolic adaptations occur primarily at the transcriptional level through the coordinated upregulation of enzymes and proteins in key metabolic pathways. A prominent example in this case is the nuclear receptor peroxisome proliferator-activated receptor alpha (PPARα), which is a key regulator of myocardial fatty acid uptake, oxidation, and storage.[68] In diabetes mellitus, PPARα activity is increased, leading to an upregulation in genes controlling fatty acid uptake and oxidation.[69] In contrast, in dilated cardiomyopathy PPARα activity is reduced, leading to

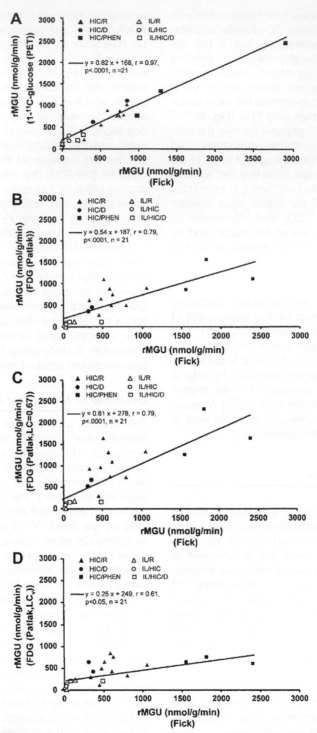

Fig. 4. Correlation in dog hearts between Fick-derived (x-axis) measurements of the rate of myocardial glucose use (rMGU) and PET-derived (y-axis) rMGU using (*A*) 1-^{11}C-glucose, (*B*) FDG before correcting PET values for the lumped constant (LC), (*C*) FDG after correcting PET values by the LC, and (*D*) FDG after correcting PET values by a variable LC (LC$_v$) that accounts for varying substrate, hormonal, and work environments. Correlation with Fick-derived values was significantly close when 1-^{11}C-glucose (*A*), as opposed to ^{18}F-FDG was used, regardless of whether or what type of LC was used (*B–D*). (*From* Herrero P, Sharp TL, Dence C, et al. Comparison of 1-(11)C-glucose and (18)F-FDG for quantifying myocardial glucose use with PET. J Nucl Med 2002;43(11):1530–41; with permission.)

a down-regulation of genes controlling fat metabolism, which in turn leads to an upregulation of glucose use.[70] These chronic adaptations can induce numerous detrimental effects that extend beyond alterations in energy production and may include increases in oxygen free radical production, impaired energetics, increases in apoptosis, and the induction of left ventricular dysfunction. Subsequent sections discuss how metabolic imaging has helped characterize this loss of metabolic flexibility due to these chronic adaptations in various disease processes.

Research Applications

Gender and aging
Both gender and aging impact the myocardial metabolic phenotype. Results of studies in animal models show that there are sex differences in myocardial substrate metabolism, with female rats exhibiting less myocardial glucose and more fatty acid metabolism.[71,72] Recently, using PET with ^{11}C-glucose and ^{11}C-palmitate in humans, women exhibited lower levels of glucose metabolism compared with men.[73] These gender differences in substrate metabolism become more pronounced as one transitions to more pathologic conditions, such as obesity.[74]

In various experimental models of aging, the contribution of fatty acid oxidation to overall myocardial substrate metabolism declines with age.[75,76] Using the PET approaches described above, it has been shown that a similar metabolic shift occurs in healthy older humans.[77] Moreover, older individuals are not able to increase glucose use in response to β-adrenergic stimulation with dobutamine to the same extent as younger individuals. However, this impairment in metabolic reserve can be ameliorated by endurance exercise training in older subjects.[78] Although requiring further study, these gender and age differences in metabolism may provide a partial explanation for the gender- and age-related outcome differences for various cardiovascular diseases in which altered myocardial metabolism plays a role.

Myocardial ischemia
Under conditions of mild-to-moderate myocardial ischemia, β-oxidation ceases and anaerobic metabolism supervenes. Glucose becomes the primary substrate for increased anaerobic glycolysis and for continued, albeit diminished, oxidative metabolism.[79] It appears that these abnormalities in myocardial substrate metabolism may persist well after the resolution of ischemia, so-called "ischemic memory." Demonstration of accelerated myocardial glucose metabolism using FDG has been used to document this phenomenon.

For example, it has been shown that PET myocardial FDG uptake is increased in subjects who have unstable angina during pain-free episodes.[80] Moreover, in subjects who have stable angina, increased FDG uptake was demonstrated following exercise-induced ischemia in the absence of either perfusion deficits or electrocardiographic abnormalities.[81] Metabolic imaging with FDG has also been used for direct ischemia detection during stress testing.[82] However numerous questions still remain regarding optimization of the imaging protocols, whether added diagnostic and prognostic information is provided over perfusion imaging, and if this information alters clinical management.

Left ventricular hypertrophy
There is a well-established link between abnormalities in myocardial substrate metabolism and left ventricular hypertrophy with a metabolic phenotype typified by a decrease in fatty acid metabolism and an overdependence on myocardial glucose use. Indeed, in an animal model of hypertrophy,[83] PET with FDG demonstrated myocardial glucose uptake tracked directly with increasing hypertrophy. Similar results have been found in humans. PET with ^{11}C-palmitate in humans has shown the reduction in myocardial fatty acid oxidation is an independent predictor of left ventricular mass in hypertension.[84] Combining measurements of left ventricular myocardial external work (either by echocardiography or MR imaging) with measurements of MVO_2 performed by PET with ^{11}C-acetate or ^{15}O-oxygen, it is possible to estimate cardiac efficiency.[38,85] Using this approach in subjects who have hypertension-induced left ventricular hypertrophy has shown that the decline in myocardial fatty acid metabolism is associated with a decline in efficiency, a condition that may increase the potential for the development of heart failure. More recently, metabolic studies with PET have been used to phenotype subjects who have hypertrophic cardiomyopathy attributable to a known specific variant in the α-tropomyosin gene.[86]

Nonischemic dilated cardiomyopathy
As mentioned previously, the overdependence on glucose metabolism typifies the myocardial metabolic phenotype in dilated cardiomyopathy. This metabolic pattern has been well documented using PET. For example, PET using ^{11}C-palmitate and ^{11}C-glucose demonstrated that myocardial fatty acid uptake and oxidation are lower in subjects who have nonischemic dilated cardiomyopathy when compared with age-matched controls. In contrast, myocardial glucose use

was higher in the cardiomyopathic subjects (**Fig. 5**).[56] PET has also been used to provide mechanistic insights into the myocardial metabolic perturbations associated with heart failure. For example, in normal subjects, abrupt lowering of fatty acid delivery with acipimox results in reduced fatty acid uptake, MVO_2, and cardiac work, and no change in cardiac efficiency.[87] In contrast, subjects who have nonischemic dilated cardiomyopathy exhibited a decrease in myocardial fatty acid uptake and cardiac work, no change in MVO_2, and a decline in efficiency. These results appear to reinforce to the central role of loss flexibility in myocardial substrate metabolism in the pathogenesis of heart failure with even minor changes in substrate delivery having detrimental consequences on cardiac energy transduction.

Obesity and insulin resistance

The study of experimental models of obesity demonstrate that a significant increase in body mass index (BMI) induces marked increases in myocardial fatty acid metabolism.[88,89] Imaging of obese young women with PET and ^{11}C-acetate and ^{11}C-palmitate has confirmed this observation in humans as an increase in BMI is associated with a shift in myocardial substrate metabolism toward greater fatty acid use. Moreover, this dependence on myocardial fatty acid metabolism increases with worsening insulin resistance.[58] Of note, little change in myocardial glucose metabolism is observed. Using similar PET techniques, it has been recently demonstrated that in contrast to obese women, obese men had a greater impairment in myocardial glucose metabolism per level of plasma insulin, suggesting greater myocardial insulin resistance. In addition, obesity has less effect on myocardial fatty acid metabolism in men. Thus, there appears to be a complex interplay between gender and obesity in influencing myocardial substrate metabolism.

Diabetes mellitus

Small animal imaging has helped clarify the mechanisms responsible for the metabolic alterations that occur in diabetes mellitus. For example,

mice with cardiac-restricted overexpression of PPARα demonstrate a metabolic phenotype that is similar to diabetic hearts.[90] Small animal PET studies with ^{11}C-palmitate and FDG in these mice demonstrate a relative increase in fatty acid uptake and oxidation and an abnormal suppression of glucose uptake. In contrast, in mice with cardiac-restricted overexpression of PPARβ/δ, small animal PET measurements demonstrated a relative increase glucose uptake and reduced fatty acid uptake and oxidation.[91] Taken in sum these observations demonstrate that PPARα and PPARβ/δ control different metabolic regulatory programs and that imaging can help characterize genetic manipulations in mouse heart. Quantitative measures of myocardial substrate metabolism are now possible in rat heart as rates of myocardial glucose uptake correlate directly and closely and GLUT 4 gene expression in the Zucker-diabetic-fat (ZDF) rat, a model of type-2 diabetes mellitus.[92] Moreover, PET studies have confirmed the importance of increased fatty acid delivery to the development of the myocardial metabolic phenotype in type-2 diabetes mellitus (**Fig. 6**A, B).

PET studies in subjects who have diabetes mellitus have confirmed the same metabolic phenotype is present in humans. PET with either FDG or ^{11}C-glucose has documented a reduction in myocardial glucose uptake in diabetic subjects. Moreover, the metabolic fate of extracted glucose is impaired in diabetes, with reduced rates of glycolysis and glucose oxidation that become more pronounced with increases in cardiac work induced by dobutamine.[93] In contrast, both myocardial fatty acid uptake and oxidation are increased in diabetics based on studies using PET with ^{11}C-palmitate. The increase fatty acid metabolism is due primarily to an increase in plasma fatty acid levels secondary to peripheral insulin resistance. The increase in plasma fatty acids are an attractive target to reduce the overdependence of the myocardium on fatty acid metabolism. Indeed, PET studies in subjects who have type-2 diabetes mellitus have confirmed that reducing fatty acid delivery therapeutically improves myocardial metabolism.[94,95]

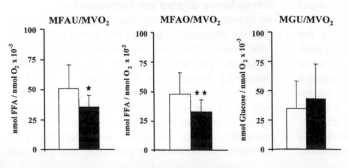

Fig. 5. Myocardial fatty acid and glucose metabolism in idiopathic dilated cardiomyopathy (IDCM). (*From* Davila-Roman VG, Vedala G, Herrero P, et al. Altered myocardial fatty acid and glucose metabolism in idiopathic dilated cardiomyopathy. J Am Coll Cardiol 2002;40(2):271–7; with permission.)

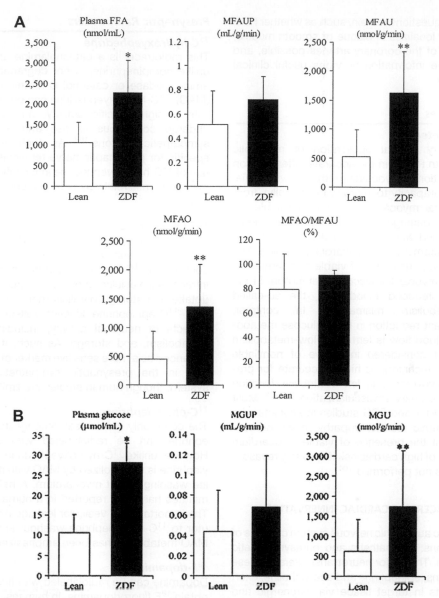

Fig. 6. (*A*) Fatty acid metabolism measurements obtained in ZDF (*closed*) and lean (*open*) rats by compartmental modeling of 1-^{11}C-palmitate PET data. *Abbreviations:* MFAO, myocardial fatty acid oxidation; MFAO/MFAU, myocardial fatty acid that was oxidized; MFAU, myocardial fatty acid use; MFAUP, myocardial fatty acid uptake. (*B*) Glucose metabolism measurements obtained in ZDF (*closed*) and lean (*open*) rats by compartmental modeling of 1-^{11}C-glucose PET data. *Abbreviations:* MGU, myocardial glucose use; MGUP, myocardial glucose uptake.

Beyond the myocardium – vascular imaging

Inflammation is a key component of atherosclerosis. Moreover, it is an important and likely contributor to rupture of a coronary artery plaque, which leads to myocardial infarction and, frequently, sudden cardiac death. Despite the plethora of currently available imaging tools to detect and characterize the extent and severity coronary atherosclerosis, none of them identify patients with active disease and who are at risk of plaque rupture. Consequently, FDG is being evaluated for the detection of biologically "active" atherosclerosis based on the premise that the tracer accumulates in activated macrophages, which are a key inflammatory component of atherosclerotic plaque. The increased uptake has been noted in animal models of atherosclerosis, and demonstrated in humans with atherosclerosis of the carotid artery and aorta.[96–99] A decrease in carotid artery FDG uptake has been observed following treatment with cholesterol-lowering agents[98] Despite these early successes, numerous questions remain, such as whether FDG radiotracer localizes in plaque or smooth muscle, is imaging of the coronary arteries possible, and whether the information provides useful clinical information.

Clinical Uses

Viability detection

The primary clinical application of metabolic imaging with PET is in the accurate differentiation of dysfunctional myocardium that is viable (ie, retains the capacity to improve functionally), from dysfunctional myocardium that is nonviable (ie, irreversibly damaged).[100] Viability assessments are performed with PET and FDG in conjunction with measurements of myocardial perfusion. The typical pattern indicative of viable myocardium is preserved myocardial glucose metabolism in the setting of reduced blood flow, the so-called "flow-metabolism mismatch." In contrast, a concordant reduction in both glucose metabolism and blood flow is termed a flow-metabolism match and considered indicative of nonviable tissue. The technique is highly accurate for predicting improvement in left ventricular function following coronary revascularization.[101,102] Most important, PET and FDG studies in subjects who have ischemic cardiomyopathy have demonstrated that the presence of viable myocardium is a marker of high cardiac risk if coronary revascularization is not performed.[101]

RADIOTRACERS OF CARDIAC INNERVATION

The cardiac autonomic nervous system consists of two divisions: sympathetic and parasympathetic innervation. The major neurotransmitters of these two divisions, epinephrine and acetylcholine, exert their effects in target tissue via adrenergic and muscarinic receptors, respectively. The sympathetic nervous system is the predominant autonomic component in the ventricles, whereas parasympathetic fibers predominantly innervate the atria and are less abundant overall. Radiotracers to evaluate cardiac innervations are summarized in **Table 1**.

The Cardiac Sympathetic Nervous System

Radiopharmaceuticals for imaging the cardiac sympathetic nervous system are divided into those that image the presynaptic sympathetic nerve terminals and those that target postsynaptic adrenergic receptors. Presynaptic radiotracers can either be radiolabeled catecholamines or radiolabeled catecholamine analogs.

Presynaptic Radiotracers

11C-hydroxyephedrine

This radiotracer is a catecholamine analog that, unlike norepinephrine, is not degraded by monamine oxidase or catechol O-methyl transferase (MAO). 11C-hydroxyephedrine can be synthesized with a high specific activity, and appears to undergo continuous release and reuptake by sympathetic neurons.[103] As such, it is highly specific for presynaptic nerve terminals. Distribution of 11C-hydroxyephedrine in the left ventricular myocardium is relatively homogenous and can be quantified.[104,105]

11C-epinephrine

This radiotracer a true neurotransmitter that is also synthesized with a high specific activity. In contrast to 11C-hydroxyephedrine, it is stored in intracellular vesicles and thus cleared slowly. Its uptake and storage parallels that of norepinephrine. 11C-epinephrine kinetics reflect the many aspects of neuronal activity, including uptake, metabolism, and storage. As such, it has been advanced as a more sensitive marker of abnormalities in the presynaptic sympathetic nervous system, though human studies are limited.[106,107]

11C-phenylephrine

The commonly used nasal decongestant phenylephrine can be radiolabeled with carbon-11. However unlike 11C-hydroxyephedrine, 11C-phenylephrine is metabolized by MAO with its metabolite washing out of myocardium. A half-life of 60 minutes has been reported in a human study.[105] The importance of vesicular leakage as a contributor to 11C-phenylephrine washout in addition to MAO metabolism has been emphasized.[108]

18F-dopamine

Dopamine can be radiolabeled with fluorine-18 to obtain 18F fluorodopamine. In humans, 18F-fluorodopamine imaging has been used to assess sympathetic innervation in the heart.[109] Because of the nature of the radiolabel and the similarity of the metabolic pathways compared with the endogenous norepinephrine, 18F-fluorodopamine can assess the uptake and clearance of this neurotransmitter. Because of the complex fate of dopamine in the plasma and the heart, it is not widely used as the tracer of choice in assessing cardiac neuronal function.

Postsynaptic Radiotracers

A variety of post-ynaptic adrenergic receptor tracers have been tested, but most are limited by their nonspecific binding. 11C-CGP12177 is fairly specific for β-receptors and has the most extensive clinical use, but its use is limited by its difficult synthesis.[110] ^{11}C-CGP12388 is easier to synthesize, but has limited use in humans. Finally, a prazosin derivative, ^{11}C-GB67, has limited use in humans for imaging the α_1 receptor.[111]

The Cardiac Parasympathetic Nervous System

Presynaptic binding with ^{18}F-fluoroethoxybenzo-vesamicol has been performed in rats, but has been greatly limited by the low density of cholinergic neurons in the ventricles, nonspecific binding and rapid degradation.[112] Postsynaptic binding of the muscarinic receptors has been performed in humans in a limited number of studies with ^{11}C-methylquinuclidinyl benzilate.[113–115]

Research Applications

The autonomic nervous system of the heart plays a major role in the regulation of myocardial function, metabolism, and blood flow, both in the normal heart and in various pathologic processes that include ischemic heart disease, heart failure, sudden death, and diabetes. Detailed below are some research applications of neuronal imaging using PET.

Myocardial infarction and ischemia

It has been hypothesized that sympathetic neurons are more sensitive to ischemia. In clinical studies of nontransmural myocardial infarction, the area of reduced ^{11}C-hydroxyephedrine retention is greater than the perfusion defect.[116] Moreover, in subjects who have CAD but no evidence of myocardial infarction, there are regional reductions in ^{11}C-hydroxyephedrine retention.[117] A reduction in ^{18}F-fluorodopamine washout in infarct areas was associated with an improvement in heart rate variability.[118] Further investigation of the sympathetic nervous system using PET tracers could potentially link sympathetic denervation with a higher incidence of ventricular arrhythmias.

Heart transplantation

The sympathetic reinnervation that occurs late after cardiac transplantation serves as useful model to study the effect of autonomic function on myocardial function. Allograft reinnervation, as measured by PET with ^{11}C-hydroxyephedrine, begins approximately 1 year after surgery and increases in extent and intensity until year 12 (**Fig. 7**). It begins in the basal anterior and septal walls and progresses toward the apex and lateral walls, seemingly along the distribution of the left anterior descending coronary artery. Reinnervation has been associated with improved endothelial-dependent vasodilation, a metabolic switch from the use of glucose to free fatty acids, and improved exercise performance.[119,120] Exercise

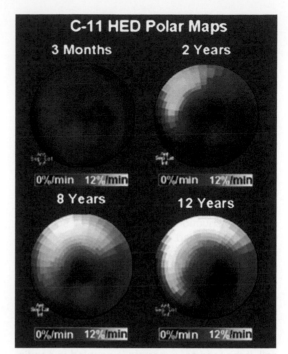

Fig. 7. Polar maps of myocardial retention of C-11 hydroxyephedrine (HED) in four cardiac transplant recipients at different times after surgery, illustrating time course and regional extent of sympathetic reinnervation. *Ant*, anterior; *Sep*, septal; *Lat*, lateral; *Inf*, inferior. (*From* Bengal FM, Schwaiger M. Assessment of cardiac sympathetic neuronal function using PET imaging. J Nucl Cardiol 2004;11:603–16; with permission.)

performance was also regionally improved with reinnervation as measured by contractile function and heart rate response.[121]

Heart Failure/Cardiomyopathy

Heart failure is associated with a hyperadrenergic state and resultant down-regulation of β-adrenergic receptors. In vivo studies with PET and ^{11}C-CGP12177 have confirmed this down-regulation, which is associated with decreased responsiveness to dobutamine.[122] By contrast, muscarinic receptor density is increased and may be an adaptive mechanism.[115] Presynaptic cardiac innervation, as quantified with ^{11}C-meta-hydroxyephedrine, is also reduced, and the degree of this reduced retention is an independent predictor of adverse outcomes.[123] Furthermore, serial cardiac neuronal mapping has been used to assess the beneficial effects of exercise training on global ^{11}C-metahydroxyephedrine retention in tandem with a functional improvement in autonomic nervous system control.[124]

Diabetes mellitus

Diabetes mellitus is characterized by cardiac autonomic neuropathy.[125–129] Similarly, PET with ^{11}C-hydroxyephedrine has been used to demonstrate relationships between myocardial neuropathy, blood flow regulation, and outcome in diabetic subjects but the incremental clinical significance of these findings have yet to be demonstrated.[130–135]

Molecular Imaging Radiotracers

Imaging is now extending beyond the assessments of morphology, function, physiology, and biochemistry to the study of specific cellular and subcellular processes such as gene expression, signal transduction pathways and cell survival or what is now called molecular imaging. Examples of PET radiotracers for molecular imaging are summarized in **Table 1**. One of the most commonly used applications is to measure gene expression using reporter gene technology. The product of the reporter gene is often an enzyme that selectively converts a reporter substrate to a metabolite that is trapped within the transduced cell. If the reporter substrate is coupled to a radiotracer, then an in vivo assay is created that can be used to measure the regulation and expression of various endogenous or transfected genes as well as signal transduction pathways in a noninvasive, repetitive, and quantitative manner. The most common type of enzyme-based reporter gene is the herpes simplex virus type-1 thymidine kinase. This gene can be transfected in line with a therapeutic gene. The resultant gene product is an enzyme that phosphorylates reporter probes such as the thymidine analog 5-iodo-2′-fluoro-2′deoxy-1-β-D-arabinofuranosyluracil or a guanine analog 9-(4-fluoro-3-hydroxymethylbutyl) guanine. This approach has been used to track both the fate and survival of stem cell therapy.[136,137] Another example of molecular imaging is the use of nanoparticle strategies to target the inflammatory component of atherosclerosis.[138] Thus, molecular imaging probes such as these demonstrate the potential of molecular imaging to permit delineation of cardiovascular disease processes and therapeutic interventions with a level of biologic resolution not achievable with current radiotracers.

FUTURE DIRECTIONS

Continued advances in PET radiotracer design are needed and will likely fall into two broad but still related categories. First, radiotracers must be developed to measure key metabolic and neuronal pathways radiolabeled with either F-18 or I-123 and to readily export image analysis schemes. In

this way, appropriately powered clinical trials can be performed that answer key questions about the utility of these measurements for diagnosis, risk stratification, and monitoring of therapy in specific patient populations. In parallel, there needs to be development of novel molecular imaging probes that permit interrogation of cellular and subcellular processes relevant to cardiovascular disease and provide the specificity necessary for the transition to more personalized approaches for medical care.

REFERENCES

1. Herrero P, Markham J, Shelton ME, et al. Implementation and evaluation of a two-compartment model for quantification of myocardial perfusion with rubidium-82 and positron emission tomography. Circ Res 1992;70:496–507.
2. Lautamaki R, George RT, Kitagawa K, et al. Rubidium-82 PET-CT for quantitative assessment of myocardial blood flow: validation in a canine model of coronary artery stenosis. Eur J Nucl Med Mol Imaging 2009;36(4):576–86.
3. Schelbert HR, Phelps ME, Huang SC, et al. N-13 ammonia as an indicator or myocardial blood flow. Circulation 1981;63:1259–72.
4. Shah A, Schelbert HR, Schwaiger M, et al. Measurement of regional myocardial blood flow with N-13 ammonia and positron-emission tomography in intact dogs. J Am Coll Cardiol 1985;5:92–100.
5. Muzik O, Beanlands RS, Hutchins GD, et al. Validation of nitrogen-13-ammonia tracer kinetic model for quantification of myocardial blood flow using PET. J Nucl Med 1993;34:83–91.
6. Hutchins GD, Schwaiger M, Rosenspire KC, et al. Noninvasive quantification of regional blood flow in the human heart using N-13 ammonia and dynamic positron emission tomographic imaging. J Am Coll Cardiol 1990;15(5):1032–42.
7. Gropler RJ, Siegel BA, Geltman EM. Myocardial uptake of carbon-11-acetate as an indirect estimate of regional myocardial blood flow. J Nucl Med 1991;32(2):245–51.
8. Sun KT, Yeatman A, Buxton DB, et al. Simultaneous measurement of myocardial oxygen consumption and blood flow using [1-carbon-11] acetate. J Nucl Med 1998;39(2):272–80.
9. Yu M, Guaraldi MT, Mistry M, et al. BMS-747158-02: a novel PET myocardial perfusion imaging agent. J Nucl Cardiol 2007;14(6):789–98.
10. Huisman MC, Higuchi T, Reder S, et al. Initial characterization of an ^{18}F-labeled myocardial perfusion tracer. J Nucl Med 2008;49(4):630–6.
11. Nekolla SG, Reder S, Saraste A, et al. Evaluation of the novel myocardial perfusion positron-emission

tomography tracer ^{18}F-BMS-747158-02: comparison to ^{13}N-ammonia and validation with microspheres in a pig model. Circulation 2009;119(17): 2333–42.

12. Kety SS. The theory and applications of the exchange of inert gas at the lungs and tissues. Pharmacol Rev 1951;3:1–41.

13. Kety SS. Measurement of local blood flow by the exchange of an inert, diffusible substance. Methods Med Res 1960;8:228–36.

14. Araujo LI, Lammertsma AA, Rhodes CG, et al. Noninvasive quantification of regional myocardial blood flow in coronary artery disease with oxygen-15-labeled carbon dioxide inhalation and positron emission tomography. Circulation 1991; 83:875–85.

15. Bergmann SR. Quantification of myocardial perfusion with positron emission tomography. In: Bergmann SR, Sobel BE, editors. Positron emission tomography of the heart. Mount Kisco (NY): Futura; 1992. p. 97–127.

16. Bergmann SR, Fox KA, Rand AL, et al. Quantification of regional myocardial blood flow in vivo with H215O. Circulation 1984;70:724–33.

17. Bergmann SR, Herrero P, Markham J, et al. Noninvasive quantitation of myocardial blood flow in human subjects with oxygen-15-labeled water and positron emission tomography. J Am Coll Cardiol 1989;14:639–52.

18. Tripp MR, Meyer MW, Einzig S, et al. Simultaneous regional myocardial blood flows by tritiated water in microspheres. Am J Physiol Heart Circ Physiol 1977;232:H173–90.

19. Rahimtoola SH. A perspective on the three large multicenter randomized clinical trials of coronary bypass surgery for chronic stable angina. Circulation 1985;72:V123–35.

20. Rahimtoola SH. The hibernating myocardium. Am Heart J 1989;117:211–21.

21. Convercano A, Walsh JF, Gellman EM, et al. Delineation of myocardial stunning and hibernation by positron emission tomgraphy in advanced coronary artery disease. Am Heart J 1996;131:440–50.

22. Baller D, Notohamiprodjo G, Gleichmann U, et al. Improvement in coronary flow reserve determined by positron emission tomography after 6 months of cholesterol-lowering therapy in patients with early stages of coronary atherosclerosis. Circulation 1999;99:2871–5.

23. Soto PF, Herrero P, Baumstark JM, et al. Endurance exercise training improves endothelial function in older individuals [abstract]. Circulation 2004;110: III-560.

24. Hamasaki S, Suwaidi JA, Higano ST, et al. Attenuated coronary flow reserve and vascular remodeling in patients with hypertension and left ventricular hypertrophy. J Am Coll Cardiol 2000;35:1654–60.

25. Treasure CB, Klein JL, Vita JA, et al. Hypertension and left ventricular hypertrophy are associated with impaired endothelium-mediated relaxation in human coronary resistance vessels. Circulation 1993;87:86–93.

26. Jorg-Ciopor M, Namdar M, Turina J, et al. Regional myocardial ischemia in hypertrophic cardiomyopathy: impact of myomectomy. J Thorac Cardiovasc Surg 2004;128(2):163–9.

27. Rajappan K, Rimoldi OE, Camici PG, et al. Functional changes in coronary microcirculation after valve replacement in patients with aortic stenosis. Circulation 2003;107:3170–5.

28. Rechavia E, Araujo LI, de Silva R, et al. Dipyridamole vasodilator response after human orthotopic heart transplantation: quantification by oxygen-15-labeled water and positron emission tomography. J Am Coll Cardiol 1992;19(1):100–6.

29. Senneff MJ, Hartman J, Sobel BE, et al. Persistence of coronary vasodilator reserve after cardiac transplantation. Am J Cardiol 1993;71(4):333–8.

30. Krivokapich J, Stevenson LW, Kobashigawa J, et al. Quantification of absolute myocardial blood flow at rest and during exercise with positron emission tomography after human cardiac transplantation. J Am Coll Cardiol 1991;18:512–7.

31. Hickey KT, Sciacca RR, Bokhari S, et al. Assessment of cardiac wall motion and ejection fraction with gated PET using N-13 ammonia. Clin Nucl Med 2004;29:243–8.

32. Sampson UK, Dorbala S, Limaye A, et al. Diagnostic accuracy of rubidium-82 myocardial perfusion imaging with hybrid positron emission tomography/computed tomography in the detection of coronary artery disease. J Am Coll Cardiol 2007;49(10):1052–8.

33. Stewart RE, Schwaiger M, Molina E, et al. Comparison of rubidium-82 positron emission tomography and thallium-201 SPECT imaging for detection of coronary artery disease. Am J Cardiol 1991; 67(16):1303–10.

34. Bateman TM, Heller GV, McGhie AI, et al. Diagnostic accuracy of rest/stress ECG-gated Rb-82 myocardial perfusion PET: comparison with ECG-gated Tc-99m sestamibi SPECT. J Nucl Cardiol 2006;13(1):24–33.

35. Marwick TH, Shan K, Patel S, et al. Incremental value of rubidium-82 positron emission tomography for prognostic assessment of known or suspected coronary artery disease. Am J Cardiol 1997;80(7): 865–70.

36. Schenker MP, Dorbala S, Hong EC, et al. Interrelation of coronary calcification, myocardial ischemia, and outcomes in patients with intermediate likelihood of coronary artery disease: a combined positron emission tomography/computed tomography study. Circulation 2008;117(13):1693–700.

37. Iida H, Rhodes CG, Araujo LI, et al. Noninvasive quantification of regional myocardial metabolic rate for oxygen by use of $^{15}O_2$ inhalation and positron emission tomography. Theory, error analysis, and application in humans. Circulation 1996; 94(4):792–807.

38. Laine H, Katoh C, Luotolahti M, et al. Myocardial oxygen consumption is unchanged but efficiency is reduced in patients with essential hypertension and left ventricular hypertrophy. Circulation 1999; 100(24):2425–30.

39. Yamamoto Y, de Silva R, Rhodes CG, et al. Noninvasive quantification of regional myocardial metabolic rate of oxygen by $^{15}O_2$ inhalation and positron emission tomography. Experimental validation. Circulation 1996;94(4):808–16.

40. Armbrecht JJ, Buxton DB, Schelbert HR. Validation of [1-11C]acetate as a tracer for noninvasive assessment of oxidative metabolism with positron emission tomography in normal, ischemic, postischemic, and hyperemic canine myocardium. Circulation 1990;81(5):1594–605.

41. Brown M, Marshall DR, Sobel BE, et al. Delineation of myocardial oxygen utilization with carbon-11-labeled acetate. Circulation 1987;76(3):687–96.

42. Brown MA, Myears DW, Bergmann SR. Noninvasive assessment of canine myocardial oxidative metabolism with carbon-11 acetate and positron emission tomography. J Am Coll Cardiol 1988; 12(4):1054–63.

43. Buck A, Wolpers HG, Hutchins GD, et al. Effect of carbon-11-acetate recirculation on estimates of myocardial oxygen consumption by PET. J Nucl Med 1991;32(10):1950–7.

44. Choi Y, Hawkins RA, Huang SC, et al. Parametric images of myocardial metabolic rate of glucose generated from dynamic cardiac PET and 2-[^{18}F]fluoro-2-deoxy-d-glucose studies. J Nucl Med 1991;32(4):733–8.

45. Gambert S, Vergely C, Filomenko R, et al. Adverse effects of free fatty acid associated with increased oxidative stress in postischemic isolated rat hearts. Mol Cell Biochem 2006; 283(1–2):147–52.

46. Iozzo P, Chareonthaitawee P, Di Terlizzi M, et al. Regional myocardial blood flow and glucose utilization during fasting and physiological hyperinsulinemia in humans. Am J Physiol Endocrinol Metab 2002;282(5):E1163–71.

47. Krivokapich J, Huang SC, Selin CE, et al. Fluoro-deoxyglucose rate constants, lumped constant, and glucose metabolic rate in rabbit heart. Am J Physiol 1987;252(4 Pt 2):H777–87.

48. Botker HE, Bottcher M, Schmitz O, et al. Glucose uptake and lumped constant variability in normal human hearts determined with [^{18}F]fluorodeoxyglucose. J Nucl Cardiol 1997;4(2 Pt 1):125–32.

49. Hariharan R, Bray M, Ganim R, et al. Fundamental limitations of [^{18}F]2-deoxy-2-fluoro-D-glucose for assessing myocardial glucose uptake. Circulation 1995;91(9):2435–44.

50. Hashimoto K, Nishimura T, Imahashi KI, et al. Lumped constant for deoxyglucose is decreased when myocardial glucose uptake is enhanced. Am J Physiol 1999;276(1 Pt 2):H129–33.

51. Herrero P, Sharp TL, Dence C, et al. Comparison of 1-(11)C-glucose and (18)F-FDG for quantifying myocardial glucose use with PET. J Nucl Med 2002;43(11):1530–41.

52. Herrero P, Weinheimer CJ, Dence C, et al. Quantification of myocardial glucose utilization by PET and 1-carbon-11-glucose. J Nucl Cardiol 2002;9(1): 5–14.

53. Herrero P, Kisrieva-Ware Z, Dence CS, et al. PET measurements of myocardial glucose metabolism with 1-11C-glucose and kinetic modeling. J Nucl Med 2007;48(6):955–64.

54. Herrero P, Dence CS, Coggan AR, et al. L-3-11C-lactate as a PET tracer of myocardial lactate metabolism: a feasibility study. J Nucl Med 2007; 48(12):2046–55.

55. Bergmann SR, Weinheimer CJ, Markham J, et al. Quantitation of myocardial fatty acid metabolism using PET. J Nucl Med 1996;37(10):1723–30.

56. Davila-Roman VG, Vedala G, Herrero P, et al. Altered myocardial fatty acid and glucose metabolism in idiopathic dilated cardiomyopathy. J Am Coll Cardiol 2002;40(2):271–7.

57. Herrero P, Peterson LR, McGill JB, et al. Increased myocardial fatty acid metabolism in patients with type 1 diabetes mellitus. J Am Coll Cardiol 2006; 47(3):598–604.

58. Peterson LR, Herrero P, Schechtman KB, et al. Effect of obesity and insulin resistance on myocardial substrate metabolism and efficiency in young women. Circulation 2004;109(18):2191–6.

59. DeGrado TR. Synthesis of 14(R, S)-[^{18}F]fluoro-6-thia-heptadecanoic acid (FTHA). J Labelled Comp Radiopharm 1991;29:989–95.

60. DeGrado TR, Coenen HH, Stocklin G. 14(R, S)-[^{18}F]fluoro-6-thia-heptadecanoic acid (FTHA): evaluation in mouse of a new probe of myocardial utilization of long chain fatty acids. J Nucl Med 1991;32(10):1888–96.

61. Schulz G, von Dahl J, Kaiser HJ, et al. Imaging of beta-oxidation by static PET with 14(R, S)-[^{18}F]-fluoro-6-thiaheptadecanoic acid (FTHA) in patients with advanced coronary heart disease: a comparison with 18FDG-PET and 99Tcm-MIBI SPET. Nucl Med Commun 1996;17(12):1057–64.

62. Taylor M, Wallhaus TR, Degrado TR, et al. An evaluation of myocardial fatty acid and glucose uptake using PET with [^{18}F]fluoro-6-thia-heptadecanoic

acid and [^{18}F]FDG in patients with congestive heart failure. J Nucl Med 2001;42(1):55–62.

63. DeGrado TR, Wang S, Holden JE, et al. Synthesis and preliminary evaluation of (18)F-labeled 4-thia palmitate as a PET tracer of myocardial fatty acid oxidation. Nucl Med Biol 2000;27(3):221–31.

64. DeGrado TR, Kitapci MT, Wang S, et al. Validation of ^{18}F-fluoro-4-thia-palmitate as a PET probe for myocardial fatty acid oxidation: effects of hypoxia and composition of exogenous fatty acids. J Nucl Med 2006;47(1):173–81.

65. Shoup TM, Elmaleh DR, Bonab AA, et al. Evaluation of trans-9-^{18}F-fluoro-3,4-Methyleneheptadecanoic acid as a PET tracer for myocardial fatty acid imaging. J Nucl Med 2005;46(2):297–304.

66. Bing RJ. The metabolism of the heart. Harvey Lect 1955;50:27–70.

67. Neely JR, Morgan HE. Relationship between carbohydrate and lipid metabolism and the energy balance of heart muscle. Annu Rev Physiol 1974;36:413–59.

68. Kelly DP. PPARs of the heart: three is a crowd. Circ Res 2003;92(5):482–4.

69. Finck BN, Han X, Courtois M, et al. A critical role for PPARalpha-mediated lipotoxicity in the pathogenesis of diabetic cardiomyopathy: modulation by dietary fat content. Proc Natl Acad Sci U S A 2003;100(3):1226–31.

70. Depre C, Shipley GL, Chen W, et al. Unloaded heart in vivo replicates fetal gene expression of cardiac hypertrophy. Nat Med 1998;4(11):1269–75.

71. Desrois M, Sidell RJ, Gauguier D, et al. Gender differences in hypertrophy, insulin resistance and ischemic injury in the aging type 2 diabetic rat heart. J Mol Cell Cardiol 2004;37(2):547–55.

72. Dyck JR, Lopaschuk GD. Glucose metabolism, H+ production and Na+/H+-exchanger mRNA levels in ischemic hearts from diabetic rats. Mol Cell Biochem 1998;180(1–2):85–93.

73. Peterson LR, Soto PF, Herrero P, et al. Sex differences in myocardial oxygen and glucose metabolism. J Nucl Cardiol 2007;14(4):573–81.

74. Peterson LR, Soto PM, Herrero P, et al. Impact of gender on the myocardial metabolic response to obesity. JACC Cardiovasc Imaging 2008;1:424–33.

75. Abu-Erreish GM, Neely JR, Whitmer JT, et al. Fatty acid oxidation by isolated perfused working hearts of aged rats. Am J Physiol 1977;232(3):E258–62.

76. McMillin JB, Taffet GE, Taegtmeyer H, et al. Mitochondrial metabolism and substrate competition in the aging Fischer rat heart. Cardiovasc Res 1993;27(12):2222–8.

77. Kates AM, Herrero P, Dence C, et al. Impact of aging on substrate metabolism by the human heart. J Am Coll Cardiol 2003;41:293–9.

78. Soto PF, Herrero P, Schechtman KB, et al. Exercise training impacts the myocardial metabolism of

older individuals in a gender-specific manner. Am J Physiol Heart Circ Physiol 2008;295(2):H842–50.

79. Lopaschuk G. Regulation of carbohydrate metabolism in ischemia and reperfusion. Am Heart J 2000; 139(2 Pt 3):S115–9.

80. Araujo LI, Camici P, Spinks TJ, et al. Abnormalities in myocardial metabolism in patients with unstable angina as assessed by positron emission tomography. Cardiovasc Drugs Ther 1988;2(1):41–6.

81. Camici P, Araujo LI, Spinks T, et al. Increased uptake of ^{18}F-fluorodeoxyglucose in postischemic myocardium of patients with exercise-induced angina. Circulation 1986;74(1):81–8.

82. He ZX, Shi RF, Wu YJ, et al. Direct imaging of exercise-induced myocardial ischemia with fluorine-18-labeled deoxyglucose and Tc-99m-sestamibi in coronary artery disease. Circulation 2003;108(10): 1208–13.

83. Handa N, Magata Y, Mukai T, et al. Quantitative FDG-uptake by positron emission tomography in progressive hypertrophy of rat hearts in vivo. Ann Nucl Med 2007;21(10):569–76.

84. de las Fuentes L, Herrero P, Peterson LR, et al. Myocardial fatty acid metabolism: independent predictor of left ventricular mass in hypertensive heart disease. Hypertension 2003;41(1):83–7.

85. de las Fuentes L, Soto PF, Cupps BP, et al. Hypertensive left ventricular hypertrophy is associated with abnormal myocardial fatty acid metabolism and myocardial efficiency. J Nucl Cardiol 2006; 13(3):369–77.

86. Tuunanen H, Kuusisto J, Toikka J, et al. Myocardial perfusion, oxidative metabolism, and free fatty acid uptake in patients with hypertrophic cardiomyopathy attributable to the Asp175Asn mutation in the alpha-tropomyosin gene: a positron emission tomography study. J Nucl Cardiol 2007;14(3): 354–65.

87. Tuunanen H, Engblom E, Naum A, et al. Decreased myocardial free fatty acid uptake in patients with idiopathic dilated cardiomyopathy: evidence of relationship with insulin resistance and left ventricular dysfunction. J Card Fail 2006;12(8):644–52.

88. Commerford SR, Pagliassotti MJ, Melby CL, et al. Fat oxidation, lipolysis, and free fatty acid cycling in obesity-prone and obesity-resistant rats. Am J Physiol Endocrinol Metab 2000;279(4):E875–85.

89. Zhou YT, Grayburn P, Karim A, et al. Lipotoxic heart disease in obese rats: implications for human obesity. Proc Natl Acad Sci U S A 2000;97(4): 1784–9.

90. Finck BN, Lehman JJ, Leone TC, et al. The cardiac phenotype induced by PPARalpha overexpression mimics that caused by diabetes mellitus. J Clin Invest 2002;109(1):121–30.

91. Burkart EM, Sambandam N, Han X, et al. Nuclear receptors PPARbeta/delta and PPARalpha direct

distinct metabolic regulatory programs in the mouse heart. J Clin Invest 2007;117(12):3930–9.

92. Shoghi KI, Gropler RJ, Sharp T, et al. Time course of alterations in myocardial glucose utilization in the Zucker diabetic fatty rat with correlation to gene expression of glucose transporters: a small-animal PET investigation. J Nucl Med 2008;49(8):1320–7.

93. Herrero P, McGill JB, Lesniak D, et al. Pet dection of the impact of dobutamine on myocardial glucose metabolism in women with type 1 diabetes mellitus. J Nucl Cardiol 2008;15(6):598–604.

94. Hallsten K, Virtanen KA, Lonnqvist F, et al. Enhancement of insulin-stimulated myocardial glucose uptake in patients with Type 2 diabetes treated with rosiglitazone. Diabet Med 2004; 21(12):1280–7.

95. van der Meer RW, Rijzewijk LJ, de Jong HW, et al. Pioglitazone improves cardiac function and alters myocardial substrate metabolism without affecting cardiac triglyceride accumulation and high-energy phosphate metabolism in patients with well-controlled type 2 diabetes mellitus. Circulation 2009;119(15):2069–77.

96. Ogawa M, Ishino S, Mukai T, et al. (18)F-FDG accumulation in atherosclerotic plaques: immunohisto-chemical and PET imaging study. J Nucl Med 2004;45(7):1245–50.

97. Rudd JH, Warburton EA, Fryer TD, et al. Imaging atherosclerotic plaque inflammation with [18F]-fluo-rodeoxyglucose positron emission tomography. Circulation 2002;105(23):2708–11.

98. Tahara N, Kai H, Ishibashi M, et al. Simvastatin attenuates plaque inflammation: evaluation by fluo-rodeoxyglucose positron emission tomography. J Am Coll Cardiol 2006;48(9):1825–31.

99. Tawakol A, Migrino RQ, Bashian GG, et al. In vivo 18F-fluorodeoxyglucose positron emission tomog-raphy imaging provides a noninvasive measure of carotid plaque inflammation in patients. J Am Coll Cardiol 2006;48(9):1818–24.

100. Gropler RJ, Bergmann SR. Myocardial viability. What is the definition? J Nucl Med 1991;32:10–2.

101. Allman KC, Shaw LJ, Hachamovitch R, et al. Myocardial viability testing and impact of revascu-larization on prognosis in patients with coronary artery disease and left ventricular dysfunction: a meta-analysis. J Am Coll Cardiol 2002;39(7): 1151–8.

102. Bax JJ, Poldermans D, Elhendy A, et al. Sensitivity, specificity, and predictive accuracies of various noninvasive techniques for detecting hibernating myocardium. Curr Probl Cardiol 2001;26(2): 141–86.

103. DeGrado TR, Hutchins GD, Toorongian SA, et al. Myocardial kinetics of carbon-11-meta-hydroxye-phedrine: retention mechanisms and effects of norepinephrine. J Nucl Med 1993;34:1287–93.

104. Caldwell JH, Kroll K, Li Z, et al. Quantitation of presynaptic cardiac sympathetic function with carbon-11-meta-hydroxyephedrine. J Nucl Med 1998;39:1327–34.

105. Raffel DM, Corbett JR, del Rosario RB, et al. Clin-ical evaluation of carbon-11-pheynylephrine: MAO-sensitive marker of cardiac sympathetic ner-uons. J Nucl Med 1996;37(12):1923–31.

106. Munch G, Nguyen NT, Nekolla S, et al. Evaluation of sympathetic nerve terminals with 11C-epineph-rine and 11C-hydroxyephedrine and positron emis-sion tomography. Circulation 2000;101:516–23.

107. Chakraborty PK, Gildersleeve DL, Jewett DM, et al. High yield synthesis of high specific activity R-(-)-[11C]epinephrine for routine PET studies in humans. Nucl Med Biol 1993;20:939–44.

108. Raffel DM, Corbett JR, del Rosario RB, et al. Sensi-tivity of [11C]phenylephrine kinetics to monoamine oxidase activity in normal human heart. J Nucl Med 1999;40(2):232–8.

109. Tipre DN, Goldstein DS. Cardiac and extracardiac sympathetic denervation in Parkinson's disease with orthostatic hypotension and in pure autonomic failure. J Nucl Med 2005;46(11):1775–81.

110. Elsinga PH, van Waarde A, Vaalburg W. Receptor imaging in the thorax with PET. Eur J Pharmacol 2004;499(1–2):1–13.

111. Law MP, Osman S, Pike VW. Evaluation of 11C BG67, a novel radioligand for imaging myocardial alpha 1-adrenoreceptors with positron emission tomography. Eur J Nucl Med 2000;27:7–17.

112. DeGrado TR, Mulholland GK, Wieland DM, et al. Evaluation of [11F]fluoroethoxybenzovesamicol as a new PET tracer of cholinergic neurons of the heart. Nucl Med Biol 1994;21:189–95.

113. Delahaye N, Le Guludec D, Dinanian S, et al. Myocardial muscarinic receptor upregulation and normal respsonse to isoproterenol in denervated hearts by familial amyloid polyneuropathy. Circula-tion 2001;104:2911–6.

114. Le Guludec D, Delforge J, Syrota A, et al. In vivo quantification of myocardial muscarinic receptors in heart transplant patients. Circulation 1994;90:172–8.

115. Le Guludec D, Cohen-Solal A, Delforge J, et al. Increased myocardial muscarinic receptor density in idiopathic dilated cardiomyopathy: an in vivo PET study. Circulation 1997;96:3416–22.

116. Allman KC, Wieland DM, Muzik O, et al. Carbon-11 hydroxyephedrine with positron emission tomog-raphy for serial assessment of cardiac adrenergic neuronalo function after acute myocardial infarction in humans. J Am Coll Cardiol 1993;22:368–75.

117. Bulow HP, Stahl F, Lauer B, et al. Alterations of myocardial presynaptic sympathetic innervation in patients with multi-vessel coronary artery disease but without history of myocardial infarction. Nucl Med Commun 2003;24:233–9.

118. Fallen EL, Coates G, Nahmias C, et al. Recovery rates of regional sympathetic reinnervation and myocardial blood flow after acute myocardial infarction. Am Heart J 1999;137:863–9.

119. Bengel FM, Ueberfuhr P, Ziegler SI, et al. Non-invasive assessment of the effect of cardiac sympathetic innervation on metabolism of the human heart. Eur J Nucl Med 2000;27(11):1650–7.

120. Di Carli MF, Tobes MC, Mangner T, et al. Effects of cardiac sympathetic innervation on coronary blood flow. N Engl J Med 1997;336:1208–16.

121. Bengel FM, Ueberfuhr P, Schiepel N, et al. Effect of sympathetic reinnervation on cardiac performance after heart transplantation. N Engl J Med 2001;345:731–8.

122. Merlet P, Delforge J, Syrota A, et al. Positron emission tomography with 11C CGP-12177 to assess beta-adrenergic receptor concentration in idiopathic dilated cardiomyopathy. Circulation 1993;87:1169–78.

123. Pietila M, Malminiemi K, Ukkonen H, et al. Reduced myocardial carbon-11 hydroxyephedrine retention is associated with poor prognosis in chronic heart failure. Eur J Nucl Med 2001;28(3):373–6.

124. Pietila M, Malminiemi K, Veselainen R, et al. Exercise training in chronic heart failure: beneficial effects on cardiac ^{11}C-hydroxyephedrine PET, autonomic nervous control, and ventricular repolarization. J Nucl Med 2002;43(6):773–9.

125. Calkins H, Allman K, Bolling S, et al. Correlation between scintigraphic evidence of regional sympathetic neuronal dysfunction and ventricular refractoriness in the human heart. Circulation 1993;88:172–9.

126. Calkins H, Lehmann MH, Allman K, et al. Scintigraphic pattern of regional cardiac sympathetic innervation in patients with familial long QT syndrome using positron emission tomography. Circulation 1993;87:1616–21.

127. Mazzadi AN, Andre-Fouet X, Duisit J, et al. Cardiac retention of ^{11}C HED in genotyped long QT patients: a potential amplifier role for severity of the disease. Am J Physiol Heart Circ Physiol 2003;285:H1286–93.

128. Schafers M, Lerch H, Wichter T, et al. Cardiac sympathetic innervation in patinets with idiopathic right ventricular outflow tract tachycardia. J Am Coll Cardiol 1998;32:181–6.

129. Wichter T, Schafers M, Rhodes CG, et al. Abnormalities of cardiac sympathetic innervation in arrhythmogenic right ventricular cardiomyopathy: quantitative assessment of presynaptic norepinephrine reuptake and postsynaptic beta-adrenergic receptor density with positron emission tomography. Circulation 2000;101:1552–8.

130. Allman KC, Stevens MJ, Wieland DM, et al. Noninvasive assessment of cardiac diabetic neuropathy by carbon-11 hydroxyephedrine and positron emission tomography. J Am Coll Cardiol 1993;22:1425–32.

131. Di Carli MF, Bianco-Batlles D, Landa ME, et al. Effects of autonomic neuropathy on coronary blood flow in patients with diabetes mellitus. Circulation 1999;100:813–9.

132. Stevens MJ, Dayanikli F, Raffel DM, et al. Scintigraphic assessment of regionalized defects in myocardial sympathetic innervation and blood flow regulation in diabetic patients with autonomic neuropathy. J Am Coll Cardiol 1998;31:1575–84.

133. Stevens MJ, Raffel DM, Allman KC, et al. Cardiac sympathetic dysinnervation in diabetes. Circulation 1998;98:961–8.

134. Stevens MJ, Raffel DM, Allman KC, et al. Regression and progression of cardiac sympathetic dysinnervation complicating diabetes: an assessment by C-11 hydroxyephedrine and positron emission tomography. Metabolism 1999;48:92–101.

135. Schmid H, Forman LA, Cao X, et al. Heterogeneous cardiac sympathetic denervation and decreased myocardial nerve growth factor in streptozotocin-induced diabetic rates: implications for cardiac sympathetic dysinnervation complicating diabetes. Diabetes 1999;48:603–8.

136. Wu JC, Chen IY, Sundaresan G, et al. Molecular imaging of cardiac cell transplantation in living animals using optical bioluminescence and positron emission tomography. Circulation 2003;108:1302–5.

137. Wu JC, Inubushi M, Sundaresan G, et al. Positron emission tomography imaging of cardiac reporter gene expression in living rats. Circulation 2002;106:180–3.

138. Nahrendorf M, Zhang H, Hembrador S, et al. Nanoparticle PET-CT imaging of macrophages in inflammatory atherosclerosis. Circulation 2008;117(3):379–87.

Clinical Perspective and Recent Development of PET Radioligands for Imaging Cerebral Nicotinic Acetylcholine Receptors

Andrew G. Horti, PhD[a],*, Dean F. Wong, MD, PhD[b]

KEYWORDS

- Positron emission tomography • PET • nAChR
- Nicotine • Radioligands

IMAGING NICOTINIC ACETYLCHOLINE RECEPTORS WITH PET IN HUMAN SUBJECTS

There have been a number of attempts to study the nicotinic cholinergic system in the human brain and the only successful approaches have been for the $\alpha_4\beta_2$ subtype of the nicotinic acetylcholine receptor (nAChR), the main cerebral nAChR subtype. The first and perhaps the most straight-forward approach was to study the active and less active isomers of [11C]nicotine [(−)-enantiomers (Fig. 1) and (+)-enantiomers, respectively].[1] These were among the earliest PET tracers to be used in human beings because of the known toxicology of nicotine and their ease of radiolabeling. Several efforts have been made to quantify [11C](−)-nicotine and use the less active [11C](+)-nicotine to assist in measuring nonspecific binding. Measures of perfusion with [15O]water have also been used to aid in the quantification of nAChR binding.[2] However, a number of investigators[2–4] have concluded that, although specific binding could be measured, there were large changes in specific binding reflected by small changes in distribution volume and that neither the (−)- nor the (+)-[11C]nicotine were very suitable radiotracers.

In subsequent years, fluorinated derivatives of A-85380 labeled in both the 2 and the 6 position of the pyridine ring have been considered as promising radiotracers for imaging $\alpha_4\beta_2$-nAChRs (see Fig. 1).

One of the most popular, 2-[18F]FA (see Figs 1 and 2, Table 1), has been shown to have a radiation effective dose of 39.6 mSv/MBq and radiation dose-equivalent value for the critical organ urinary bladder of 461 μSv/MBq.[19] This allows at least two or more injections using typical state-of-the-art PET cameras and setting five Rem as the effective dose for an annual occupational limit. Toxicology studies with 2-FA typically show safety margins in excess of 1,000-fold with no change in blood pressure or heart rate.[19] Unlike the very toxic epibatidine derivatives, which were initially considered for [18F] radiolabeling for human use and studied in primates,[20–25] 2-[18F]FA and the related derivative 6-[18F]FA have provided the field with radiopharmaceutics for multiple brain applications that have acceptable toxicity and low radiation risk.

This research was supported by National Institutes of Health Grants MH079017 and DA020777 and by the Division of Nuclear Medicine of the Johns Hopkins School of Medicine.
a Division of Nuclear Medicine, Department of Radiology, PET Center, The Johns Hopkins School of Medicine, 600 North Wolfe Street, Nelson B1-122, Baltimore, MD 21287-0816, USA
b Radiology, Psychiatry and Environmental Health Sciences, The Johns Hopkins School of Medicine, JHOC Building Room 3245, 601 N, Caroline Street, Baltimore, MD 21287, USA
* Corresponding author.
E-mail address: ahorti1@jhmi.edu (A.G. Horti).

PET Clin 4 (2009) 89–100
doi:10.1016/j.cpet.2009.04.014

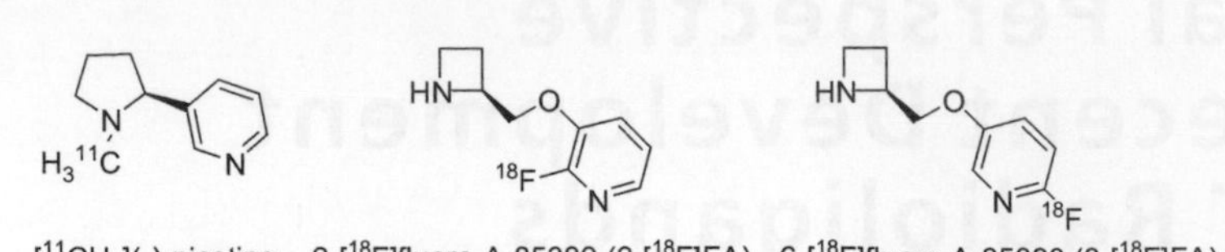

[^{11}CH$_3$](-)-nicotine   2-[^{18}F]fluoro-A-85380 (2-[^{18}F]FA)   6-[^{18}F]fluoro-A-85380 (6-[^{18}F]FA)

Fig. 1. The currently available nAChR PET radioligands for human studies.

2-[^{18}F]FA is not entirely ideal because it does not reach a steady state for several hours after injection, but it can be quantified by number of procedures in the human brain. Some of these have included dynamic PET scans over 2 hours followed by repeat scans an hour later. With arterial sampling and compartmental modeling, this technique has provided quantifiable measures of distribution volume that is regionally specific and stable in the brain.[7,8] Bolus injection studies have employed a scanning time of only 140 minutes and two-tissue compartmental models but do require arterial blood sampling. Other methods, such as

those employed by Brody and colleagues[26] and Kimes and colleagues[9] have performed 2-[^{18}F]FA studies using bolus-plus-infusion methods with a duration of 6 to 8 hours (K$_{bolus}$ = 500 minutes). Similarly, both bolus and continuous infusion methods have been performed with the single-photon emission computed tomography nAChR radioligand 5-[^{123}I]IA.[18,27]

A number of attempts have been made to simplify the 2-[^{18}F]FA studies. For example, a simplified distribution volume determined by the ratio of the tissue to the metabolite corrected plasma and using a single 90- to 120-minute PET

Radioligand	Name	logD$_{7.4}$	K$_i$, nM	BP	Peak time in thalamus (required scanning time), min
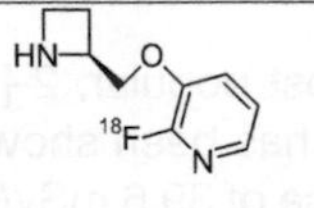	2-[^{18}F]FA	-1.4	0.1 - 1.3	2	120 (480)
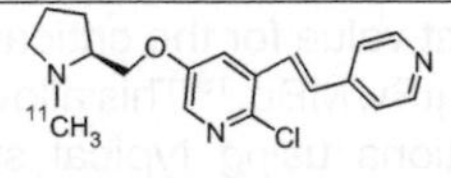	[^{11}C]Me-PVC	2	0.06	1.7	20 (90)
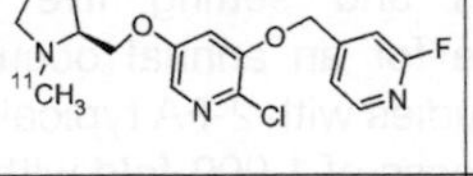	[^{11}C]JHU85208	1.8	0.06	0.7	10 (120)
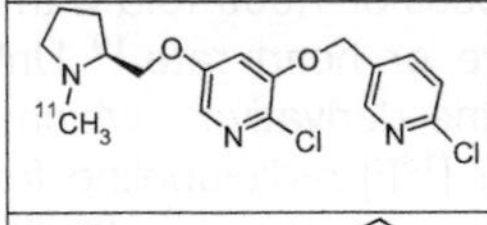	[^{11}C]JHU85157	2.2	0.05	0.8	10 (120)
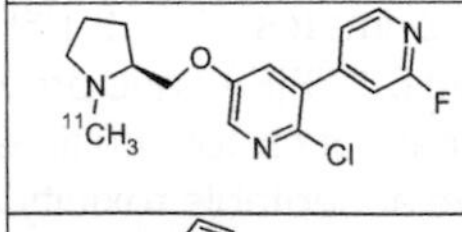	[^{11}C]JHU85270	1.6	0.06	0.7	30 (120)
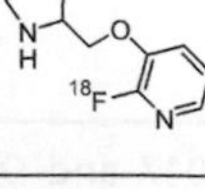	[^{18}F]Nifene	-0.5	0.5	1.1	5 (90)
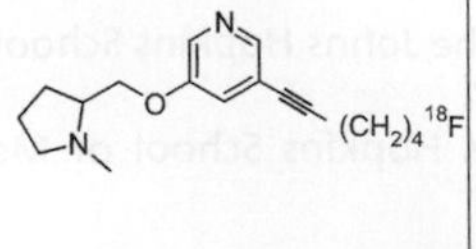	(S)-3-(6-[^{18}F]fluorohex-1-ynyl)-5-((1-methylpyrrolidin-2-yl)methoxy)pyridine	1.4	1	1[a]	4 (60)

Fig. 2. 2-[^{18}F]FA and its new analogs with improved imaging properties. [a]High accumulation of radioactivity in striatum suggests the presence of active radio-labeled metabolites.

Table 1
PET Imaging of nAChR in human subjects

PET/SPECT Radiotracer	Number of Patients	Single Scan or Dynamic	Arterial Line	Bolus or Continuous Infusion	Reference
(−)- [^{11}C] nicotine	5 subjects	Dynamic: baseline and challenge	Yes	Bolus	3
2- [^{18}F]FA	6 healthy controls	Single whole-body scan and dynamic brain scan	No	Bolus	5
2- [^{18}F]FA	3 healthy controls	Single whole-body scan	No	Bolus	6
2- [^{18}F]FA	7 healthy controls	Dynamic	Yes	Bolus	7,8
2- [^{18}F]FA	8; 4 of which were smokers	Dynamic	Yes	Bolus plus infusion	9
2- [^{18}F]FA	97 (12 healthy controls)	Single	Yes	Bolus	10
2- [^{18}F]FA	15 AD patients; 14 age-matched controls	Single scan	No	Slow intravenous bolus injection	11,12
2-FA	10 normal volunteers	Dynamic	Yes	Bolus	13
2- [^{18}F]FA; [^{18}F]FDG	8 nonsmoking ADNFLE patients; 7 age-matched controls. 5 patients underwent additional FDG PET experiment	Dynamic	No	Bolus	14
2- [^{18}F]FA	17 AD patients; 6 w/amnestic MCI; 10 normal aged healthy controls	Dynamic	Yes	Bolus	15
2- [^{18}F]FA	7 smokers; 7 nonsmokers	Dynamic	Yes	Continuous infusion	16
6- [^{18}F]FA	5 nonsmokers	Dynamic (2-hour scan) 4-hour study	Yes	Bolus	17
5- [^{123}I]IA	6 nonsmokers, 6 light smokers	Dynamic	Yes	Bolus and continuous infusion	18

Abbreviations: AD, Alzheimer's disease; ADNFLE, autosomal dominant nocturnal frontal lobe epilepsy; FDG, [^{18}F]-2-fluoro deoxy-D-glucose; MCI, mild cognitive impairment; SPECT, single-photon emission computed tomography.

acquisition appeared to correlate reasonably well with graphical methods and two compartmental models in cortical regions. Lower correlations were found in regions with higher binding of nicotinic cholinergic receptors, such as the thalamus. This lower correlation in higher binding regions is not unexpected because the time to achieve steady-state conditions is even slower than in the lower binding regions.[13]

In addition to the extensive use 2-[^{18}F]FA, there is increasing interest in derivatives such as 6-[^{18}F]FA.[28] Based on nonhuman primate studies, some centers believe that 6-[^{18}F]FA shows more reversible kinetics and higher specific binding than 2-[^{18}F]FA.[29] The initial studies with 6-[^{18}F]FA[17] in five human subjects suggested some reversibility in various brain regions, with the radiotracer peaking at 1 to 2 hours in the thalamus. The half-life for clearance was about 4 hours. Cortical binding peaked early in less than 60 minutes, but there was lower—but persistent—uptake in white matter. Retest studies ranged from as low as 0.5% to as high as 14% in various brain regions. Relatively high toxicity of 6-FA is an obstacle for more wide use of 6-[^{18}F]FA as a PET radioligand for human studies.[30]

Given the success with both 2-[^{18}F]FA and 6-[^{18}F]FA, a number of successful applications have been performed. Among the first, not surprisingly, were studies of cigarette smokers. For example, a recent study[26] demonstrated that there was a dose-dependent effect of smoking from one puff, to three puffs, to a full cigarette or to satiety (around ~3 cigarettes), demonstrating a dose-dependent occupancy in nAChR-rich regions. Most importantly, it suggested that one to two puffs of the cigarette resulted in 15% occupancy for more than 3 hours after smoking. A full cigarette resulted in greater than 88% occupancy, and the investigators concluded that daily smoking results in near complete occupancy of nAChRs, suggesting that tobacco-dependent smokers maintain almost full occupancy throughout the day.

Another example of an application in patients includes 2-[^{18}F]FA PET images of medial frontal-lobe epilepsy demonstrating a significant increase in the distribution volume in the mesencephalon, pons, and cerebellum when compared with controls. This, together with FDG measurements, suggested that the mesencephalon might be related to arousal.[14]

Because of the importance of nicotine and memory, and the known $\alpha_4\beta_2$ abnormalities seen in postmortem studies, 2-[^{18}F]FA studies have been explored in Alzheimer's disease.[11,12,15] One example[11,12] was unable to demonstrate loss of nAChRs in vivo in early Alzheimer's disease, in spite of the fact that these patients showed significant cognitive impairment. Although this could be related to the sensitivity of the technique, it could also illustrate the ability of the technique to separate a lack of change in spite of cognitive decline in Alzheimer's disease patients versus controls. This is in contrast to postmortem studies, where the decline was always demonstrated, but perhaps at a later stage in the disease. Other studies, such as those of patients with mild dementia and mild cognitive impairment, demonstrate a reduction of nAChRs in some subjects with early Alzheimer's disease and mild cognitive impairment, as expected. There was considerable overlap of the extent of binding between patients with mild cognitive impairment and controls. Some investigators have even suggested (albeit without definitive evidence) that 2- [^{18}F]FA might have a predictive potential in patients with mild cognitive impairment at risk for developing Alzheimer's disease. The evidence for this is not yet available, however.

Studies investigating 2-[^{18}F]FA continue, with attempts being made to improve the measurements of metabolites. A recent study[10] showed that solid-phase extraction methods are less time consuming than high-performance liquid chromatography and might be more suitable for 2-[^{18}F]FA measurements during long PET investigations.

THE NEED FOR NEW NAChR RADIOLIGANDS FOR THALAMIC AND EXTRATHALAMIC BINDING

There are two main considerations for the need for new tracers beyond 2-[^{18}F]FA and 6-[^{18}F]FA. First, the widest used nicotinic cholinergic radiotracer at present, 2-[^{18}F]FA, which has a reasonable binding potential value of approximately 2 in the thalamus, displays the highest binding region for $\alpha_4\beta_2$-nAChRs, but below 1 for cortical and subcortical regions. This quantification would be further compromised in the absence of up-regulation of the nicotinic cholinergic system by smoking or a reduction in binding in a neurodegenerative disorder, such as Alzheimer's disease.

A further problem is the kinetics of the radiotracer in cortical, subcortical (striatal), and thalamic brain areas. For example, with 2-[^{18}F]FA the radiotracer reaches steady state either with a bolus or definitively with constant-infusion methods. However, in the thalamic areas, which are of considerable interest in some disorders, including smoking, there is a need for long infusions. Sometimes it takes up to 6 or 8 hours to reach the steady state, and bolus-injection studies—while performed for as little as 2 to 3 hours—are not ideal and undoubtedly include compromises in the mathematical modeling of the thalamic regions.

New radiotracers to study the thalamus are needed that are more reversible during reasonable PET scan times, such as 90 minutes to 2 hours. Similarly, in the cortical region, higher binding potentials are needed even if they reach a steady state during this time. Examples of some approaches include radiotracers such as [^{18}F]NIDA522131, which was designed to image extra thalamic regions.[31,32] In comparisons, this radiotracer had higher in vitro affinity and increased uptake with greater distribution volumes than 2-[^{18}F]FA, especially in extra thalamic areas. The increase in brain binding of [^{18}F]NIDA522131 was about four times greater than 2-[^{18}F]FA in multiple brain regions, including the cingulate cortex, frontal cortex, thalamus, mid-brain and, to a less extent, putamen. However, [^{18}F]NIDA522131 exhibits evidence for even less-reversible binding than that of 2-[^{18}F]FA and requires more than 6 hours of scanning.

It has been hypothesized[20] that some of the slow entry into the brain of radiotracers, such as 2-[^{18}F]FA or 6-[^{18}F]FA, may be related to lipophicity, affinity, and possibly a slow-off rate. It was documented that although peak activity may occur between 80 and 100 minutes in the brain with 2-[^{18}F]FA, there was still a slow approach to steady state (tissue plasma ratios). Five hours after injection, a steady state still was not reached in the thalamus. Similarly, 6-[^{18}F]FA required at least 4 hours of scanning time and 5-[^{123}I]IA at least 4 hours. All suffer from failure to achieve a steady state in various brain regions of interest.

It has been proposed[20] that two classes of radiotracers for nAChR are needed. These would include one group with relatively rapid brain kinetics to allow facile quantitation in the brain regions with the highest binding, such as the thalamus. A second group would require high binding in extra thalamic regions, presumably by using higher affinity radioligands. This latter group would be unlikely to reach a steady state in higher binding regions, but would be more useful in regions such as the cortex. The radiopharmaceutics in the second group would be used for studies of neurodegenerative disorders, such as Alzheimer's disease, where cortical changes are most important. The radiopharmaceutics in the first group would have higher binding in the thalamus and might play an important role in nicotine addiction.

PET NACHR RADIOLIGANDS WITH OPTIMIZED BRAIN KINETICS

Development of nAChR PET radioligands has a long history and it has been reviewed in several publications.[20–25,33,34] In summary, at the moment [^{11}C]nicotine, 2-[^{18}F]FA, and 6-[^{18}F]FA are the only available radioligands for imaging of nAChRs in human subjects. [^{11}C]Nicotine is not a very suitable radioligand for PET quantification of nAChRs because of its low specific and high nonspecific binding and its very rapid metabolism. The slow brain kinetics of 2-[^{18}F]FA and 6-[^{18}F]FA lead to lengthy and expensive imaging studies that cannot be tolerated by patients and afforded by most PET centers. In addition, 2-[^{18}F]FA and 6-[^{18}F]FA exhibit relatively low binding potential values in animal and human brains.

The drawbacks of existing nAChR radioligands hamper the PET imaging research of $\alpha_4\beta_2$-nAChR, the major class of cerebral receptors that is directly linked to various central nervous system (CNS) disorders. On the other hand, these drawbacks are the driving force of development of better PET radioligands for imaging nAChRs. The aim of these recent studies is to synthesize radioligands with an adequately high binding-potential value (BP^{Thalamus} ≥ 2) that is normally considered a minimum requirement for quantitative PET studies. Most importantly, the expected radioligands have to rapidly reach a steady state in various brain regions and require a scanning time

of less than or equal to 2 hours, which is regarded as the most practical time for human application.

The development of nAChR radioligands that are superior to 2-[^{18}F]FA was based on the idea that the binding affinity (K$_i$) and lipophilicity (logD) values are the two major factors that affect the brain kinetics and binding potentials of in vivo CNS nAChR radioligands. The most interesting results in the last few years involved the radiolabeled analogs of (i) A-84,543/A-85,380, high-affinity nAChR ligands that have been synthesized by Abbott Laboratories[35] and (ii) epibatidine, a very high affinity nAChR agonist that was discovered by National Institutes of Health scientists in Ecuadorian frogs (**Fig. 3**).[36]

Radiolabeled Analogs of A-84,543 and A-85,380

Structurally similar pyridyl ethers A-84,543 and A-85,380 were attractive leads for discovery of new nAChR radioligands because these leads exhibit high binding affinity and excellent $\alpha_4\beta_2$-nAChR subtype selectivity. 2-[^{18}F]FA and 6-[^{18}F]FA (see **Fig. 1**), the only available nAChR radioligands that are approved for human studies, are derivatives of A-84,543 and A-85,380, suggesting that new analogs of these leads will be sufficiently safe for human application.

[^{11}C]Me-PVC

(S,E)-2-chloro-5-((1-[^{11}C]methylpyrrolidin-2-yl)methoxy)-3-(2-(pyridin-4-yl)vinyl)pyridine ([^{11}C]Me-PVC) (see **Fig. 2**)[37–39] was one of the first attempts to resolve the issue of the slow brain kinetics of 2-[^{18}F]FA, which were thought to be because of its high polarity. [^{11}C]Me-PVC exhibits substantially greater lipophilicity than 2-[^{18}F]FA and was expected to display better blood-brain barrier permeability. Because of the high binding affinity of [^{11}C]Me-PVC, this radioligand specifically labels nAChRs in vivo with a reasonable binding-potential value. In the Rhesus monkey, the brain kinetics of [^{11}C]Me-PVC are optimally reversible (see **Fig. 2**). After a bolus injection of [^{11}C]Me-PVC, only 90 to 120 minutes of scanning is necessary to obtain quantifiable PET data in a Rhesus monkey.[39] Despite the promising results in

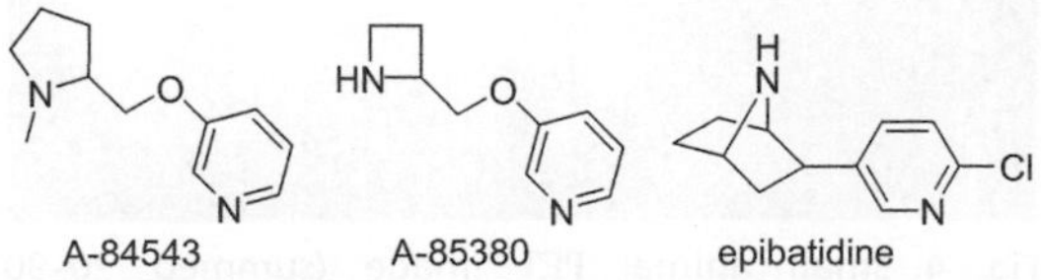

Fig. 3. Lead compounds for the recent development of nAChR radioligands.

animals, [^{11}C]Me-PVC has never been used in human subjects because its binding potential value is slightly lower than that of 2-[^{18}F]FA and the authors have chosen to hunt for a radioligand with equally optimal brain kinetics but greater binding potential.

[^{11}C]JHU85208, [^{11}C]JHU85157 and [^{11}C]JHU85270

As an attempt to overcome the problem of the low binding-potential value of [^{11}C]Me-PVC, three analogs of this compound ([^{11}C]JHU85208, [^{11}C]JHU85157, and [^{11}C]JHU85270) (see **Fig. 2**) have been synthesized.[40,41] All three have better binding affinity and slightly lower lipophilicity than [^{11}C]Me-PVC. All three radioligands demonstrated excellent imaging properties in rodents with high accumulation of radioactivity in the nAChR-rich thalamus, moderate uptake in the cortex, a region with a medium density of nAChRs, and lowest uptake in the nAChR-poor cerebellum (**Fig. 4**).

Inspired by the successful rodent imaging results, the Johns Hopkins group studied these three radioligands, [^{11}C]JHU85208, [^{11}C]JHU85157, and [^{11}C]JHU85270 in baboons.[40] The kinetics of the radioligands in the baboon brain were reversible (see **Fig. 2**) and only 2 hours were required for the radioligands to reach a steady state in the baboon thalamus. Unexpectedly, the thalamic binding potentials of [^{11}C]JHU85208, [^{11}C]JHU85157, and [^{11}C]JHU85270 were lower than that of 2-[^{18}F]FA (0.7–0.8 versus 2). Metabolite analysis of [^{11}C]JHU85208, [^{11}C]JHU85157, and [^{11}C]JHU85270 demonstrated that, like their analog [^{11}C](–)nicotine that metabolizes to lipophilic [^{11}C]cotinine, in baboon plasma all three ^{11}C-radioligands generated oxidative lipophilic metabolites that are likely to penetrate the blood-brain barrier and increase nonspecific binding. Because the binding-potential values are relatively low there are no current plans to pursue

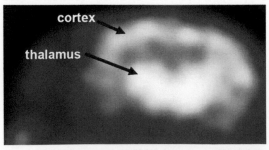

Fig. 4. Small animal PET image (summed 20–90 minutes) of [^{11}C]JHU85157 in the rat brain. *Courtesy of* C.J. Endres, PhD, Baltimore, MD.

[^{11}C]JHU85208, [^{11}C]JHU85157, and [^{11}C]JHU85270 as radioligands for human imaging.

[^{18}F]Nifene

The development of 3-((2,5-dihydro-1H-pyrrol-2-yl)methoxy)-2- [^{18}F]fluoropyridine ([^{18}F]nifene)[42,43] was justified by the hypothesis that an analog of 2-[^{18}F]FA with slightly reduced binding affinity might display more rapid brain kinetics. The binding affinity of [^{18}F]nifene is lower than that of 2-[^{18}F]FA (see **Fig. 2**). As was expected, the brain kinetics of [^{18}F]nifene in the Rhesus monkey brain is highly reversible (see **Fig. 2**). Unfortunately, the moderate thalamus/cerebellum ratio value of 2.2 of [^{18}F]nifene in monkey is the price paid for the rapid brain kinetics of this radioligand with relatively low binding affinity. The authors are not aware of any further in vivo studies with [^{18}F]nifene in animals or human subjects.

[^{18}F]- and [^{11}CH$_3$]-(S)-3-(6-fluorohex-1-ynyl)-5-((1-methylpyrrolidin-2-yl)methoxy) pyridines

The title isotopomer-radioligands (see **Fig. 2**) was a part of a medicinal chemistry project directed toward the synthesis of ligands with high β_2/β_4-nAChR subtype selectivity ($K_i^{\alpha4\beta2}$ = 0.95 nM, $K_i^{\alpha3\beta4}$ = 88,000 nM).[44] In baboon PET imaging studies, the radioligands[45] specifically labeled nAChRs in the nAChR-rich thalamus with optimally reversible brain kinetics (see **Fig. 2**). The thalamus/cerebellum ratio reached a value of 2.5 at 1 hour after injection. It is unlikely that [^{18}F]- or [^{11}CH$_3$]-(S)-3-(6-fluorohex-1-ynyl)-5-((1-methyl-pyrrolidin-2-yl)methoxy)pyridines will be useful for $\alpha_4\beta_2$-subtype nAChR imaging because both radioligands manifested high uptake of radioactivity in the nAChR-poor striatum. After injection of the radioligands into baboons, the uptake of the radioactivity in the striatum was not diminished by injection of nicotine. This observation suggests that striatum binding is not mediated by nAChRs and can be explained by the appearance of radiolabeled metabolites that are ligands of another CNS receptor.

Radiolabeled Analogs of Epibatidine

Epibatidine is a very high affinity agonist of nAChRs that exhibits little nAChR-subtype selectivity and is notorious for its acute toxicity. In the past, many PET-labeled epibatidine analogs have been developed (see for review[20]). Several of these compounds exhibited excellent imaging properties but they were too toxic for human application. The recent success in the development of radiolabeled analogs of epibatidine for PET imaging of nAChRs is largely indebted to the discovery of derivatives of epibatidine analogs with properties of antagonists of nAChR.[46,47] This discovery initiated a series of research studies by several groups that are described below.

(±)- [11C]NMI-EPB

The synthesis of 7-methyl-2-exo-(3'-iodo-5'-pyridinyl)-7-azabicyclo[2.2.1]heptane ((±)-NMI-EPB) was first published by Carroll and colleagues.[47] Unlike many other epibatidine analogs that are highly toxic nAChR agonists, (±)-NMI-EPB with a bulky substituent in position 5 of the pyridine ring is a nAChR antagonist with high binding affinity[47] (**Fig. 5**). Being a nAChR antagonist, (±)-NMI-EPB should not be as toxic as epibatidine. It was expected that (±)-NMI-EPB would be sufficiently safe for in vivo experiments. Thus, in the functional in vivo studies[47] up to 0.8 mg/kg (1,250 nmol/kg –2500 nmol/kg) of (±)-NMI-EPB was injected into mice. In further experiments the same group radiolabeled (±)-NMI-EPB with ^{11}C and [11C](±)-NMI-EPB has been studied by PET in baboon.[48] The radioligand specifically labeled nAChRs in the baboon brain with a very good ratio of specific/nonspecific binding (see **Fig. 5**). Because the time-uptake curves in the baboon brain regions exhibit a 5-minute peak, it was reasonable to hypothesize that [11C](±)-NMI-EPB might manifest rapid brain equilibrium and that the radioligand would potentially be more advantageous than 2-[18F]FA and 6-[18F]FA.

The binding affinity of enantiomers of N-methylepibatidine manifests little enantioselectivity,[49] but the analogs of N-methylepibatidine with large substituents in the pyridine ring are highly enantioselective.[50] Therefore, one could anticipate that (–)- and (+)-enantiomers of (±)-NMI-EPB should be enantioselective and a more potent enantiomer of ^{11}C-NMI-EPB might exhibit better PET imaging properties than those of [11C](±)-NMI-EPB. Preparation of (+)-NMI-EPB and (–)-NMI-EPB was reported and the binding affinity of (–)-NMI-EPB was 30 times greater than that of (+)-NMI-EPB.[51] A rodent study with [11C](–)-NMI-EPB has confirmed that the radioligand labels cerebral nAChRs with a high level of specificity.[51] Unfortunately, the baseline baboon PET imaging showed that [11C](–)-NMI-EPB does not reach a steady state in the thalamus within 90 minutes after administration and its kinetics are too slow for a ^{11}C-radioligand with a 20-minute half-life. The previously described rapid brain kinetics of [11C](±)-NMI-EPB are likely to correspond to the superimposition of the slow kinetics of [11C](–)-NMI-EPB and very fast nonspecific uptake of

less active [11C](+)-NMI-EPB. Therefore, the authors of the article suggested that neither [11C](–)-NMI-EPB nor [11C](±)-NMI-EPB are suitable for quantitative human PET imaging.[51]

[18F]FPhEP and [18F]F2PhEP

Two more $\alpha_4\beta_2$-nAChR selective[52] epibatidine analogs from Carroll and colleagues,[53] 2-(6-fluoro-5-phenylpyridin-3-yl)-7-aza-bicyclo[2.2.1]heptane, FPhEP (K_i = 240 PM) and 2-(6-fluoro-5-(4-fluorophenyl)pyridin-3-yl)-7-aza-bicyclo[2.2.1]heptane, F2PhEP (K_i = 29 PM) (see **Fig. 5**) were of interest for PET.[52,54,55] The researchers from Orsay radiolabeled both compounds with ^{18}F and studied [18F]FPhEP and [18F]F2PhEP in baboons.[54,55] Both radioligands readily penetrated the blood-brain barrier, showing more rapid brain kinetics than those of 2-[18F]FA. As evidence of the specific in vivo binding of [18F]FPhEP in the baboon brain, its uptake was blocked by injection of nicotinic ligands. Unfortunately, the binding-potential value of [18F]FPhEP (see **Fig. 5**) was too low for further investment in this radioligand.

The binding affinity of F2PhEP is one order of magnitude greater than that of FPhEP, but [18F]F2PhEP has thalamic uptake that is lower than of [18F]FPhEP.[54,55] In contrast, the shape of the time-activity curves in different brain regions reflected the affinity of the ligands. [18F]FPhEP displayed similar time-activity curves in all regions of interest (except white matter), whether or not the region is receptor rich or poor, whereas for [18F]F2PhEP uptake was substantially greater in the thalamus than in the cerebellum. Surprisingly, the uptake of [18F]F2PhEP in the cortex, the region with substantial density of nAChRs, was lower than uptake in the nAChR-poor cerebellum. The radioligand [18F]F2PhEP also presented another surprise in the blocking studies when it did not show a significant reduction of radioactivity accumulation after injection of nicotine. The authors of the article[54] concluded that the radiotracers did not fulfill the widely adopted criteria for a quality PET radioligand. It is likely that both radioligands are too lipophilic (see **Fig. 5**) and their nonspecific binding is too high for a successful radioligand.

[18F](–)NCFHEB

Enantiomers of the radiofluorinated homolog of epibatidine, 6-(6- [18F]fluoropyridin-3-yl)-8-aza-bicyclo[3.2.1]octane, (see **Fig. 5**), (–)- [18F]NCFHEB, and (+)-NCFHEB were reported in several recent publications.[56–58] Both compounds display high $\alpha_4\beta_2$-nAChR and low $\alpha_3\beta_4$-nAChR in vitro binding affinity and excellent specific radiolabeling of nAChRs in mice.[56] The same group performed a substantial number of PET studies and

Radiolabeled analog of epibatidine	Code name	$logD_{7.4}$[c]	K_i, nM[d]	BP	Peak time in thalamus (required scanning time), min
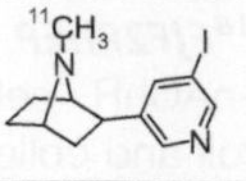	(±)-NMI-EPB	1.1	0.03	1.5-2.5[Th]	5 (>90-120)[a]
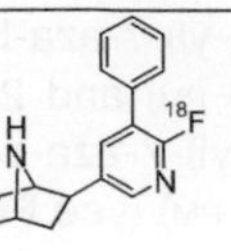	[^{18}F]FPhEP	2.9	0.24	~0.5[Th]	20 (~90-120)[a]
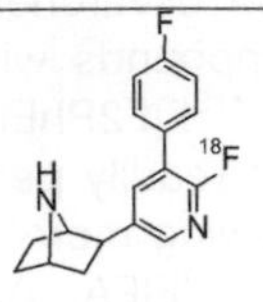	[^{18}F]F2PhEP	3.0	0.03	~2[Th]	45 (~180)[a]
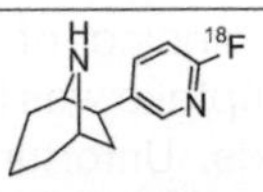	[^{18}F](+)-NCFHEB	-1.4	0.06	7.6[Th]	142 (~300)[b]
	[^{18}F](-)-NCFHEB		0.1	2.5[Th]	80 (~100)[b]
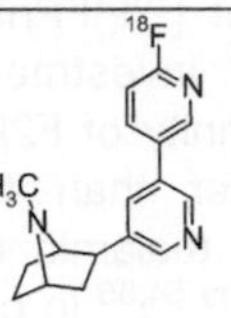	[^{18}F](-)-JHU86358	0.5	0.05	>7[Th] 1.1[Cx]	>180 (>180)[a]
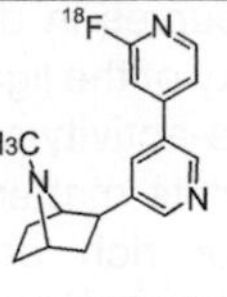	[^{18}F](-)-JHU86430	0.7	0.05	>7[Th] 1.0[Cx]	160 (>180)[a]
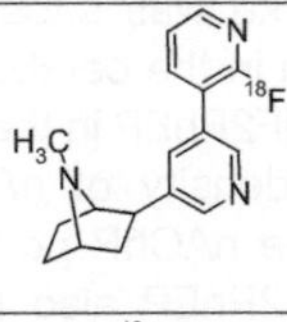	[^{18}F](-)-JHU86428 ([^{18}F]XTRA)	0.7	0.1	7.3[Th] 1.3[Cx]	65 (120-150)[a]
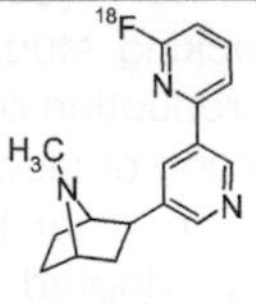	[^{18}F](-)-JHU87522 ([^{18}F]AZAN)	1.0	0.3	2.1-4.8[Th] 0.6-1.0[Cx]	10-25 (90)[a]

Fig. 5. PET imaging properties of new radiolabeled analogs of epibatidine. [a]Baboon; [b]Piglets; [c]Lipophilicity value (logarithm of partition coefficient between n-octanol and water at pH 7.4); [d]Inhibition binding affinity. Cx = cortex, Th = thalamus.

compared the porcine brain kinetics of (–)-[^{18}F]NCFHEB and (+)-NCFHEB with 2-[^{18}F]FA to evaluate the potential of the new radioligands for human neuroimaging. Several animals received an additional intravenous injection of the nAChR agonist A81418 to confirm the specific binding of the radioligands. Both enantiomers of [^{18}F]NCFHEB showed a higher brain uptake and better binding-potential values than 2-[^{18}F]FA (see **Fig. 5**). In the piglet thalamus (+)-[^{18}F]NCFHEB, (–)- [^{18}F]NCFHEB and 2-[^{18}F]FA manifest a peak uptake at 142 minutes, 80 minutes, and 68 minutes, correspondingly, suggesting relatively slow brain kinetics of the new radioligands. Interestingly, the thalamus/olfactory bulb ratio had reached its peak for (–)-[^{18}F]NCFHEB earlier than for 2-[^{18}F]FA. This observation led the investigators to the opinion that the equilibrium of specific binding of (−)- [^{18}F]NCFHEB was reached earlier than that of 2-[^{18}F]FA and, therefore, PET imaging properties of (−)-[^{18}F]NCFHEB may be potentially superior to 2-[^{18}F]FA. The authors look forward to further development of (−)- [^{18}F]NCFHEB for PET imaging of nAChRs in nonhuman primates and, perhaps, in human subjects.

Development of [^{18}F]AZAN ([^{18}F]JHU87522)

High demand for a better radioligand for imaging $\alpha_4\beta_2$-nAChRs inspired the authors group to exert a major synthetic effort to develop a nicotinic-receptor ligand with optimized imaging properties. As the result of these studies, an ^{18}F-labeled nAChR antagonist (−)-2-(6- [^{18}F]fluoro-2,3′-bipyridin-5′-yl)-7-methyl-7-aza-bicyclo[2.2.1]heptane ([^{18}F]JHU87522 or [^{18}F]AZAN) was obtained that showed evidence of better PET imaging properties than 2-[^{18}F]FA. These properties include brain kinetics that require only 1.5 hours of data acquisition after bolus administration, good binding-potential values (2.5–4), very high total brain uptake, absence of lipophilic metabolites, a good safety profile, and simple radiosynthesis, with more details shown below.

The preliminary studies[50] suggested that ^{18}F-radiolabeled derivatives of dipyridyl analogs of epibatidine show excellent potential for PET. The structure-activity relationship studies demonstrated that the high binding-affinity value of dipyridyl analogs of epibatidine can be optimized within the subnanomolar range by modification of substituents in the external pyridine ring, and by the change of the connecting position of the ring. Because of this, the authors had a large degree of freedom in optimization of binding affinity and lipophilicity. The authors were convinced that the best preliminary radioligand, [^{18}F](−)-JHU86358, which displayed very high binding affinity and binding potential but relatively slow brain kinetics, could be optimized toward a compound with faster brain kinetics and a sufficient binding potential value if the binding affinity was slightly reduced. Three additional isomers of [^{18}F](−)-JHU86358, namely [^{18}F](−)-JHU86430, [^{18}F](−)-JHU86428, and [^{18}F](−)-JHU87522 with similar physical-chemical properties but reduced binding affinities (see **Fig. 5**) have been synthesized. [^{18}F](−)-JHU86430 exhibited almost the same K_i value as that of [^{18}F](−)-JHU86358 and both radioligands showed comparable PET imaging properties.

The next isomer, [^{18}F](−)-JHU86428 ((-)-2-(2′-[^{18}F]fluoro-3,3′-bipyridin-5-yl)-7-methyl-7-aza-bicyclo[2.2.1]heptane, [^{18}F]XTRA) with slightly reduced binding affinity (see **Fig. 5**), peaked in the baboon thalamus at 75 minutes after injection. This compound had excellent binding-potential values and required about 2.5 hours scanning in thalamus and 1.5 hours scanning in the cortex after bolus injection.[59] [^{18}F]XTRA holds promise for imaging extrathalamic nAChRs in human beings.

The isomer [^{18}F](−)-JHU87522[59] ((−)-2-(6-[^{18}F]fluoro-2,3′-bipyridin-5′-yl)-7-methyl-7-aza-bicyclo[2.2.1]heptane, [^{18}F]AZAN) had the lowest binding affinity within the series (see **Fig. 5**) and gave the most interesting results in baseline and blockade baboon PET studies. The radioligand requires only 90 minutes of scanning to reach a steady state. In addition to the rapid brain kinetics, [^{18}F]AZAN displays a higher binding-potential value than 2-FA. [^{18}F]AZAN also exhibits a 200% greater total brain uptake than 2-[^{18}F]FA and an absence of lipophilic metabolites. The radiosynthesis of [^{18}F]AZAN is a one-step radiolabeling that is simpler than the two-step radiosynthesis of 2-[^{18}F]FA.

The inhibition binding assay studies with various nAChR subtypes demonstrated that AZAN is a highly selective $\alpha_4\beta_2$-nAChR ligand, whereas a functional assay in vitro showed that AZAN exhibits properties of a potent antagonist of the $\alpha_4\beta_2$-nAChR subtype. Preliminary behavioral toxicologic studies in mice demonstrated that AZAN exhibits acute toxicity comparable to that of 2-FA.[59] Radiation dosimetry and toxicology studies with AZAN will establish whether or not [^{18}F]AZAN is safe for PET imaging in human beings.

SUMMARY

PET imaging of $\alpha_4\beta_2$-nAChRs in human subjects is a vibrant field of contemporary neuroscience and nuclear medicine. Nicotinic imaging studies in smoking, epilepsy, attention deficit hyperactivity disorder, depression, schizophrenia, cognition, behavior, memory, and in research of aging, cognitive impairments, and dementia attract the attention of many researchers. The nAChR radioligands that are currently available for PET manifest slow brain kinetics and low binding potentials that prevent widespread use of PET imaging research of nAChR in human beings.

To address the problems with existing PET radioligands for imaging of nAChRs, especially the most common one 2-[^{18}F]FA, several research groups have worked to develop novel compounds with improved brain kinetics. One new compound is (−)-[^{18}F]NCFHEB, which demonstrated PET imaging properties that are superior to 2- [^{18}F]FA in pigs. Further experiments with this radioligand that include PET imaging in nonhuman primates and safety studies are needed to qualify

(−)-[¹⁸F]NCFHEB as a potential candidate for human imaging.

The most recent candidate, radioligand [¹⁸F](−)-JHU87522 ([¹⁸F]AZAN), exhibited all the necessary properties that are required for a successful PET radiotracer for imaging of nAChRs.[59] [¹⁸F]AZAN specifically labels cerebral nAChRs with high binding potential and its brain uptake is substantially greater than that of 2-[¹⁸F]FA. Most importantly, [¹⁸F]AZAN requires only 90 to 100 minutes of PET scanning to obtain quantifiable receptor data. In addition, [¹⁸F]AZAN is a β₂-subtype selective nAChR antagonist with low acute side effects in animals. The radiosynthesis of [¹⁸F]AZAN is simpler than that of 2-[¹⁸F]FA. All of these properties suggest that [¹⁸F]AZAN is a substantially better radioligand than 2-[¹⁸F]FA, the most popular radioligand for PET imaging of nAChRs in the human brain. The safety studies currently being performed with [¹⁸F]AZAN will determine whether [¹⁸F]AZAN can replace 2-[¹⁸F]FA in the PET clinic.

ACKNOWLEDGMENTS

We thank Mrs. Judy Buchanan for editorial help.

REFERENCES

1. Nordberg A, Hartvig P, Lundqvist H, et al. Uptake and regional distribution of (+)-(R)- and (−)-(S)-N-[methyl-¹¹C]-nicotine in the brains of rhesus monkey. An attempt to study nicotinic receptors in vivo. J Neural Transm Park Dis Dement Sect 1989;1(3):195–205.

2. Lundqvist H, Nordberg A, Hartvig P, et al. (S)-(-)-[¹¹C]nicotine binding assessed by PET: a dual tracer model evaluated in the rhesus monkey brain. Alzheimer Dis Assoc Disord 1998;12(3):238–46.

3. Muzic RF Jr, Berridge MS, Friedland RP, et al. PET quantification of specific binding of carbon-11-nicotine in human brain. J Nucl Med 1998;39(12):2048–54.

4. Grunwald F, Biersack HJ, Kuschinsky W. Nicotine receptor mapping. Eur J Nucl Med 1996;23(8):1012–4.

5. Kimes AS, Horti AG, London ED, et al. 2-[¹⁸F]F-A85380: PET imaging of brain nicotinic acetylcholine receptors and whole body distribution in humans. FASEB J 2003;17(10):1331–3.

6. Bottlaender M, Valette H, Roumenov D, et al. Biodistribution and radiation dosimetry of ¹⁸F-fluoro-A-85380 in healthy volunteers. J Nucl Med 2003;44(4):596–601.

7. Gallezot JD, Bottlaender MA, Delforge J, et al. Quantification of cerebral nicotinic acetylcholine receptors by PET using 2-[(¹⁸)F]fluoro-A-85380 and the multiinjection approach. J Cereb Blood Flow Metab 2007;28:172–89.

8. Gallezot JD, Bottlaender M, Gregoire MC, et al. In vivo imaging of human cerebral nicotinic acetylcholine receptors with 2-¹⁸F-fluoro-A-85380 and PET. J Nucl Med 2005;46(2):240–7.

9. Kimes AS, Chefer SI, Matochik JA, et al. Quantification of nicotinic acetylcholine receptors in the human brain with PET: bolus plus infusion administration of 2-[¹⁸F]F-A85380. Neuroimage 2008;39(2):717–27.

10. Sorger D, Becker GA, Patt M, et al. Measurement of the alpha4beta2* nicotinic acetylcholine receptor ligand 2-[(18)F]Fluoro-A-85380 and its metabolites in human blood during PET investigation: a methodological study. Nucl Med Biol 2007;34(3):331–42.

11. Ellis JR, Nathan PJ, Villemagne VL, et al. Galantamine-induced improvements in cognitive function are not related to alterations in alpha(4)beta(2) nicotinic receptors in early Alzheimer's disease as measured in vivo by 2-[(18)F]Fluoro-A-85380 PET. Psychopharmacology (Berl) 2009 Jan;202(1–3):79–91 Epub 2008 Oct 24.

12. Ellis JR, Villemagne VL, Nathan PJ, et al. Relationship between nicotinic receptors and cognitive function in early Alzheimer's disease: a 2-[¹⁸F]fluoro-A-85380 PET study. Neurobiol Learn Mem 2008;90(2):404–12.

13. Mitkovski S, Villemagne VL, Novakovic KE, et al. Simplified quantification of nicotinic receptors with 2[¹⁸F]F-A-85380 PET. Nucl Med Biol 2005;32(6):585–91.

14. Picard F, Bruel D, Servent D, et al. Alteration of the in vivo nicotinic receptor density in ADNFLE patients: a PET study. Brain 2006;129(Pt 8):2047–60.

15. Sabri O, Kendziorra K, Wolf H, et al. Acetylcholine receptors in dementia and mild cognitive impairment. Eur J Nucl Med Mol Imaging 2008;35(Suppl 1):S30–45.

16. Wullner U, Gundisch D, Herzog H, et al. Smoking upregulates alpha4beta2* nicotinic acetylcholine receptors in the human brain. Neurosci Lett 2008;430(1):34–7.

17. Ding YS, Fowler JS, Logan J, et al. 6-[¹⁸F]Fluoro-A-85380, a new PET tracer for the nicotinic acetylcholine receptor: studies in the human brain and in vivo demonstration of specific binding in white matter. Synapse 2004;53(3):184–9.

18. Brasic JR, Zhou Y, Musachio JL, et al. Single photon emission computed tomography experience with (S)-5-[(¹²³)I]iodo-3-(2-azetidinylmethoxy)pyridine in the living human brain of smokers and nonsmokers. Synapse 2009;63(4):339–58.

19. Vaupel DB, Tella SR, Huso DL, et al. Pharmacological and toxicological evaluation of 2-fluoro-3-(2(S)-azetidinylmethoxy)pyridine (2-F-A-85380), a ligand for imaging cerebral nicotinic acetylcholine receptors with positron emission tomography. J Pharmacol Exp Ther 2005;312(1):355–65.

20. Horti AG, Villemagne VL. The quest for Eldorado: development of radioligands for in vivo imaging of

20. nicotinic acetylcholine receptors in human brain. Curr Pharm Des 2006;12(30):3877–900.

21. Gundisch D. Nicotinic acetylcholine receptors and imaging. Curr Pharm Des 2000;6(11):1143–57.

22. Sihver W, Langstrom B, Nordberg A. Ligands for in vivo imaging of nicotinic receptor subtypes in Alzheimer brain. Acta Neurol Scand Suppl 2000;176: 27–33.

23. Sihver W, Nordberg A, Langstrom B, et al. Development of ligands for in vivo imaging of cerebral nicotinic receptors. Behav Brain Res 2000;113(1–2):143–57.

24. Volkow ND, Ding YS, Fowler JS, et al. Imaging brain cholinergic activity with positron emission tomography: its role in the evaluation of cholinergic treatments in Alzheimer's dementia. Biol Psychiatry 2001;49(3):211–20.

25. Ding YS, Fowler J. New-generation radiotracers for nAChR and NET. Nucl Med Biol 2005;32(7):707–18.

26. Brody AL, Mandelkern MA, London ED, et al. Cigarette smoking saturates brain alpha 4 beta 2 nicotinic acetylcholine receptors. Arch Gen Psychiatry 2006;63(8):907–15.

27. Fujita M, Al-Tikriti MS, Tamagnan G, et al. Influence of acetylcholine levels on the binding of a SPECT nicotinic acetylcholine receptor ligand [123I]5-I-A-85380. Synapse 2003;48(3):116–22.

28. Horti AG, Chefer SI, Mukhin AG, et al. 6-[18F]fluoro-A-85380, a novel radioligand for in vivo imaging of central nicotinic acetylcholine receptors. Life Sci 2000;67(4):463–9.

29. Ding YS, Liu N, Wang T, et al. Synthesis and evaluation of 6-[18F]fluoro-3-(2(S)-azetidinylmethoxy)pyridine as a PET tracer for nicotinic acetylcholine receptors. Nucl Med Biol 2000;27(4):381–9.

30. Scheffel U, Horti AG, Koren AO, et al. 6-[18F]Fluoro-A-85380: an in vivo tracer for the nicotinic acetylcholine receptor. Nucl Med Biol 2000;27(1):51–6.

31. Chefer SI, Pavlova OA, Zhang Y, et al. NIDA522131, a new radioligand for imaging extrathalamic nicotinic acetylcholine receptors: in vitro and in vivo evaluation. J Neurochem 2008;104:306–15.

32. Zhang Y, Pavlova OA, Chefer SI, et al. 5-substituted derivatives of 6-halogeno-3-((2-(S)-azetidinyl)methoxy)pyridine and 6-halogeno-3-((2-(S)-pyrrolidinyl)methoxy)pyridine with low picomolar affinity for alpha4beta2 nicotinic acetylcholine receptor and wide range of lipophilicity: potential probes for imaging with positron emission tomography. J Med Chem 2004;47(10):2453–65.

33. Paterson D, Nordberg A. Neuronal nicotinic receptors in the human brain. Prog Neurobiol 2000; 61(1):75–111.

34. Villemagne VL, Musachio JL, Scheffel U. Nicotine and related compounds as PET and SPECT ligands. In: Arneric SP, Brioni JD, editors. Neuronal nicotinic receptors, pharmacology and therapeutic opportunities. New York: Johns Wiley & Sons; 1999. p. 235–50.

35. Abreo MA, Lin NH, Garvey DS, et al. Novel 3-pyridyl ethers with subnanomolar affinity for central neuronal nicotinic acetylcholine receptors. J Med Chem 1996;39(4):817–25.

36. Spande TF, Garraffo HM, Edwards MW, et al. Epibatidine: a novel (chloropyridyl)azabicycloheptane with potent analgesic activity from an Ecuadoran poison frog. J Am Chem Soc 1992;114(9):3475–8.

37. Brown LL, Pavlova O, Mukhin A, et al. Radiosynthesis of 5-[2-(4-pyridinyl)vinyl]-6-chloro-3-[(1-[11C]methyl-2-(S)-pyrrolidinyl)methoxy]pyridine, a high affinity ligand for studying nicotinic acetylcholine receptors by positron emission tomography. Bioorg Med Chem 2001;9(11):3055–8.

38. Brown LL, Kulkarni S, Pavlova OA, et al. Synthesis and evaluation of a novel series of 2-chloro-5-(1-methyl-2-(S)-pyrrolidinyl)methoxy)-3-(2-(4-pyridinyl)vinyl) pyridine analogues as potential positron emission tomography imaging agents for nicotinic acetylcholine receptors. J Med Chem 2002;45(13):2841–9.

39. Brown L, Chefer S, Pavlova O, et al. Evaluation of 5-(2-(4-pyridinyl)vinyl)-6-chloro-3-(1-methyl-2-(S)-pyrrolidinylmethoxy)pyridine and its analogues as PET radioligands for imaging nicotinic acetylcholine receptors. J Neurochem 2004;91(3):600–12.

40. Gao Y, Ravert HT, Kuwabara H, et al. Synthesis and biological evaluation of novel carbon-11 labeled pyridyl ethers: candidate ligands for in vivo imaging of nicotinic acetylcholine receptors (nAChRs) with positron emission tomography. Bioorg Med Chem 2009 Jul 1;17(13):4367–77 Epub 2009 May 15.

41. Gao Y, Ravert HT, Holt D, et al. 6-Chloro-3-(((1-[11C]methyl)-2-(S)-pyrrolidinyl)methoxy)-5-(2-fluoropyridi n-4-yl)pyridine ([11C]JHU85270), a potent ligand for nicotinic acetylcholine receptor imaging by positron emission tomography. Appl Radiat Isot 2007;65(8):947–51.

42. Easwaramoorthy B, Pichika R, Collins D, et al. Effect of acetylcholinesterase inhibitors on the binding of nicotinic alpha4beta2 receptor PET radiotracer, (18)F-nifene: a measure of acetylcholine competition. Synapse 2007;61(1):29–36.

43. Pichika R, Easwaramoorthy B, Collins D, et al. Nicotinic alpha4beta2 receptor imaging agents: part II. Synthesis and biological evaluation of 2-[18F]fluoro-3-[2-((S)-3-pyrrolinyl)methoxy]pyridine (18F-nifene) in rodents and imaging by PET in nonhuman primate. Nucl Med Biol 2006;33(3):295–304.

44. Wei ZL, Xiao Y, Yuan H, et al. Novel pyridyl ring C5 substituted analogues of epibatidine and 3-(1-methyl-2(S)-pyrrolidinylmethoxy)pyridine (A-84543) as highly selective agents for neuronal nicotinic acetylcholine receptors containing beta2 subunits. J Med Chem 2005;48(6):1721–4.

45. Kozikowski AP, Chellappan SK, Henderson D, et al. Acetylenic pyridines for use in PET imaging of nicotinic receptors. ChemMedChem 2006;2(1):54–7.

46. Spang JE, Bertrand S, Westera G, et al. Chemical modification of epibatidine causes a switch from agonist to antagonist and modifies its selectivity for neuronal nicotinic acetylcholine receptors. Chem Biol 2000;7(7):545–55.

47. Carroll FI, Ma W, Yokota Y, et al. Synthesis, nicotinic acetylcholine receptor binding, and antinociceptive properties of 3′-substituted deschloroepibatidine analogues. Novel nicotinic antagonists. J Med Chem 2005;48(4):1221–8.

48. Ding YS, Kil KE, Lin KS, et al. A novel nicotinic acetylcholine receptor antagonist radioligand for PET studies. Bioorg Med Chem Lett 2006;16(4): 1049–53.

49. Badio B, Shi D, Garraffo HM, et al. Antinociceptive effects of the alkaloid epibatidine—further-studies on involvement of nicotinic receptors. Drug Dev Res 1995;36(1):46–59.

50. Gao Y, Horti AG, Kuwabara H, et al. Derivatives of (-)-7-methyl-2-(5-(pyridinyl)pyridin-3-yl)-7-azabicyclo[2.2.1]heptane are potential ligands for positron emission tomography imaging of extrathalamic nicotinic acetylcholine receptors. J Med Chem 2007; 50(16):3814–24.

51. Gao Y, Horti AG, Kuwabara H, et al. New synthesis and evaluation of enantiomers of 7-methyl-2-exo-(3′-iodo-5′-pyridinyl)-7-azabicyclo[2.2.1]heptane as stereoselective ligands for PET imaging of nicotinic acetylcholine receptors. Bioorg Med Chem Lett 2008;18(23):6168–70.

52. Huang Y, Zhu Z, Xiao Y, et al. Epibatidine analogues as selective ligands for the alpha(x)beta2-containing subtypes of nicotinic acetylcholine receptors. Bioorg Med Chem Lett 2005;15(19):4385–8.

53. Carroll FI, Ware R, Brieaddy LE, et al. Synthesis, nicotinic acetylcholine receptor binding, and antinociceptive properties of 2′-fluoro-3′-(substituted phenyl)deschloroepibatidine analogues. Novel nicotinic antagonist. J Med Chem 2004;47(18):4588–94.

54. Valette H, Dolle F, Saba W, et al. [^{18}F]FPhEP and [^{18}F]F2PhEP, two new epibatidine-based radioligands: evaluation for imaging nicotinic acetylcholine receptors in baboon brain. Synapse 2007;61(9):764–70.

55. Roger G, Saba W, Valette H, et al. Synthesis and radiosynthesis of [(^{18})F]FPhEP, a novel alpha(4)-beta(2)-selective, epibatidine-based antagonist for PET imaging of nicotinic acetylcholine receptors. Bioorg Med Chem 2006;14(11):3848–58.

56. Deuther-Conrad W, Patt JT, Lockman PR, et al. Norchloro-fluoro-homoepibatidine (NCFHEB) - a promising radioligand for neuroimaging nicotinic acetylcholine receptors with PET. Eur Neuropsychopharmacol 2008;18(3):222–9.

57. Brust P, Patt JT, Deuther-Conrad W, et al. In vivo measurement of nicotinic acetylcholine receptors with [^{18}F]norchloro-fluoro-homoepibatidine. Synapse 2008;62(3):205–18.

58. Deuther-Conrad W, Patt JT, Feuerbach D, et al. Norchloro-fluoro-homoepibatidine: specificity to neuronal nicotinic acetylcholine receptor subtypes in vitro. Farmaco 2004;59(10):785–92.

59. Gao Y, Kuwabara H, Spivak CE, et al. Discovery of (−)-7-methyl-2-exo-[3′-(6-[^{18}F]fluoropyridin-2-yl)-5′-pyridinyl]-7-azabicyclo[2.2.1]heptane, a radiolabeled antagonist for cerebral nicotinic acetylcholine receptor (alpha4beta2-nAChR) with optimal positron emission tomography imaging properties. J Med Chem 2008;51(15):4751–64.

Fluorine-18 Radiolabeled PET Tracers for Imaging Monoamine Transporters: Dopamine, Serotonin, and Norepinephrine

Jeffrey S. Stehouwer, PhD, Mark M. Goodman, PhD*

KEYWORDS

- Fluorine-18 PET • Tropanes • Dopamine transporter
- Serotonin transporter • Norepinephrine transporter

The dopamine transporter (DAT), serotonin transporter (SERT), and norepinephrine transporter (NET) are plasma membrane biogenic monoamine transporters that belong to the family of Na^+/Cl^--dependent transporters.[1–8] In the central nervous system the DAT, SERT, and NET are located on presynaptic neurons and function to remove their respective neurotransmitter from the synapse thereby terminating the action of that neurotransmitter. These three transporters have each been implicated in numerous psychiatric disorders, such as depression, suicide, schizophrenia, Parkinson's disease (PD), and attention-deficit–hyperactivity disorder and are also the target of drugs of abuse, such as cocaine, amphetamines, and 3,4-methylenedioxymethamphetamine (Ecstasy). As such, these transporters have become therapeutic targets to treat psychiatric disorders and drug addiction.[9–11] The ability to image the DAT, SERT, and NET with PET or single-photon emission computed tomography (SPECT) may aid in the diagnosis and management of psychiatric disease by providing a means to measure the density of these transporters in specific brain regions.[12–17] Additionally, the availability of radiolabeled tracers for these transporters may aid in the development of new therapeutics by enabling the occupancy of the therapeutic to be measured.[18–24]

Numerous PET tracers for the DAT, SERT, and NET have been developed that are radiolabeled with carbon-11, but these are limited to use in the location where they are prepared and only allow for imaging times of up to about 2 hours because of the short half-life of ^{11}C ($t_{1/2} = 20.4$ minutes).[25–27] The longer half-life of ^{18}F ($t_{1/2} = 109.8$ minutes) allows for longer synthesis times and imaging sessions and for the transport of the ^{18}F-labeled tracer to locations away from the cyclotron facility, which allows for PET imaging centers without onsite cyclotrons to use these tracers. In addition to the longer half-life of ^{18}F, the positrons emitted from ^{18}F-nuclides have a lower maximum energy (0.64 MeV)[26] than the positrons emitted from ^{11}C-nuclides (0.97 MeV), which deposits less energy into tissue and also results in a shorter linear range that allows for higher spatial resolution.[28,29] Radiolabeling tracers with

Department of Radiology, Center for Systems Imaging, Emory University School of Medicine, Atlanta, GA 30329, USA

Department of Radiology, Wesley Woods Health Centers, 2nd Floor, WWHC # 209, 1841 Clifton Road NE, Atlanta, GA 30329, USA

* Corresponding author. Department of Radiology, Wesley Woods Health Centers, 2nd Floor, 1841 Clifton Road NE, Atlanta, GA 30329, USA.

E-mail address: mgoodma@emory.edu (M.M. Goodman).

PET Clin 4 (2009) 101–128

doi:10.1016/j.cpet.2009.05.006

[11]C is convenient because of the ubiquitous nature of carbon in organic compounds, whereas fluorine is far less common. Fluorine, however, has been shown to impart unique properties to organic molecules and is now being exploited extensively in medicinal chemistry.[30–36] Thus, numerous methods have been developed to introduce ^{18}F or ^{19}F into molecules.[37–41] This article focuses on fluorine-18 radiolabeled PET tracers for imaging the DAT, SERT, and NET. Several carbon-11 PET tracers are also included to allow for comparisons in instances where a tracer can be radiolabeled with either isotope or where fluorinated analogs of existing ^{11}C-labeled tracers have been developed.

There are several performance criteria that should be met for a candidate brain PET tracer to become a useful tracer. High binding affinity to the target, especially if the target is of low density, enables highly specific and selective binding to the target. The goal is to obtain the highest possible target-to-nontarget uptake ratios which will result in PET images with high signal-to-noise ratios. If the tracer does not bind strong enough to the target, then the tracer is not retained in the tissue of interest and just passes through. If the tracer binds too strongly, then it does not dissociate from the target during the course of the PET study and accumulates in the tissue of interest and only blood flow is measured. A balance must be obtained that allows for the achievement of peak uptake in the target tissue in a short time frame (^{18}F allows for longer time frames compared with ^{11}C) followed by a steady washout to allow for kinetic modeling of the behavior of the tracer.[42–47] Moderate lipophilicity in the range of log$P$ = approximately 1 to 3 is necessary to allow for rapid entry into the brain and to limit nonspecific binding.[48–50] Low binding to plasma proteins is necessary to make as many tracer molecules as possible available for brain entry. Metabolism of the tracer is unavoidable but the resulting metabolites that are generated in the periphery, if they are radiolabeled, should be hydrophilic so that they cannot enter the brain. The generation of radiolabeled metabolites in the brain is also undesirable and any radiolabeled metabolites that are produced should have little or no affinity for the target of interest. As will become apparent below, meeting all of these criteria simultaneously is a difficult task.

DOPAMINE TRANSPORTER

The human DAT is a 620–amino acid transmembrane protein that is 98.9% homologous to the monkey DAT and 92% homologous to the rat DAT.[4,51–53] The DAT is found in high densities in the caudate, putamen, nucleus accumbens, and olfactory tubercle with lower densities in the substantia nigra, amygdala, and hypothalamus.[54–57] The DAT has been associated with numerous neuropsychiatric diseases including PD,[58–60] supranuclear palsy,[59] attention-deficit–hyperactivity disorder,[61] and Tourette's syndrome.[62] The ability to image the DAT with PET may aid in the diagnosis, monitoring, and treatment of these diseases.[13,15,17,63]

Early work toward developing an ^{18}F-labeled DAT imaging agent focused on the GBR-compounds[64,65] [^{18}F]1 and [^{18}F]2 (Fig. 1).[66–71] PET imaging with [^{18}F]2 in monkeys[72] showed rapid uptake into the striatum and cerebellum with maximum levels achieved within 2 to 3 minutes followed by a slow but steady washout. Washout was faster from the cerebellum than the striatum, which resulted in a striatum-to-cerebellum ratio of 1.76 at the end of the study. Radiotracer uptake was highest in the liver and kidneys because of metabolism of the tracer but low bone uptake indicated that the aryl-fluorine bond was stable to metabolic defluorination. The imaging results with [^{18}F]2 were promising but the tracer still suffered from high lipophilicity and nonspecific binding. The synthesis and radiolabeling of the GBR-derivatives [^{18}F]3 and [^{18}F]4 has

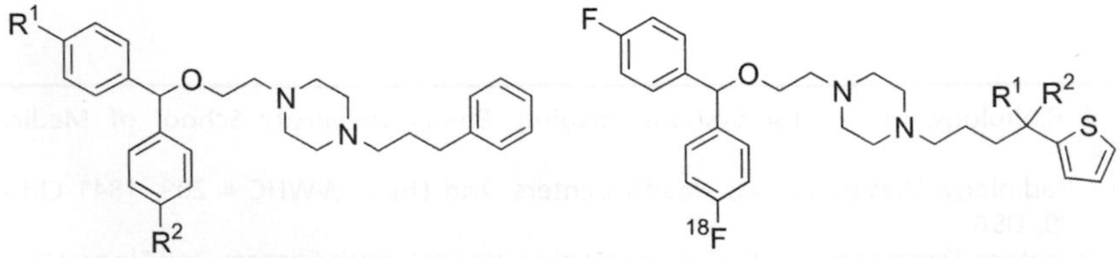

[^{18}F]1 R^1 = F, R^2 = [18]F (GBR 12909)
[^{18}F]2 R^1 = H, R^2 = [18]F (GBR 13119)

[^{18}F]3 R^1,R^2 = O (NNC 12-0817)
[^{18}F]4 R^1 = H, R^2 = OH (NNC 12-0818)

Fig. 1. Structures of GBR-based DAT PET tracers.

also been reported but imaging data were not included.[73]

Cocaine (5) (**Fig. 2**, **Table 1**) binds to the DAT, SERT, and NET[74,75] but the DAT was initially implicated as the site related to substance abuse.[76–78] As a tool to study cocaine addiction [^{11}C]cocaine PET imaging has been used[79–83] but imaging times are limited because of the short half-life of ^{11}C. 4'- [^{18}F]Fluorococaine ([^{18}F]6) allows for extended imaging studies because of the longer half-life of ^{18}F and [^{18}F]6 was shown to have identical kinetic behavior to [^{11}C]cocaine in PET imaging studies.[82]

Cocaine metabolism can take several possible routes: (1) ester hydrolysis, (2) N-demethylation, (3) N-oxidation, (4) aryl hydroxylation or epoxidation, and (5) dehydrobenzoylation.[82,84–89] The benzoic ester hydrolysis route was rendered obsolete when Clarke and coworkers[90] demonstrated that replacement of the benzoyloxy group with a phenyl group attached directly to the 3β-position of the tropane skeleton produced compounds with higher binding affinities at the DAT than cocaine itself. This new class of 3β-phenyl tropanes has been exploited extensively in the search for therapeutics to treat cocaine addiction[10,11,91–95] and hundreds of compounds have already been reported in the past[96] and more continue to be reported to this day.[97,98] The structures of some of the first 3β-phenyl tropane compounds prepared (7–12) are shown in **Fig. 2** and **Table 1**.[90–92,99] The high affinity of these compounds for the DAT naturally made them candidates for use as PET tracers when labeled with ^{11}C because

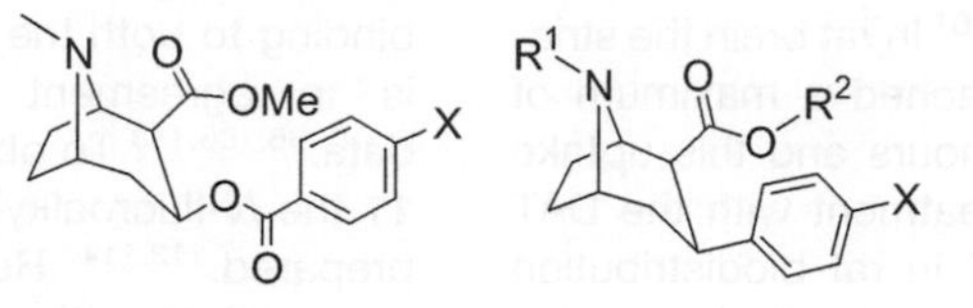

5 R = H (Cocaine)
6 R = F

Fig. 2. Structures of cocaine, 4'-fluorococaine, and 3β-phenyltropane–based DAT ligands.

Table 1
Compound numbering and substituent list for the 3β-phenyltropane structure shown in Figure 2.

	Compound	R^1=	R^2=	X=
7	WIN 35,065-2	Me	Me	H
8	WIN 35,428; β-CFT	Me	Me	F
9	RTI-31	Me	Me	Cl
10	RTI-51; CBT	Me	Me	Br
11	RTI-55; β-CIT	Me	Me	I
12	RTI-32	Me	Me	Me
13	β-CFT-FE	CH$_2$CH$_2$F	Me	F
14	β-CFT-FP	CH$_2$CH$_2$CH$_2$F	Me	F
15	FE-β-CIT; β-CIT-FE	CH$_2$CH$_2$F	Me	I
16	FP-β-CIT; β-CIT-FP	CH$_2$CH$_2$CH$_2$F	Me	I
17	—	CH$_2$CH$_2$CH$_2$F	i-Pr	I
18	FECNT	CH$_2$CH$_2$F	Me	Cl
19	FPCT	CH$_2$CH$_2$CH$_2$F	Me	Cl
20	FPCMT	CH$_2$CH$_2$CH$_2$F	Me	Me
21	FPCBT	CH$_2$CH$_2$CH$_2$F	Me	Br
22	FETT	Me	CH$_2$CH$_2$F	Me
23	FECT	Me	CH$_2$CH$_2$F	Cl
24	MCL322	Me	CH$_2$CH$_2$F	Br
25	MCL301; FE@CIT	Me	CH$_2$CH$_2$F	I

they can all be labeled on either the N-methyl group or the methyl ester.[88,100–104] Unfortunately, these ^{11}C-labeled compounds do not reach binding equilibrium during the course of the imaging study which limits their usefulness in kinetic modeling. Furthermore, compound 11 has a similar affinity for the DAT and SERT and compounds 9 and 10 are only slightly selective for the DAT over the SERT,[94,96,105] thus limiting the use of these compounds as DAT-selective imaging agents.

Out of compounds 7 to 12, only compound 8 contains a ^{19}F atom that could be replaced with [18]F. Additionally, 8 is more selective for the DAT over the SERT and NET than compounds 9 to 11,[94,96] and previous work with [^{11}C]8 had demonstrated that it was capable of imaging the DAT.[100,101] Thus, [^{18}F]8 was synthesized and evaluated by biodistribution studies in rats[106] and then by PET imaging in humans.[107] In rat brain the striatum-to-cerebellum ratio reached a maximum of approximately 9.6 after 2 hours and this uptake could be blocked by pretreatment with the DAT ligand GBR 12,909 (1).[64,65] In rat biodistribution studies the highest uptake at all times was observed in the liver and urine, whereas uptake in the kidney, spleen, and lungs was initially high but then decreased. Very little bone uptake was observed indicating that the aryl-fluorine bond of [^{18}F]8 is stable to metabolic defluorination, similar to what was observed for [^{18}F]2. In human subjects the total activity of [^{18}F]8 in the caudate and putamen peaked at 225 minutes and then slowly declined, whereas the specific binding remained at a plateau from 3 to 5 hours postinjection. Application of [^{18}F]8 to studying human subjects with early PD demonstrated that [^{18}F]8 was capable of detecting presynaptic dopaminergic hypofunction.[108]

To reduce the time required to reach peak uptake of [^{18}F]8, the N-[^{18}F]fluoroethyl[105] and N-[^{18}F]fluoropropyl[109,110] derivatives, [^{18}F]13 and [^{18}F]14, respectively, were prepared. In vitro binding assays demonstrated that both 13 and 14 had a reduced affinity for the DAT, SERT, and NET relative to 8, but 13 and 14 both had a slightly improved selectivity for the DAT over the SERT relative to 8.[105] PET imaging with [^{18}F]13 in conscious rhesus monkeys demonstrated that [^{18}F]13 reaches peak uptake after about 20 minutes followed by a washout phase, demonstrating reversible binding. A comparison study with [^{11}C]8 showed only irreversible binding during the 91-minute PET scan as the radioactivity continuously increased throughout the study. Replacing the N-methyl group of 8 with an N-fluoroethyl group as in 13 resulted in improved tracer performance. A blocking study with 1 demonstrated that [^{18}F]13 binding was DAT-specific. Metabolite analysis of [^{18}F]13 in plasma showed only polar metabolites and no lipophilic metabolites that could cross the blood-brain barrier. Compound [^{18}F]14 was evaluated ex vivo in rats and demonstrated rapid entry into the brain with a striatum-to-cerebellum ratio of approximately 3.1 after 5 minutes followed by a continuous decrease. This uptake could be blocked by pretreatment with 1. A continuous uptake was observed in the skull indicating a slow defluorination of the [^{18}F]fluoropropyl group.

Compound 11 has a nearly equal affinity for the DAT and SERT[94,96,105] and PET imaging with [^{11}C]11 showed uptake in the striatum and the thalamus and neocortex.[88,103] This uptake in the thalamus and neocortex could be displaced by the SERT ligand citalopram,[111,112] demonstrating binding to both the DAT and SERT in vivo, which is in agreement with the in vitro binding data.[96,105,113] To obtain ^{18}F-labeled derivatives of 11 the N-fluoroalkyl compounds 15 and 16 were prepared.[113,114] Replacement of the N-methyl group of 11 with an N-fluoroethyl group (15) or an N-fluoropropyl group (16) resulted in a reduced binding affinity at the DAT and NET but an increased binding affinity at the SERT relative to 11.[113] Replacement of the methyl ester group of 16 with an isopropyl ester to give 17 increased the binding affinity at the DAT relative to 11 and significantly reduced the binding affinity at both the SERT and NET.[113,115] A SPECT imaging comparison[116] of [^{123}I]15, [^{123}I]16, and [^{123}I]17 in baboons demonstrated that [^{123}I]15 and [^{123}I]16 had higher peak uptake in the striatum than [^{123}I]17, ruling out [^{123}I]17 for adaptation to PET imaging as [^{18}F]17. Additionally, [^{123}I]15 had more rapid kinetics than [^{123}I]16. Comparison between [^{123}I]11 and [^{123}I]16 in humans with SPECT imaging showed that [^{123}I]16 had higher nonspecific binding than [^{123}I]11 but a lower radiation burden to the basal ganglia.[117]

PET studies in anesthetized cynomolgus monkeys with [^{11}C]15 showed high uptake in the putamen with lesser uptake in the thalamus and neocortex.[118] A blocking study with 1 reduced the uptake of [^{11}C]15 in the putamen by 75% but did not affect the uptake in the thalamus or neocortex, indicating that SERT binding was still an issue. Compound [^{18}F]16 has been radiolabeled and evaluated in anesthetized cynomolgus monkeys[119] and conscious humans.[120] In monkeys high uptake of [^{18}F]16 was observed in the putamen (this was blockable with 1) with peak uptake achieved in 30 to 40 minutes followed by only a very slight washout. After 70 minutes the striatum-to-cerebellum ratio was 4.5 to 5. Uptake in the thalamus was at levels similar to the cerebellum demonstrating an improvement over [^{11}C]11, [^{11}C]15, and [^{11}C]16. Metabolite analysis did not detect any lipophilic metabolites but [^{18}F]fluoride was detected in plasma indicating that defluorination was occurring. Initial studies in humans with [^{18}F]16 showed high uptake in the putamen of a healthy normal volunteer, whereas uptake was reduced 65% in a PD patient.[120] Additional studies[121] in healthy normal humans with [^{18}F]16 showed that uptake in the striatum increased rapidly after injection but then leveled off after 40 minutes and did not wash out. Uptake in the thalamus peaked at approximately 20 minutes and then began to wash out. In PD patients uptake in the putamen peaked at 30 minutes and then slowly washed out. Additional studies have been performed with [^{18}F]16 to acquire data for parametric mapping,[122] dosimetry,[123] and modeling.[124] A one-step high-yield radiosynthesis of [^{18}F]16 has been developed.[125]

Compounds 18 and 19 are the N-fluoroalkyl derivatives of 9, which has been previously radiolabeled as [^{11}C]9 and evaluated in rats.[102] PET studies with [^{18}F]19 in anesthetized rhesus monkeys showed high uptake in the striatum with putamen-to-cerebellum and caudate-to-cerebellum ratios of 3.35 and 2.28, respectively, after 115 minutes.[126] The uptake in the cerebellum washed out after an initial peak at 13.5 minutes but the uptake in the caudate and putamen remained nearly constant after peaking, indicating irreversible binding to the DAT. Biodistribution studies in rats showed continuously increasing bone uptake indicating that the fluoropropyl group was not resistant to defluorination, which is in agreement with the detection of [^{18}F]fluoride in plasma reported for the metabolism of [^{18}F]16 and the observed skull uptake in studies with [^{18}F]14. PET imaging with [^{18}F]18 in an anesthetized rhesus monkey showed high uptake in the caudate and putamen (displaceable with 11) with peak uptake achieved in 60 to 75 minutes followed by washout at a rate of 8% per hour.[127] At 115 minutes the putamen-to-cerebellum ratio was 12.7 and the caudate-to-cerebellum ratio was 12.3. When an imaging study with [^{18}F]19 was performed in the same rhesus monkey the uptake in the caudate and putamen continuously increased throughout the course of the study,[127] similar to what was previously reported.[126] Thus, [^{18}F]18 displays reversible binding and can achieve binding equilibrium, whereas [^{18}F]19 binds irreversibly. Compound [^{18}F]18 has since been used to measure DAT occupancy of cocaine[128] and radiation dosimetry studies have been performed in rats

and monkeys.[129,130] Two different automated radiosynthesis methods of [^{18}F]18 have been reported.[131,132] Initial studies[133] in six healthy humans with [^{18}F]18 showed that the time for peak uptake in the caudate and putamen was in the range of 70 to 130 minutes with caudate-to-cerebellum ratios of 7.6 - 10.5 and putamen-to-cerebellum ratios of 7.1 - 9.3. Comparison of the data obtained in healthy humans with that obtained in PD patients demonstrated that [^{18}F]18 has the potential to measure DAT density in the brain and to detect the reduction in DAT density that is associated with PD. Metabolism studies in humans using arterial samples after injection of [^{18}F]18 identified a polar non–ether-extractable component.[133] Subsequent studies[134] in rats, monkeys, and humans identified this polar metabolite as either [^{18}F]fluoroethanol, [^{18}F]fluoroacetaldehyde, or [^{18}F]fluoroacetic acid (or a combination of all three as they are metabolically interchangeable). This work demonstrated that the polar metabolite is generated in the periphery but then passes into the brain and distributes evenly throughout the brain. The authors suggest that the tissue reference method should not be used for analyzing PET data obtained with [^{18}F]18 but rather an arterial input function should be used.

This N-dealkylation of [^{18}F]18 is not unique to [^{18}F]18 but has also been observed with cocaine,[84] [^{11}C]cocaine (to give [^{11}C]CO$_2$ in baboons),[79,82] and [^{11}C]11,[88] and other tracers.[135–139] Metabolic cleavage of radiolabeled N-methyl and N-fluoroethyl groups is unavoidable and it should be expected that any tracer radiolabeled with an N- [^{18}F]fluoroethyl group will be metabolized in the periphery to [^{18}F]fluoroethanol, [^{18}F]fluoroacetaldehyde, or [^{18}F]fluoroacetic acid, and such an effect has recently been reported with the amyloid imaging agent [^{18}F]FDDNP.[140] Switching to an N- [^{18}F]fluoropropyl group is not necessarily a better alternative because the N- [^{18}F]fluoropropyl group is not stable to defluorination as was demonstrated with [^{18}F]14, [^{18}F]16, and [^{18}F]19.

Compounds 20 and 21 are the N-fluoropropyl derivatives of 12 and 10, respectively. A procedure for preparing [^{18}F]20 has been reported but imaging data were not included.[141] PET imaging with [^{18}F]21 in baboons showed the highest uptake in the putamen with peak uptake achieved in 7 to 10 minutes. The washout half-life was 54 minutes for the striatum, whereas it was 19 minutes for the midbrain and 16 minutes for the cerebellum. A striatum-to-cerebellum ratio of 3.3 was achieved at 45 to 60 minutes postinjection. Metabolite analysis detected a "less-lipophilic" metabolite, which was presumed to be the 2β-carboxylic acid resulting from hydrolysis of the methyl ester.

As an alternative to radiolabeling with N-fluoroalkyl groups several compounds containing fluoroethyl esters have been prepared (22–25). Biodistribution studies in rats with [18F]22 and [18F]23 showed high uptake in the striatum and olfactory tubercles.[102] Compound [18F]23 showed higher uptake in the striatum than [18F]22 but also significantly higher liver uptake. Bone uptake was minimal for both tracers indicating that the [18F]fluoroethyl ester was stable to defluorination. An improved synthesis and metabolic stability analysis in rats of [18F]23 has recently been reported.[142] This work found that after 3 hours plasma radioactivity consisted of approximately 93% intact [18F]23 and the radioactivity in homogenized cerebrum and cerebellum extracts each consisted of approximately 96% intact [18F]23. Furthermore, there was no trace of [18F]fluoroacetaldehyde or [18F]fluoroacetic acid, which would result from hydrolysis of the [18F]fluoroethyl ester.

Compounds 24 and 25 are the fluoroethyl ester derivatives of 10 and 11, respectively.[143,144] Biodistribution studies of [18F]24 in rats showed high uptake in the striatum (blockable with 1) with peak uptake around 60 minutes followed by a slow washout.[145] Uptake in the adrenals and kidneys was initially high but then washed out, whereas uptake in the liver continuously increased throughout the study. The tracer was rapidly metabolized in rat plasma to a polar metabolite, which accounted for 85% of radioactivity in plasma after 60 minutes. In rat striatal homogenates the radioactivity was greater than 90% intact parent compound after 60 minutes. Low bone uptake in the biodistribution studies indicated that the [18F]fluoroethyl ester was stable to defluorination. The striatal uptake observed in the biodistribution studies was further confirmed by autoradiography. Micro-PET studies with [18F]24 in rats showed a steady uptake in the striatum for the first 20 minutes, which then peaked and remained stable for 30 to 100 minutes postinjection. At the end of the study (115 minutes postinjection) the striatum-to-cerebellum ratio was 2.8.

Evaluation of [18F]25 in rats showed peak uptake in the striatum at 15 minutes followed by a steady washout.[146] At 60 minutes the striatum-to-cerebellum ratio was 3.73 and the striatum-to-thalamus ratio was 2.99, whereas at 120 minutes the thalamus-to-cerebellum ratio was 1.65. High uptake in the kidneys suggested a renal excretion route, whereas low bone uptake indicated stability to defluorination. A metabolic stability study with porcine carboxyl esterase found that [18F]25 and [123I]11 have similar stabilities in regards to resistance to enzymatic hydrolysis of the ester but this stability was less than that found for [123I]16.[147] The authors suggest that the N-fluoropropyl group of [123I]16 is bulky enough to impede access to the ester bond by the enzyme, inhibiting this route of metabolism. This bulkiness of the N-[18F]fluoropropyl group and the subsequent prevention of ester hydrolysis may account for why defluorination of [18F]14, [18F]16, and [18F]19 is observed as the major metabolic route.

It had been previously shown that replacing the methyl ester of 9 with an isopropyl ester significantly reduced binding affinity at the SERT and NET, whereas only slightly reducing DAT binding affinity.[115] The fluoroisopropyl derivatives (R)-26 and (S)-26 (Fig. 3) were prepared and evaluated.[148] Competitive binding assays in murine kidney cells with transfected DAT or SERT showed that (S)-26 had a nearly fivefold higher affinity ($K_i = 0.67$ nM) than (R)-26 ($K_i = 3.2$ nM) at the DAT and a lower affinity at the SERT (K_i's = 85 nM [S] and 65 nM [R]). For comparison, 11 was included and had binding affinities of $K_i = 0.48$ nM (DAT) and $K_i = 0.67$ nM (SERT), which is in agreement with the previously reported nearly equal affinities at each transporter.[96,105,113] (S)-26 has only a slight reduction in DAT affinity compared with 11 but has a significant improvement in DAT versus SERT selectivity. Biodistribution studies in rats with [18F](R/S)-26 showed highest uptake in the liver but very little bone uptake indicating that the fluoroisopropyl ester was stable to defluorination. In rat brain biodistribution studies [18F](R)-26 reached peak uptake in the striatum at 30 minutes and had a striatum-to-cerebellum ratio of 6 at 60 minutes, whereas

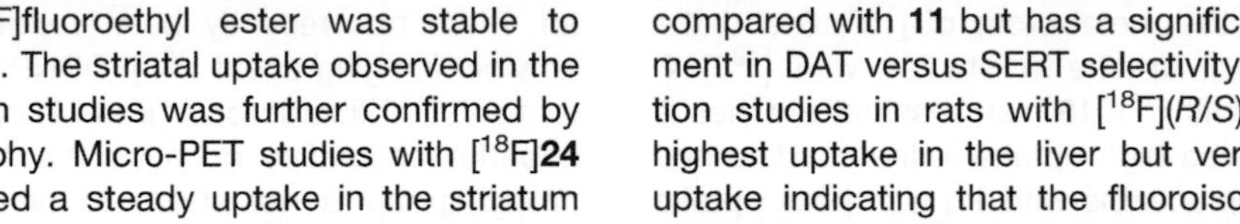

(R)-26 ((R)-FIPCT)   (S)-26 ((S)-FIPCT)   27 X = Me (FTT)
                                                     28 X = Cl (FCT)

Fig. 3. 3β-Phenyltropane–based DAT ligands.

[^{18}F](S)-**26** also reached peak uptake in the striatum at 30 minutes but at 60 minutes the striatum-to-cerebellum ratio was 11.8 and at 120 minutes it was 12.7. This higher uptake ratio for [^{18}F](S)-**26** compared with [^{18}F](R)-**26** is in agreement with the higher in vitro DAT binding affinity observed for [^{18}F](S)-**26**. PET imaging in rhesus monkeys with [^{18}F](R)-**26** and [^{18}F](S)-**26** showed that for [^{18}F](R)-**26** uptake peaked in the putamen and caudate around 45 minutes and remained nearly stable until the end of the study (115 minutes), whereas uptake of [^{18}F](S)-**26** was still increasing at 115 minutes when the study ended. At 115 minutes [^{18}F](R)-**26** had a putamen-to-cerebellum ratio of 3.5 and a caudate-to-cerebellum ratio of 2.5, whereas [^{18}F](S)-**26** had a putamen-to-cerebellum ratio of 2.5 and a caudate-to-cerebellum ratio of 2.5. Additionally, the cerebellum uptake washed out significantly faster for [^{18}F](R)-**26** than for [^{18}F](S)-**26**, which allowed [^{18}F](R)-**26** to achieve a transient equilibrium at 75 minutes. Metabolite analysis of rhesus monkey arterial plasma indicated that both [^{18}F](R)-**26** and [^{18}F](S)-**26** are metabolized to a non–ether-extractable polar compound but that [^{18}F](R)-**26** is metabolized more rapidly with 25% unmetabolized [^{18}F](R)-**26** remaining after 14 minutes but 30% unmetabolized [^{18}F](S)-**26** remaining after 30 minutes.

Other variations on the tropane structure have included the N-benzyl 2β-ethyl ketones **27** and **28**.[149] PET studies in rhesus monkeys with [^{18}F]**27** and [^{18}F]**28** demonstrated that both tracers reached peak uptake in the basal ganglia in approximately 20 minutes followed by a steady washout, indicating reversible binding. Compound [^{18}F]**28** was the superior of the two tracers with

a basal ganglia-to-cerebellum uptake ratio of 2.6 versus 1.5 for [^{18}F]**27**, presumably because of the higher affinity [^{18}F]**28** has for the DAT.[149] Both tracers were rapidly metabolized in a rhesus monkey with less than 30% [^{18}F]**27** remaining and less than 20% [^{18}F]**28** remaining after 20 minutes. Metabolite analysis of arterial plasma samples from both a rhesus monkey and rats showed that [^{18}F]**28** was metabolized to a lipophilic metabolite but this metabolite was not observed in rat whole brain samples indicating that the metabolite cannot cross the blood-brain barrier.

The N-(E)-fluorobutenyl tropanes **29–32 Fig. 4** have been previously reported.[150,151] Subsequently, the tolyl-derivative **33** was also reported.[152–156] Compounds **29–33** are the N-(E)-fluorobutenyl derivatives of **8–12**, respectively. The binding affinities of **29–32** are shown in and **Table 2**.[151] Compounds **31** and **32** have a high affinity at both the DAT and SERT with little or no selectivity, similar to what has been reported for **10** and **11**.[11,96,105,113,148] Compound **30** has a reduced affinity at the DAT and SERT relative to **31** and **32** without a significant improvement in selectivity. Compound **29** has a 10-fold lower affinity at the DAT than **32** along with a greatly reduced affinity at the SERT, which results in a significantly improved selectivity for the DAT over the SERT compared with **30** to **32**.

The PET imaging properties of [^{18}F]**29**, [^{18}F]**30** and [^{18}F]**31** have been evaluated in anesthetized cynomolgus monkeys with a microPET scanner.[157] The highest uptake of [^{18}F]**29** is seen in the putamen with peak uptake achieved after 25 minutes followed by a steady washout. Uptake in the caudate is also high but less than that seen in the putamen. This uptake in the caudate peaks

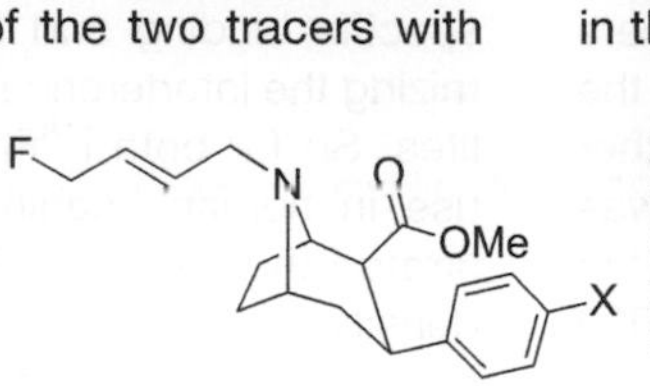

29 X = F (FBFNT)
30 X = Cl (FBClNT)
31 X = Br (FBBrNT)
32 X = I (FBINT)
33 X = Me (LBT-999)

Fig. 4. Structure of N-(E)-fluorobutenyl tropanes.

Table 2
Binding affinities of 29-32 at transfected human monoamine transporters

Compound	K_i (nM)			Selectivity	
	DAT	SERT	NET	SERT/DAT	NET/DAT
29	1.70	85.5	>10,000	50.3	>5882
30	2.54	24.2	>10,000	9.5	>3937
31	0.24	0.85	91	3.5	379
32	0.17	0.21	57	1.2	335

after approximately 30 minutes but then remains stable until approximately 100 minutes postinjection followed by only a slight washout. Uptake in the substantia nigra peaks after 10 minutes and then slowly washes out, whereas uptake in the cerebellum peaks after 10 minutes and rapidly washes out. Injection of the DAT ligand RTI-113[158–161] at 90 minutes postinjection completely displaces [^{18}F]29 from the caudate and the putamen. Compound [^{18}F]30 shows a rapid uptake in the putamen with peak uptake achieved after 20 minutes followed by only a slight washout. Uptake in the caudate increases rapidly for the first 20 minutes, then increases slowly for 20 to 90 minutes, and then remains level for 90 to 235 minutes. The uptake in the caudate is less than that observed in the putamen and remains less than in the putamen even after the slight washout of activity from the putamen. The uptake in the substantia nigra peaks after 15 minutes and then washes out at a slower rate than that observed for [^{18}F]29. Uptake of [^{18}F]31 in the putamen peaks after 30 minutes and only slightly washes out, whereas uptake in the caudate peaks after 30 minutes and then remains constant for 30 to 235 minutes. The initial uptake in the putamen was 1.5 times that observed in the caudate. Uptake in the substantia nigra peaked after 20 minutes and then washed out steadily but slower than that observed for [^{18}F]29. This rapid and high uptake of [^{18}F]30 and [^{18}F]31 in the putamen and the caudate followed by a lack of washout is similar to that reported for [^{11}C]33.[152,153,156]

Compounds [^{18}F]29, [^{18}F]30, [^{18}F]31, and [^{11}C]33 all show higher uptake in the putamen than in the caudate. It has been previously shown that anesthesia can influence the behavior of PET tracers and can cause trafficking of the DAT to the plasma membrane.[162–168] To evaluate whether the uptake observed for [^{18}F]29- [^{18}F]31 was influenced by the anesthesia used in the micro-PET studies a PET study with [^{18}F]29 was performed in an awake rhesus monkey on a high-resolution research tomograph.[157] The uptake of [^{18}F]29 in the caudate and putamen was equal in each hemisphere of the brain in the awake rhesus monkey, indicating that the higher uptake in the putamen relative to the caudate observed in the micro-PET studies with [^{18}F]29- [^{18}F]31 was most likely an anesthesia effect. This is presumably also the cause of the higher uptake observed in the putamen than in the caudate with [^{11}C]33 in an anesthetized baboon and the reported putamen-to-cerebellum and caudate-to-cerebellum uptake ratios of 30 and 24.6, respectively, in one study[152] and 28.9 and 23.6, respectively, in another

study.[153] The uptake of [^{18}F]29 in the putamen and the caudate of the awake rhesus monkey peaked at 30 minutes and then slowly washed out until the end of the study (85 minutes), whereas the uptake ratios peaked around 60 minutes and then began to decline. Thus, [^{18}F]29 is able to achieve peak uptake, reversible binding, and attain a transient equilibrium in an acceptable time frame while also achieving excellent uptake ratios versus cerebellum uptake in an awake state.

The micro-PET images obtained with [^{18}F]29-[^{18}F]31 and the PET images obtained with [^{18}F]29 all show skull uptake indicating defluorination of the [^{18}F]-(E)-fluorobutenyl group. To bypass this [^{18}F]-defluorination and eliminate bone uptake of [^{18}F]fluoride the authors are currently working toward radiolabeling [^{18}F]29 on the aromatic ring similar to what has been reported for [^{18}F]1-[^{18}F]4, [^{18}F]6, and [^{18}F]8. Skull uptake of [^{18}F]fluoride resulting from defluorination of [^{18}F]33 can be avoided by using [^{11}C]33 but both [^{18}F]33 and [^{11}C]33 presumably will still suffer from benzylic hydroxylation and the generation of radiolabeled metabolites similar to what has recently been reported for [^{11}C]PE2I.[139,147] It is expected that the size of the N-(E)-fluorobutenyl group will prevent enzymatic hydrolysis of the methyl ester similar to what has been previously reported.[147]

Extensive research over the past 20 years directed at developing fluorine-18 radiolabeled PET tracers for imaging the DAT has identified numerous potential candidates from the 3β-phenyl tropane class. The most promising are those that can achieve reversible binding and a transient equilibrium in a short time frame along with high specific binding and selectivity while also minimizing the interference from radiolabeled metabolites. So far both [^{18}F]16 and [^{18}F]18 have found use in human imaging and both have demonstrated their use in detecting a reduction of DAT density in human PD subjects. Both compounds, however, show a slower washout than may be desirable and both suffer from complications caused by metabolism. Compound [^{18}F]29 offers improved kinetics but it needs to be radiolabeled on the aromatic ring to avoid the skull uptake that results from defluorination of the [^{18}F]fluoro-butenyl group.

SEROTONIN TRANSPORTER

The human SERT is a 630–amino acid protein[6] that is 98.6% homologous to rhesus monkey SERT, 93% homologous to mouse SERT, and 90% homologous to rat SERT.[4,169] The SERT is found in high densities in the dorsal and median raphe nuclei, putamen, caudate, thalamus, hypothalamus, and amygdala, with lower levels in the cortex and still lower levels in the cerebellar cortex.[170–177] The serotonin system has been associated with numerous psychiatric conditions including PD,[178,179] obsessive-compulsive and panic disorders,[180] stress,[181] and depression and suicide.[182–184] A reduced density of SERT has been observed postmortem in depressed individuals and victims of suicide.[185–187] The SERT is the target of the selective serotonin reuptake inhibitor (SSRI) class of antidepressants.[111,112] The availability of specific and selective SERT PET tracers would allow for the measurement of SERT density in the brain and may allow for the detection and diagnosis of SERT-related psychiatric illness and a means of measuring SSRI occupancy and the monitoring of SSRI therapy.[16,188–192]

The SSRI fluoxetine 34 (Fig. 5)[193] has been radiolabeled with both [11]C[194] and [18]F.[195] In both cases the uptake of the tracer was characterized by nonspecific binding and high lipophilicity. A PET study with [18F]34 in rhesus monkeys showed uptake in all brain regions and an autoradiographic study in rats demonstrated irreversible binding caused by subcellular uptake of the tracer.

The antidepressant (+)-McN5652[196] 35 has been radiolabeled with ^{11}C and evaluated in rats and mice[197] and in humans.[198] In the human brain the uptake of [11C]35 in the midbrain reached a plateau after approximately 90 minutes but did not wash out before the end of the study (115 minutes), necessitating the need for the longer-lived [18]F. The fluorinated derivatives 36 and 37 were therefore prepared and evaluated. Ex vivo autoradiography with [18F]37 in mice showed accumulation in the hypothalamus, substantia nigra, and raphe nuclei but whole-brain uptake, specific binding, and tissue-to-cerebellum ratios were significantly less than that observed for [11C]35. Replacement of the methyl group of 35

with a fluoromethyl group to give 36 resulted in about a threefold loss in binding affinity at the SERT.[199] Biodistribution studies in rats with [18F]36 showed uptake in the raphe nuclei, substantia nigra, locus coeruleus, hypothalamus, thalamus, and amygdala, and this uptake could be blocked with 34.[200] The uptake in these regions washed out slower than cerebellum washout and this resulted in uptake ratios of 7 to 9 after 3 hours. High uptake was also observed in the adrenal gland, lung, intestine, spleen, kidney, liver, and bone marrow. A continuous increase of radioactivity in the skull indicated that [18F]36 was not stable to defluorination in rats. Additional studies with [18F]36 were performed in pigs.[201–203]

The fluorinated derivatives of 6-nitroquipazine,[204] 38 and 39, have been prepared and evaluated as possible SERT PET tracers.[205,206] In rats [18F]38 rapidly entered the brain and showed the highest accumulation in the frontal and posterial cortex followed by the striatum and this uptake could be reduced 10% to 20% with the SSRI citalopram.[111,112] Lesser uptake was observed in the thalamus but this uptake could be reduced 20% to 30% with citalopram. PET imaging in a monkey showed rapid uptake into the brain with a frontal cortex-to-cerebellum ratio of 1.53 and a striatum-to-cerebellum ratio of 1.25 at 80 minutes postinjection. The uptake in the thalamus was less than that observed in the cerebellum indicating that [18F]38 was not a good candidate for imaging the SERT. Biodistribution studies in mice with [18F]39 showed the highest uptake after 60 minutes in the frontal cortex and the lowest uptake in the cerebellum. High uptake was also observed in the olfactory tubercle, hypothalamus, thalamus, hippocampus, and striatum. Continuous bone uptake was also observed indicating a slow defluorination of the fluoropropyl group.

The diphenylsulfide 40 (Fig. 6) has been previously reported to be an inhibitor of the SERT and NET.[207,208] Numerous compounds have now

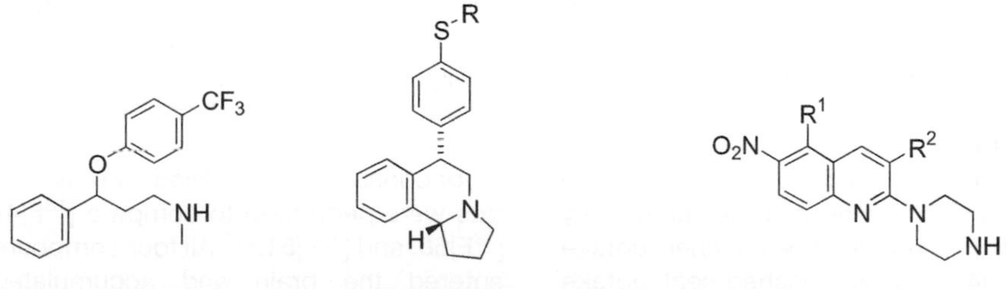

34 (Fluoxetine)

35 R = Me ((+)-McN5652)
36 R = CH₂F ((+)-FMe-McN5652)
37 R = CH₂CH₂F ((+)-FEt-McN5652)

38 R¹ = F, R² = H
39 R¹ = H, R² = CH₂CH₂CH₂F

Fig. 5. SERT ligands.

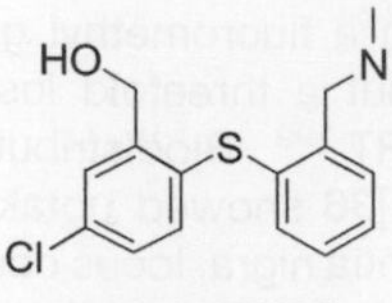

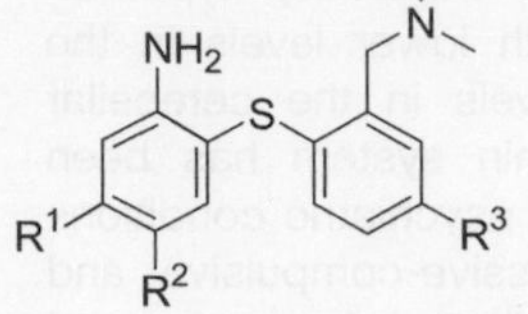

Fig. 6. Structure of diaryl sulfide–based SERT ligands.

Table 3
Compound numbering, substituent list, and binding affinities for the diaryl sulfide structure shown in Figure 6

Compound		R^1	R^2	R^3	K_i (nM)			Ref
					SERT	DAT	NET	
41	ADAM	I	H	H	0.013	840	699	221
42	DASB	CN	H	H	1.10	1423	1350	222
43	DAPP	OMe	H	H	1.89	2651	1992	222
44	DAPA	Br	H	H	0.38	N/A	N/A	209
45	HOMADAM	CH$_2$OH	H	H	0.57	>1000	144	210
46	EADAM	Et	H	H	0.17	>1000	367	211
47	AFA,	F	H	H	1.46	>10,000	141.7	212,213
	4-F-ADAM	F	H	H	0.08	2267	117	
48	—	CF$_3$	H	H	0.33	2038	1205	208
49	AFM	CH$_2$F	H	H	1.04	>10,000	664	214
50	AFE	CH$_2$CH$_2$F	H	H	1.80	>10,000	946	215
51	AFP	CH$_2$CH$_2$CH$_2$F	H	H	3.58	>10,000	505	216
52	5-F-ADAM	H	F	H	0.47	N/A	N/A	217
53	ACF	Cl	F	H	0.05	3020	650	218
54	—	H	H	OCH$_2$CH$_2$F	0.25	340	7.5	219
55	—	F	H	OCH$_2$CH$_2$F	0.10	>1000	37	219
56	—	Cl	H	OCH$_2$CH$_2$F	0.03	.847	97	219
57	—	Br	H	OCH$_2$CH$_2$F	0.05	>1000	114	219
58	—	H	H	OCH$_2$CH$_2$CH$_2$F	1.4	299	12	219
59	—	F	H	OCH$_2$CH$_2$CH$_2$F	0.95	>1000	95	219
60	—	Br	H	OCH$_2$CH$_2$CH$_2$F	0.15	>1000	>1000	219
61	—	CH$_2$OH	H	F	1.26	>2000	618	220

been reported that exploit the diphenylsulfide motif (**Fig. 6**, **Table 3**) to take advantage of its high binding affinity at the SERT and compounds **41** to **51** have been radiolabeled with [11]C.[209–212,214,215,221–224] Comparison of [11C]**35**, [11C]**41**, [11C]**42**, [11C]**44**, and [11C]**49** indicated that [11C]**42** had the fastest kinetics, whereas [11C]**49** had the highest signal-to-noise ratio.[209] Comparison between [11C]**42** and [11C]**45** in the same anesthetized rhesus monkey indicated that [11C]**45** achieved higher uptake ratios than [11C]**42** and also reached peak uptake faster.[210] Both [11C]**42** and [11C]**45** have been used in humans[225–227] and both have demonstrated that they are valuable tracers for imaging the SERT with PET, but both are ^{11}C-labeled and

are still limited to use where they are prepared and to imaging sessions of less than 2 hours.

Compounds **47**, **49**, and **50** all have a high affinity for the SERT and are selective for the SERT over the DAT and NET. Compound **51** has a slightly reduced SERT affinity but still shows selectivity over the DAT and NET.[216] Compounds [11C]**47**, [11C]**49**, and [11C]**50** have been evaluated in baboons.[212,214,215] Biodistribution studies in rats were performed to compare [18F]**47**, [18F]**49**, [18F]**50**, and [18F]**51**.[216] All four compounds rapidly entered the brain and accumulated in the thalamus, hypothalamus, frontal cortex, striatum, and hippocampus. This uptake could be blocked with citalopram, demonstrating SERT-specific binding. Compound [18F]**49** reached peak uptake after 30 minutes followed by washout and this uptake was the highest among the four tracers. Compounds [^{18}F]**47**, [^{18}F]**50**, and [^{18}F]**51** all reached peak uptake after 10 minutes followed by washout, whereas the highest uptake observed was with [^{18}F]**47**. PET imaging comparisons in the same baboon with [^{18}F]**47**, [^{18}F]**49**, and [^{18}F]**50** showed that [^{18}F]**47** and [^{18}F]**50** reached peak uptake in the thalamus in 15 to 35 minutes, whereas [^{18}F]**49** reached peak uptake in 40 to 60 minutes but showed significantly higher specific binding.[228] Another reported biodistribution study in rats with [^{18}F]**47** had shown peak uptake at 30 minutes followed by washout.[213] This study also showed that [^{18}F]**47** accumulated rapidly in the muscle, lung, liver, and kidney but then cleared, whereas bone uptake continuously increased indicating that, at least in rats, defluorination was a problem. In a PET study with [^{18}F]**47** in a baboon the radioactivity in the skull did not increase with time suggesting that defluorination was isolated to rats.[213] In this PET study peak uptake in the midbrain and striatum was reached in approximately 30 to 40 minutes with midbrain-to-cerebellum ratios of 3.2 at 2 hours and 4.2 at 3 hours and striatum-to-cerebellum ratios of 2.4 at 2 hours and 2.7 at 3 hours.

Compound **52** is an isomer of **47** where the fluorine atom has been moved from the 4-position (*para* to the sulfur atom) to the 5-position (*meta* to the sulfur atom). This change resulted in a significant loss in affinity for the SERT[217] compared with **47**[213] and a slight decrease in lipophilicity ($\log P = 2.47$ versus 2.73). Biodistribution studies in rats with [^{18}F]**52** showed an initial high uptake in the lungs, kidneys, and heart but this cleared quickly, whereas bone uptake continued to increase indicating defluorination.[229] Brain uptake was rapid with peak uptake at 2 minutes followed by a fast washout. The hypothalamus-to-cerebellum ratio was 2.97 at 60 minutes, which is less than that observed with [^{18}F]**47**. Thus, changing the position of the fluorine-atom did not produce an improvement in imaging properties compared with [^{18}F]**47**.

Compound **53** retains the fluorine atom in the 5-position and places a chlorine atom in the 4-position, which produced a compound with a high SERT affinity and selectivity.[218] Biodistribution studies with [^{18}F]**53** in rats showed initial high accumulation in lung, muscle, liver, kidney, and skin, which then declined.[218] Bone uptake was slightly less than that observed with [^{18}F]**52**[229] and significantly less than that observed with [^{18}F]**47**.[213] Brain uptake of [^{18}F]**53** was rapid with the highest uptake observed at 2 minutes followed by washout. At 60 minutes the hypothalamus-to-cerebellum ratio was 3.5 (compared with 3 for [^{18}F]**52**) and the

striatum-to-cerebellum ratio was 2.9. Thus, [^{18}F]**52** and [^{18}F]**53** behave similarly in rats with regards to uptake ratios and defluorination but both have too rapid of kinetics when compared with [^{18}F]**47**.

The fluoroalkyl ethers **54** to **60** have a high affinity for the SERT but **54** and **58** also have an appreciable affinity for the NET,[219] which may cause interference in PET imaging if the cerebellum was to be used as the reference region. In rat biodistribution studies [^{18}F]**55** to [^{18}F]**57**, [^{18}F]**59**, and [^{18}F]**60** showed high brain uptake but slow washout, whereas [^{18}F]**54** and [^{18}F]**58** also showed high brain uptake but a faster washout. Of compounds [^{18}F]**54** to [^{18}F]**60**, the highest hypothalamus-to-cerebellum ratios were observed with [^{18}F]**54** and [^{18}F]**58** (approximately 7.8 and approximately 7.7, respectively, at 120 minutes) because of the faster washout of these compounds.[219] Additional rat biodistribution studies with [^{18}F]**58** showed initial high uptake in the lung, skin, muscle, liver, and kidney, which then slowly declined.[230] Bone uptake was high and remained high indicating defluorination. Brain uptake was rapid followed by a steady washout. Autoradiography showed uptake in the olfactory tubercles, thalamic nuclei, hypothalamic nuclei, substantia nigra, superior colliculus, dorsal raphe, medial raphe, and locus coeruleus, all of which could be blocked with the SSRI escitalopram[231,232] except for the locus coeruleus, which could be blocked with the NET ligand nisoxetine.[233,234] Some NET binding in the locus coeruleus is observed in conjunction with the desired binding in the SERT-rich brain regions when performing autoradiography but uptake in the cerebellum was not observed in the rat when PET imaging was performed with [^{18}F]**58**, which allows for use of the cerebellum as the reference region. In the rat PET images obtained with [^{18}F]**58**, clear localization was observed in the thalamus, midbrain, and striatum with peak uptake achieved in 10 to 20 minutes followed by a steady washout.[230] The region-to-cerebellum ratios peaked at 100 to 110 minutes with a value of approximately 4 followed by a slow decline. The uptake in the midbrain, thalamus, and striatum could be displaced by escitalopram (2 mg/kg) but also, to a lesser extent, by nisoxetine (10 mg/kg). A similar displacement of the SERT PET tracer [^{11}C]*m*ZIENT during a chase study with the NET ligand (±)-reboxetine·mesylate (1 mg/kg) has also been observed.[235] Both nisoxetine and reboxetine[236] have a weak affinity for the SERT ($K_i = 30$ and 60 nM, respectively) but are selective for the NET over the SERT (21.4 and 6.7, respectively).[237] This weak binding to the

SERT may be the cause of the observed displacement of these two tracers but alternatively, the displacement may be an indirect effect mediated through interactions between the noradrenergic and serotonergic systems.[238–240]

Compound **61** is a fluorinated derivative of **45**.[220] Introduction of the fluorine atom resulted in a slight reduction in SERT affinity but also a reduction in DAT and NET affinity, which produced similar selectivities for the SERT over the DAT and NET. The presence of the fluorine atom also increased the lipophilicity somewhat ($\log P_{7.4}$ = 2.06 and 1.60, respectively). Micro-PET imaging with [^{11}C]**61** in an anesthetized cynomolgus monkey showed high uptake in the midbrain, pons, thalamus, and medulla with little uptake in the frontal cortex and cerebellum. No uptake was observed in the caudate or putamen, which is surprising because this brain region does contain SERT.[177] Peak uptake of [^{11}C]**61** in the midbrain occurred between 12.5 and 27.5 minutes postinjection followed by a steady washout. At 85 minutes the midbrain-to-cerebellum ratio was 3.4 and the thalamus-to-cerebellum ratio was 2.3. The observed uptake was displaceable with (R/S)-citalopram•HBr demonstrating SERT-selective binding. These promising results suggest that [^{18}F]**61** may be a viable SERT PET tracer.

Replacement of one of the N-methyl groups of **41** with a fluoroethyl group resulted in a significant loss of SERT affinity (K_i = approximately 19 nM versus 0.4 nM for **41**)[241] indicating that functionalizing this position was detrimental to binding. Nevertheless, the para-fluorobenzyl derivatives **62** (SERT K_i = approximately 4 nM) and **63** (SERT K_i = approximately 510 nM) were prepared and evaluated (**Fig. 7**).[242] As seen from the SERT binding affinities the large p-fluorobenzyl group can be tolerated to a certain extent if the nitrogen atom is substituted secondarily (**62**) but replacement of the hydrogen atom with a methyl group (**63**) completely abolished any affinity for the SERT. Biodistribution studies in rats with [^{18}F]**63**

showed low brain uptake and low selectivity in SERT-rich brain regions. Placement of the p-fluorobenzyl group on the anilino-nitrogen (**64**) produced a compound with moderate SERT affinity (K_i = approximately 10 nM) and replacement of the p-fluorobenzyl group with a p-fluorobenzoyl group (**65**) further reduced the SERT affinity (K_i = approximately 14 nM).[243]

During the search for tropane-based cocaine addiction therapeutics it was discovered that removal of the N-methyl group of a tropane to give a nortropane produced compounds with enhanced SERT and NET affinity.[244] Numerous compounds have been prepared to obtain SERT-selective nortropane derivatives[245–251] and several have been radiolabeled with ^{11}C.[235,252–255] The fluoroethyl ester nortropanes **66** and **67** (**Fig. 8**) have been reported but, similar to **11**, the affinities for the SERT and DAT were nearly equal.[144]

The results of micro-PET and high-resolution research tomograph PET imaging in monkeys with the meta- and para-vinyl iodides [^{18}F]**68** and [^{18}F]**69**, respectively, have recently been reported.[256,257] Both **68** and **69** have a high affinity for the SERT (K_i = 0.43 and 0.08 nM, respectively) but substitution in the para-position provides about a fivefold higher affinity. These differences in binding affinity to the SERT translate into significant differences in the imaging behavior of the compounds. Micro-PET imaging with [^{18}F]**68** and [^{18}F]**69** was performed in anesthetized cynomolgus monkeys (**Fig. 9**) and PET imaging on a high-resolution research tomograph with [^{18}F]**68** and [^{18}F]**69** was performed in an awake rhesus monkey (**Fig. 10**). The time required to reach peak uptake is significantly different for the two isomers with the stronger binding para-isomer [^{18}F]**69** taking longer to reach peak uptake. Also, the times required for each tracer to reach peak uptake are about the same in both the anesthetized and awake states indicating that anesthesia does not significantly affect the performance of these tracers. After reaching peak uptake the activity of [^{18}F]**68** in the midbrain, putamen, thalamus, medulla, and

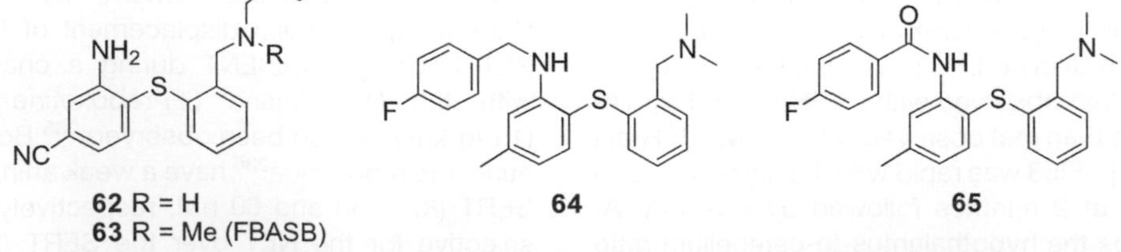

62 R = H
63 R = Me (FBASB)

64

65

Fig. 7. Diaryl sulfide–based SERT ligands.

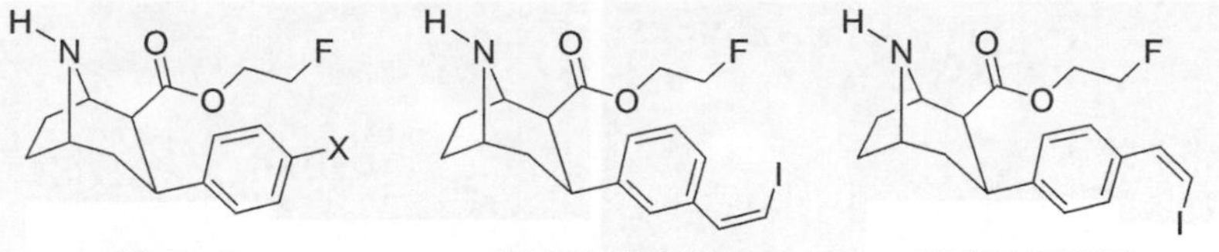

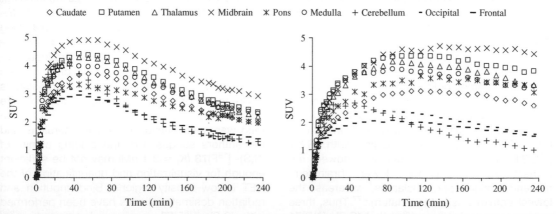

66 X = Br
67 X = I

68 (FE*m*ZIENT)

69 (FE*p*ZIENT)

Fig. 8. Fluoroethyl ester nortropane–based SERT ligands.

caudate remains nearly steady for about 20 minutes followed by a constant washout during which time (65–175 minutes postinjection) a pseudoequilibrium is achieved. Compound [18F]**69** takes significantly longer to reach peak uptake in the SERT-rich brain regions and then only slightly washes out. The uptake of [18F]**69** in the cerebellum reaches peak uptake after 45 minutes followed by a steady washout, which provides ever increasing tissue-to-cerebellum ratios as the study progresses. Because the washout of [18F]**68** from the SERT-rich brain regions is nearly parallel to the washout from the cerebellum the tissue-to-cerebellum ratios for [18F]**68** slowly increase throughout the course of the study. Thus, [18F]**68** provides superior imaging kinetics and achieves a pseudoequilibrium, whereas [18F]**69** provides higher uptake ratios. Both of the tracers can be displaced with citalopram but the observed displacement is significantly greater for [18F]**69** because of the minor washout that occurs (under baseline conditions) after peak uptake is achieved, which results in only slightly declining time-activity curves. When a citalopram chase is then performed the slope of the time-activity curves of [18F]**69** changes drastically. Each of these tracers is a promising candidate for human use because each has its own unique imaging properties.

Compound [18F]**68** can be used for kinetic analysis because of its ability to achieve a pseudoequilibrium, whereas compound [18F]**69** can be used for SSRI occupancy studies because of the large change in slope of the time-activity curves that occurs when an SSRI is administered.

The goal of developing an 18F-radiolabeled PET tracer for imaging the SERT has benefited from the availability of high affinity and selective compounds from both the diphenylsulfide and nortropane classes. Compounds [11C]**42** and [11C]**45** have both demonstrated their use in imaging normal human volunteers but the adaptation of these compounds to 18F-labeled tracers has so far proved difficult. The 18F-labeled nortropanes [18F]**68** and [18F]**69** have been shown to have improved kinetics relative to their 11C-labeled counterparts, [11C]*m*ZIENT[235] and [11C]*p*ZIENT,[255] respectively, and the authors look forward to evaluating [18F]**68** and [18F]**69** in healthy human volunteers.

NOREPINEPHRINE TRANSPORTER

The human NET is a 617–amino acid transmembrane protein and is 98.9% homologous to the monkey NET.[4,174,258] The NET is found in high densities in the locus coeruleus, cerebellum,

◇ Caudate   □ Putamen   △ Thalamus   ✕ Midbrain   ✳ Pons   ○ Medulla   + Cerebellum   - Occipital   — Frontal

Fig. 9. Micro-PET time-activity curves obtained by injection of [18F]**68** (*left*) and [18F]**69** (*right*) into anesthetized cynomolgus monkeys.

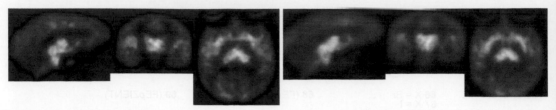

Fig. 10. High-resolution research tomograph PET images obtained by injection of [^{18}F]**68** (*left*) and [^{18}F]**69** (*right*) into an awake rhesus monkey.

dorsal raphe nuclei, thalamus, and hypothalamus.[233,234,239,259,260] The norepinephrine system has been associated with a variety of neuropsychiatric diseases including PD,[261] attention-deficit–hyperactivity disorder,[262,263] posttraumatic stress disorder,[264] depression and anxiety,[240,265–267] and seizure,[268] and a reduction in NET density has been demonstrated postmortem in depressed subjects.[269] The availability of specific and selective NET PET imaging agents allows for density measurements of the NET and may help to clarify the role of the NET in certain psychiatric diseases and help to identify and evaluate NET therapeutics.[270–272]

The antidepressant reboxetine **70 (Fig. 11, Table 4)** is a selective norepinephrine reuptake inhibitor that is marketed as the racemic mixture.[236,273,274] The ethyl group of **70** has been replaced with a [^{11}C]methyl group to give [^{11}C]**71** and PET imaging comparisons in baboon between *racemic*- [^{11}C]**71**, (*S,S*)- [^{11}C]**71**, and (*R,R*)- [^{11}C]**71** has shown that (*S,S*)- [^{11}C]**71** is the active isomer based on a significantly higher distribution volume in the thalamus and the ability to block the uptake of (*S,S*)- [^{11}C]**71**, but not (*R,R*)- [^{11}C]**71**, in the thalamus and cerebellum with nisoxetine.[275] The uptake of (*S,S*)- [^{11}C]**71** in the striatum could not be blocked with nisoxetine, demonstrating either low-affinity binding or nonspecific binding in this brain region. In biodistribution studies in rats (*S,S*)- [^{11}C]**71** showed a hypothalamus-to-striatum ratio of 2.5 at 60 minutes postinjection, whereas (*R,R*)- [^{11}C]**71** showed only a homogenous distribution.[276] Plasma analysis indicated that (*S,S*)- [^{11}C]**71** was metabolized rapidly in the periphery with 50% unmetabolized radiotracer remaining after 30 minutes and 20% remaining after 60 minutes but whole rat brain extracts showed that 95% of radioactivity in the brain was unmetabolized (*S,S*)- [^{11}C]**71**. PET imaging with (*S,S*)- [^{11}C]**71** in cynomolgus monkeys showed the highest uptake in the lower brainstem, mesencephalon, and thalamus, whereas the lowest uptake was in the striatum.[277] Thus, three groups independently verified that (*S,S*)- [^{11}C]**71** could be used to image the NET in vivo with

PET, although specific peak binding equilibrium is not achieved during the course of these studies. Based on these results fluoroalkyl ether derivatives of reboxetine have been developed in pursuit of an ^{18}F-labeled NET PET tracer, which would enable longer imaging times and possibly the achievement of peak specific binding equilibrium.

Compound (*S,S*)- [^{18}F]**72** is a fluorinated derivative of (*S,S*)- [^{11}C]**71** but PET imaging in a cynomolgus monkey with (*S,S*)- [^{18}F]**72** showed rapid defluorination and skull uptake. The deuterated derivative (*S,S*)- [^{18}F]**73** was developed and PET imaging showed that defluorination was reduced but not totally inhibited.[278] During PET imaging the total brain uptake of (*S,S*)- [^{18}F]**72** peaked at 8 minutes and then washed out, whereas total brain uptake of (*S,S*)- [^{18}F]**73** peaked at 12 minutes and then washed out. The uptake of both (*S,S*)- [^{18}F]**72** and (*S,S*)- [^{18}F]**73** could be blocked with desipramine but blocking with **1** or citalopram did not have any effect on the uptake of either tracer. At 110 minutes after injection of (*S,S*)- [^{18}F]**72** the tissue-to-striatum ratios were 1.2, 1.2, and 1.3 for the lower brainstem, mesencephalon, and thalamus, respectively. At 160 minutes after injection of (*S,S*)- [^{18}F]**73** the tissue-to-striatum ratios were 1.5, 1.6, 1.3, and 1.5 for the lower brainstem, mesencephalon, thalamus, and temporal cortex, respectively. Peak specific binding was achieved at 90 to 120 minutes for (*S,S*)- [^{18}F]**72** and at 120 to 160 minutes for (*S,S*)- [^{18}F]**73**. Autoradiography with (*S,S*)- [^{18}F]**73** using postmortem human brain slices showed the highest accumulation of radioactivity in the locus coeruleus with lower accumulation in the cerebellum, cortex, thalamus, and hypothalamus along with nonspecific binding in the caudate nucleus and putamen.[279] A low signal-to-noise ratio was seen outside the locus coeruleus and the authors suggest that the binding affinity of (*S,S*)- [^{18}F]**73** (K_i = 3.1 nM) may not be sufficient enough for visualization and quantification of the NET in low-density regions. Biodistribution and radiation dosimetry studies have been performed with (*S,S*)- [^{18}F]**73** in cynomolgus monkeys[280] and humans[281] and (*S,S*)- [^{18}F]**73** has been used

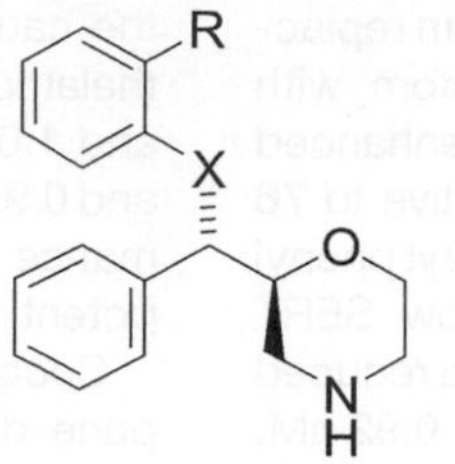

Fig. 11. Structure of (S,S)-Reboxetine derivative–based NET ligands.

Table 4
Compound numbering and substituent list for the (S,S)-Reboxetine derivative structure shown in Figure 11.

Compound		X =	R =
70	Reboxetine	O	OCH_2CH_3
71	MeNER	O	OCH_3
72	FMeNER	O	OCH_2F
73	FMeNER-D_2	O	OCD_2F
74	FERB	O	OCH_2CH_2F
75	FERB-D_2	O	OCD_2CD_2F
76	MENET	O	CH_3
77	MESNET	S	CH_3
78	FENET	O	CH_2CH_2F
79	FPNET	O	$CH_2CH_2CH_2F$
80	—	S	OCH_2CH_2F
81	—	S	$OCH_2CH_2CH_2F$

to measure the occupancy of the selective norepinephrine reuptake inhibitor atomoxetine.[282] Initial human imaging studies with (S,S)- [^{18}F]**73** have recently been reported.[283] Using four healthy male subjects the mean peak uptake in the whole brain was 2.6 ± 0.5% at 12.5 minutes after injection. Uptake in the thalamus achieved peak equilibrium with a thalamus-to-caudate ratio of 1.5. Cortical uptake was high because of high skull uptake resulting from defluorination. (S,S)-[^{18}F]**73** is a promising PET tracer for imaging the NET in humans but the inability totally to stop defluorination suggests that further structural improvements are still needed.

Compound **74** is a fluorinated derivative of **70** and compound **75** is the deuterated analog of **74**, the deuteration strategy again being used to inhibit defluorination.[284] Biodistribution studies in mice with (S,S)- [^{18}F]**74** and (S,S)- [^{18}F]**75** showed high accumulation of both tracers in the kidneys, liver, and intestines. Brain uptake was moderate and washout was slow for both (S,S)- [^{18}F]**74** and (S,S)- [^{18}F]**75**. At 2 hours postinjection the average bone uptake of (S,S)- [^{18}F]**74** was 0.83% ID/g and that of (S,S)- [^{18}F]**75** was 0.25% ID/g

demonstrating a reduction of defluorination by the deuterium isotope effect. A PET imaging comparison in baboons with (S,S)- [^{11}C]**71** and (S,S)- [^{18}F]**75** (along with several other ^{11}C-labeled NET ligands) determined that (S,S)- [^{11}C]**71** still has the best PET imaging characteristics of the prospective NET PET tracers available at that time because of the higher signal-to-noise ratio obtained with (S,S)- [^{11}C]**71** and its faster washout from the striatum.[271,285]

Compounds **76** to **81** have recently been developed as potential NET PET tracers.[286,287] Compounds **76** to **79** have directly connected the alkyl group to the aryl ring thereby eliminating the phenyl alkyl ether functionality and possibly enhancing the metabolic stability of the radiolabel. Compounds **77**, **80**, and **81** have incorporated a sulfur atom in replacement of the benzyl phenyl ether oxygen atom. Compounds **76** and **77** each have a high affinity for the NET (K_i = 1.02 ± 0.11 and 0.30 ± 0.03 nM, respectively), which is very similar to the NET affinity of **70** (K_i = 1.04 ± 0.16 nM) and **71** (0.95 ± 0.03 nM).[287] Thus, the phenyl methyl ether oxygen atom is not an important determinant of binding affinity at the NET and a slight enhancement in affinity results from replacing the benzyl phenyl ether oxygen atom with a sulfur atom. Compound **77** has an enhanced SERT affinity ($K_i = 14.8 \pm 2.83$ nM) relative to **76** ($K_i = 93 \pm 20$ nM) indicating that the benzyl phenyl ether oxygen atom is necessary for low SERT affinity. Compounds **78** and **79** each had a reduced NET affinity ($K_i = 3.14 \pm 0.17$ and 3.68 ± 0.92 nM, respectively) compared with **76** indicating that larger alkyl groups, or fluorine substitution, or both, is detrimental to the NET affinity of this series of compounds. Micro-PET imaging with [^{11}C]**76** in an anesthetized rhesus monkey showed peak uptake around 20 minutes followed by a steady washout with tissue-to-caudate ratios of 1.30, 1.45, 1.40, and 1.30 at 45 minutes postinjection and 1.30, 1.43, 1.44, and 1.25 at 85 minutes postinjection for the thalamus, midbrain, pons, and cerebellum, respectively, indicating that a quasi-equilibrium had been achieved. Micro-PET imaging with [^{11}C]**77** in an anesthetized rhesus monkey showed peak uptake around 30 to 40 minutes followed by a steady washout (but slower than that of [^{11}C]**76**) with a thalamus-to-caudate ratio of 1.34 and a midbrain-to-caudate ratio of 1.33 at 85 minutes postinjection. Because of the moderate affinity **77** has for the SERT, a chase study was performed with (R,S)-citalopram · HBr (1.5 mg/kg) at 40 minutes postinjection. The uptake of radioactivity in the caudate did not change indicating that this uptake was most likely the result of nonspecific binding rather than SERT binding. PET imaging on a high-resolution research tomograph was performed in awake rhesus monkeys with [^{11}C]**76** and [^{11}C]**77** to assess the effects of anesthesia on the performance of these tracers. With [^{11}C]**76** high uptake was observed in the thalamus, locus coeruleus, midbrain, and pons and the kinetics were very similar to that observed in the micro-PET study with an anesthetized rhesus monkey but the tissue-to-caudate ratios were slightly reduced in the awake state. Compound [^{11}C]**77**, however, showed significantly different kinetics than that observed in the micro-PET study with an anesthetized rhesus monkey with prolonged retention observed over the course of the study and very little washout. The tissue-to-caudate ratios were also slightly reduced in the awake state. It is known that the anesthetic ketamine (which is used initially to anesthetize the animal before administration of isoflurane) binds to the NET[288] and this may be the cause of the differences observed between the anesthetized and awake states. In micro-PET studies with [^{18}F]**78** and [^{18}F]**79** in anesthetized rhesus monkeys peak uptake was achieved in all regions of interest after 15 minutes followed by a fast washout. High uptake was also observed in the caudate with tissue-to-caudate ratios for the thalamus, midbrain, and cerebellum of 1.13, 1.13, and 1.05, respectively, for [^{18}F]**78** and 1.18, 1.18, and 0.95, respectively, for [^{18}F]**79**. Thus, the performance of [^{18}F]**78** and [^{18}F]**79** eliminates them as potential ^{18}F-labeled NET PET tracers.

Cocaine binds to the NET and numerous tropane derivatives have been reported as ligands for the NET.[289–294] Preliminary micro-PET evaluation of a ^{11}C-labeled NET tropane derivative showed both SERT and NET binding and a lack of NET selectivity.[295] The NET ligands talopram[296] and talsupram have been radiolabeled with ^{11}C and evaluated with PET but neither compound entered the brain in sufficient amounts to become a viable PET tracer.[297]

The goal of developing an ^{18}F-labeled PET tracer for the NET is still a work-in-progress but progress is indeed being made. The results with reboxetine derivatives demonstrate that some minor structural variation can be tolerated without a significant loss in NET affinity but it seems that placing an ^{18}F-radiolabel on the methoxy or ethoxy group does reduce the NET affinity. A similar loss in affinity was observed when going from **35** to **36**. Furthermore, defluorination also is a problem that can only be reduced, but not stopped, by incorporation of deuterium into these fluoroalkoxy groups. Defluorination was also observed with [^{18}F]**36**, which in combination with the ^{18}F-NET ligand data mentioned previously, suggests that radiolabeling with [^{18}F]methyl and [^{18}F]ethyl ethers and thioethers should be avoided if at all possible. The development of a reboxetine-based ^{18}F-labeled PET tracer for the NET may require that the ^{18}F-radiolabel be placed on one of the aromatic rings.

SUMMARY

Progress is being made toward the development of fluorine-18 radiolabeled PET tracers for the DAT, SERT, and NET. The greatest number of potential tracers developed so far has been for the DAT due to the greater number of years that have been devoted to this target but also due in part to the concurrent research effort focused on developing a cocaine addiction therapeutic based on the tropane skeleton. The development of a library of potential therapeutic tropane compounds with high DAT affinity that could be radiolabeled with ^{11}C aided in the discovery of PET tracers for the DAT and the SERT, and this knowledge was then successfully translated to ^{18}F-labeled tropane derivatives for both the DAT and SERT. The diphenylsulfide class of SERT ligands has already found success with ^{11}C-labeled PET tracers and a viable

[18]F-labeled PET tracer may soon be realized. Fewer tracers for the NET have been reported because PET imaging of the NET has received considerable less attention than the DAT or SERT but promising, although not optimal, compounds have already been reported. Further work toward this goal should also eventually provide a viable ^{18}F-labeled NET PET tracer.

It is very difficult to predict if a proposed compound will have the desired properties of a PET tracer and so numerous compounds generally have to be synthesized and evaluated. As demonstrated with [^{18}F]1- [^{18}F]4, [^{18}F]34, and [^{11}C]35, radiolabeling an antidepressant does not necessarily produce a good PET tracer. Derivatives of antidepressants may produce candidate PET tracers, however, as evidenced by the derivatives of **40** shown in **Fig. 6** and **Table 3** and the derivatives of **70** shown in **Fig. 11** and **Table 4**. High binding affinity to the target and selectivity for that target are the first requirements that need to be met and any compound that cannot meet these requirements will most likely not succeed. Compounds with a high binding affinity and selectivity must also have lipophilicity in the range of $\log P$ = approximately 1 to 3 or they will also fail. Furthermore, compounds that seem to have the appropriate affinity, selectivity, and lipophilicity can still fail because of poor kinetics or problems resulting from metabolism. The development of suitable PET tracers for the DAT, SERT, and NET is not an easy task, but with continued hard work by many research groups the goal will eventually be realized. It should be possible to develop more than one tracer for each target and, as shown above, this has already been done. Which of the available tracers is the "best" would then have to be determined from side-by-side comparisons in the same subject under the same conditions (preferably in a conscious state) while taking into consideration the influence of metabolites that are generated from each individual tracer. This has already been done with many of the tracers reported above and this should continue to be done as part of tracer development. Because the goals of different studies of the same target may vary, the availability of several different tracers with slightly different properties may be of greater benefit to the PET imaging community than having only one "best" tracer for a given target.

REFERENCES

1. Rudnick G, Clark J. From synapse to vesicle: the reuptake and storage of biogenic amine neurotransmitters. Biochim Biophys Acta 1993; 1144:249–63.
2. Nelson N. The family of Na+/Cl− neurotransmitter transporters. J Neurochem 1998;71:1785–803.
3. Eisenhofer G. The role of neuronal and extraneuronal plasma membrane transporters in the inactivation of peripheral catecholamines. Pharmacol Ther 2001;91:35–62.
4. Miller GM, Yatin SM, De La Garza R, et al. Cloning of dopamine, norepinephrine and serotonin transporters from monkey brain: relevance to cocaine sensitivity. Brain Res Mol Brain Res 2001;87: 124–43.
5. Gainetdinov RR, Caron MG. Monoamine transporters: from genes to behavior. Annu Rev Pharmacol Toxicol 2003;43:261–84.
6. Torres GE, Gainetdinov RR, Caron MG. Plasma membrane monoamine transporters: structure, regulation and function. Nat Rev Neurosci 2003;4:13–25.
7. Lester HA, Cao Y, Mager S. Listening to neurotransmitter transporters. Neuron 1996;17:807–10.
8. Melikian HE. Neurotransmitter transporter trafficking: endocytosis, recycling, and regulation. Pharmacol Ther 2004;104:17–27.
9. Iversen L. Neurotransmitter transporters: fruitful targets for CNS drug discovery. Mol Psychiatry 2000;5:357–62.
10. Carroll FI, Howell LL, Kuhar MJ. Pharmacotherapies for treatment of cocaine abuse: preclinical aspects. J Med Chem 1999;42:2721–36.
11. Carroll FI. 2002 Medicinal Chemistry Division award address: monoamine transporters and opioid receptors. Targets for addiction therapy. J Med Chem 2003;46:1775–94.
12. Volkow ND, Fowler JS, Gatley SJ, et al. PET evaluation of the dopamine system of the human brain. J Nucl Med 1996;37:1242–56.
13. Laakso A, Hietala J. PET studies of brain monoamine transporters. Curr Pharm Des 2000;6: 1611–23.
14. Jaffer FA, Weissleder R. Molecular imaging in the clinical arena. J Am Med Assoc 2005;293:855–62.
15. Hammoud DA, Hoffman JM, Pomper MG. Molecular neuroimaging: from conventional to emerging techniques. Radiology 2007;245:21–42.
16. Meyer JH. Imaging the serotonin transporter during major depressive disorder and antidepressant treatment. J Psychiatry Neurosci 2007;32:86–102.
17. Brooks DJ. Neuroimaging in Parkinson's disease. NeuroRx 2004;1:243–54.
18. Aboagye EO, Price PM, Jones T. In vivo pharmacokinetics and pharmacodynamics in drug development using positron-emission tomography. Drug Discov Today 2001;6:293–302.
19. Laruelle M, Slifstein M, Huang Y. Positron emission tomography: imaging and quantification of

neurotransporter availability. Methods 2002;27: 287–99.

20. Talbot PS, Laruelle M. The role of in vivo molecular imaging with PET and SPECT in the elucidation of psychiatric drug action and new drug development. Eur Neuropsychopharmacol 2002;12:503–11.

21. Guilloteau D, Chalon S. PET and SPECT exploration of central monoaminergic transporters for the development of new drugs and treatments in brain disorders. Curr Pharm Des 2005;11:3237–45.

22. Lee CM, Farde L. Using positron emission tomography to facilitate CNS drug development. Trends Pharmacol Sci 2006;27:310–6.

23. Hargreaves RJ. The role of molecular imaging in drug discovery and development. Clin Pharmacol Ther 2008;83:349–53.

24. Takano A, Suzuki K, Kosaka J, et al. A dose-finding study of duloxetine based on serotonin transporter occupancy. Psychopharmacology 2006;185:395–9.

25. Schlyer DJ. PET tracers and radiochemistry. Ann Acad Med Singap 2004;33:146–54.

26. Ametamey SM, Honer M, Schubiger PA. Molecular imaging with PET. Chem Rev 2008;108:1501–16.

27. Miller PW, Long NJ, Vilar R, et al. Synthesis of ^{11}C, ^{18}F, ^{15}O, and ^{13}N radiolabels for positron emission tomography. Angew Chem Int Ed Engl 2008;47:8998–9033.

28. Wernick MN, Aarsvold JN, editors. Emission tomography: the fundamentals of PET and SPECT. San Diego (CA); London, UK: Elsevier Academic Press; 2004. p. 179.

29. Levin CS, Hoffman EJ. Calculation of positron range and its effect on the fundamental limit of positron emission tomography system spatial resolution. Phys Med Biol 1999;44:781–99.

30. Smart BE. Fluorine substituent effects (on bioactivity). J Fluor Chem 2001;109:3–11.

31. Böhm HJ, Banner D, Bendels S, et al. Fluorine in medicinal chemistry. Chembiochem 2004;5:637–43.

32. DiMagno SG, Sun H. The strength of weak interactions: aromatic fluorine in drug design. Curr Top Med Chem 2006;6:1473–82.

33. Schweizer E, Hoffmann-Röder A, Schärer K, et al. A fluorine scan at the catalytic center of thrombin: C-F, C-OH, and C-OMe bioisosterism and fluorine effects on pK_a and log D values. ChemMedChem 2006;1:611–21.

34. Sun S, Adejare A. Fluorinated molecules as drugs and imaging agents in the CNS. Curr Top Med Chem 2006;6:1457–64.

35. Müller K, Faeh C, Diederich F. Fluorine in pharmaceuticals: looking beyond intuition. Science 2007; 317:1881–6.

36. Hagmann WK. The many roles for fluorine in medicinal chemistry. J Med Chem 2008;51:4359–69.

37. Prakash GKS, Hu J. Selective fluoroalkylations with fluorinated sulfones, sulfoxides, and sulfides. Acc Chem Res 2007;40:921–30.

38. Kirk KL. Fluorination in medicinal chemistry: methods, strategies, and recent developments. Org Process Res Dev 2008;12:305–21.

39. Lasne MC, Perrio C, Rouden J, et al. Chemistry of β+-emitting compounds based on fluorine-18. Top Curr Chem 2002;222:201–58.

40. Cai L, Lu S, Pike VW. Chemistry with [^{18}F]fluoride ion. Eur J Org Chem 2008;2853–73.

41. Bejot R, Fowler T, Carroll L, et al. Fluorous synthesis of ^{18}F radiotracers with the [^{18}F]fluoride ion: nucleophilic fluorination as the detagging process. Angew Chem Int Ed Engl 2009;48:586–9.

42. Logan J, Fowler JS, Volkow ND, et al. Distribution volume ratios without blood sampling from graphical analysis of PET data. J Cereb Blood Flow Metab 1996;16:834–40.

43. Morris ED, Alpert NM, Fischman AJ. Comparison of two compartmental models for describing receptor ligand kinetics and receptor availability in multiple injection PET studies. J Cereb Blood Flow Metab 1996;16:841–53.

44. Laruelle M. The role of model-based methods in the development of single scan techniques. Nucl Med Biol 2000;27:637–42.

45. Logan J. Graphical analysis of PET data applied to reversible and irreversible tracers. Nucl Med Biol 2000;27:661–70.

46. Lammertsma AA. Radioligand studies: imaging and quantitative analysis. Eur Neuropsychopharmacol 2002;12:513–6.

47. Bentourkia M, Zaidi H. Tracer kinetic modeling in PET. PET Clinics 2007;2:267–77.

48. Dischino DD, Welch MJ, Kilbourn MR, et al. Relationship between lipophilicity and brain extraction of C-11-labeled radiopharmaceuticals. J Nucl Med 1983;24:1030–8.

49. Elfving B, Bjørnholm B, Ebert B, et al. Binding characteristics of selective serotonin reuptake inhibitors with relation to emission tomography studies. Synapse 2001;41:203–11.

50. Waterhouse RN. Determination of lipophilicity and its use as a predictor of blood-brain barrier penetration of molecular imaging agents. Mol Imaging Biol 2003;5:376–89.

51. Kilty JE, Lorang D, Amara SG. Cloning and expression of a cocaine-sensitive rat dopamine transporter. Science 1991;254:578–9.

52. Shimada S, Kitayama S, Lin CL, et al. Cloning and expression of a cocaine-sensitive dopamine transporter complementary DNA. Science 1991;254: 576–8.

53. Giros B, El Mestikawy S, Godinot N, et al. Cloning, pharmacological characterization, and chromosome assignment of the human dopamine transporter. Mol Pharmacol 1992;42:383–90.

54. Ciliax BJ, Heilman C, Demchyshyn LL, et al. The dopamine transporter: immunochemical

characterization and localization in brain. J Neurosci 1995;15:1714–23.

55. Nirenberg MJ, Vaughan RA, Uhl GR, et al. The dopamine transporter is localized to dendritic and axonal plasma membranes of nigrostriatal dopaminergic neurons. J Neurosci 1996;16:436–47.

56. Ciliax BJ, Drash GW, Staley JK, et al. Immunocytochemical localization of the dopamine transporter in human brain. J Comp Neurol 1999;409:38–56.

57. Kaufman MJ, Spealman RD, Madras BK. Distribution of cocaine recognition sites in monkey brain: I. In vitro autoradiography with [3H]CFT. Synapse 1991;9:177–87.

58. Niznik HB, Fogel EF, Fassos FF, et al. The dopamine transporter is absent in parkinsonian putamen and reduced in the caudate nucleus. J Neurochem 1991;56:192–8.

59. Chinaglia G, Alvarez FJ, Probst A, et al. Mesostriatal and mesolimbic dopamine uptake binding sites are reduced in Parkinson's disease and progressive supranuclear palsy: a quantitative autoradiographic study using [3H]Mazindol. Neuroscience 1992;49:317–27.

60. Dawson TM, Dawson VL. Molecular pathways of neurodegeneration in Parkinson's disease. Science 2003;302:819–22.

61. Mazei-Robison MS, Couch RS, Shelton RC, et al. Sequence variation in the human dopamine transporter gene in children with attention deficit hyperactivity disorder. Neuropharmacology 2005;49: 724–36.

62. Singer HS, Hahn IH, Moran TH. Abnormal dopamine uptake sites in postmortem striatum from patients with Tourette's syndrome. Ann Neurol 1991;30:558–62.

63. Marek K, Jennings D, Tamagnan G, et al. Biomarkers for Parkinson's disease: tools to assess Parkinson's disease onset and progression. Ann Neurol 2008;64(Suppl):S111–21.

64. Heikkila RE, Manzino I. Behavioral proportion of GBR 12909, GBR 13069 and GBR 13098: specific inhibitors of dopamine uptake. Eur J Pharmacol 1984;103:241–8.

65. Andersen PH. The dopamine uptake inhibitor GBR 12909: selectivity and molecular mechanism of action. Eur J Pharmacol 1989;166:493–504.

66. Kilbourn MR, Haka MS, Mulholland GK, et al. Regional brain distribution of [18F]GBR 13119, a dopamine uptake inhibitor, in CD-1 and C57BL/6 mice. Eur J Pharmacol 1989;166:331–4.

67. Ciliax BJ, Kilbourn MR, Haka MS, et al. Imaging the dopamine uptake site with ex vivo [18F]GBR 13119 binding autoradiography in rat brain. J Neurochem 1990;55:619–23.

68. Haka MS, Kilbourn MR. Synthesis of [18F]GBR 12909 for human studies of dopamine reuptake sites [abstract]. J Nucl Med 1990;31(836):901.

69. Koeppe RA, Kilbourn MR, Frey KA, et al. Imaging and kinetic modeling of [F-18]GBR 12909, a dopamine uptake inhibitor [abstract]. J Nucl Med 1990; 31(55):720.

70. Van Dort ME, Chakraborty PK, Wieland DM, et al. Dopamine uptake inhibitors: comparison of 125I- and 18F-labeled ligands [abstract]. J Nucl Med 1990;31(823):898.

71. Kilbourn MR, Sherman PS, Pisani T. Repeated reserpine administration reduces in vivo [18F]GBR 13119 binding to the dopamine uptake site. Eur J Pharmacol 1992;216:109–12.

72. Kilbourn MR, Carey JE, Koeppe RA, et al. Biodistribution, dosimetry, metabolism and monkey PET studies of [18F]GBR 13119: imaging the dopamine uptake system in vivo. Nucl Med Biol (Int J Radiat Appl Instrum Part B) 1989;16:569–76.

73. Müller L, Halldin C, Foged C, et al. Synthesis of [18F]NNC 12-0817 and [18F]NNC 12-0818: two potential radioligands for the dopamine transporter. Appl Radiat Isot 1995;46:323–8.

74. Wolf WA, Kuhn DM. Cocaine and serotonin neurochemistry. Neurochem Int 1991;18:33–8.

75. Uhl GR, Hall FS, Sora I. Cocaine, reward, movement and monoamine transporters. Mol Psychiatry 2002;7:21–6.

76. Ritz MC, Lamb RJ, Goldberg SR, et al. Cocaine receptors on dopamine transporters are related to self-administration of cocaine. Science 1987;237: 1219–23.

77. Scheffel U, Boja JW, Kuhar MJ. Cocaine receptors: in vivo labeling with 3H-(-)-cocaine, 3H-WIN 35,065-2, and 3H-WIN 35,428. Synapse 1989;4: 390–2.

78. Boja JW, Kuhar MJ. [3H]Cocaine binding and inhibition of [3H]dopamine uptake is similar in both the rat striatum and nucleus accumbens. Eur J Pharmacol 1989;173:215–7.

79. Fowler JS, Volkow ND, Wolf AP, et al. Mapping cocaine binding sites in human and baboon brain in vivo. Synapse 1989;4:371–7.

80. Fowler JS, Volkow ND, MacGregor RR, et al. Comparative PET studies of the kinetics and distribution of cocaine and cocaethylene in baboon brain. Synapse 1992;12:220–7.

81. Yu DW, Gatley SJ, Wolf AP, et al. Synthesis of carbon-11 labeled iodinated cocaine derivatives and their distribution in baboon brain measured using positron emission tomography. J Med Chem 1992;35:2178–83.

82. Gatley SJ, Yu DW, Fowler JS, et al. Studies with differentially labeled [11C]cocaine, [11C]norcocaine, [11C]benzoylecgonine, and [11C]- and 4'-[18F]fluorococaine to probe the extent to which [11C]cocaine metabolites contribute to PET images of the baboon brain. J Neurochem 1994;62: 1154–62.

83. Kimmel HL, Negus SS, Wilcox KM, et al. Relationship between rate of drug uptake in brain and behavioral pharmacology of monoamine transporter inhibitors in rhesus monkeys. Pharmacol Biochem Behav 2008;90:453–62.

84. Kloss MW, Rosen GM, Rauckman EJ. N-demethylation of cocaine to norcocaine. Mol Pharmacol 1983; 23:482–5.

85. Jindal SP, Lutz T. Mass spectrometric studies of cocaine disposition in animals and humans using stable isotope-labeled analogues. J Pharm Sci 1989;78:1009–14.

86. Bergström KA, Halldin C, Kuikka JT, et al. The metabolite pattern of [^{123}I]β-CIT determined with a gradient HPLC method. Nucl Med Biol 1995;22: 971–6.

87. Potter PM, Wadkins RM. Carboxylesterases: detoxifying enzymes and targets for drug therapy. Curr Med Chem 2006;13:1045–54.

88. Lundkvist C, Halldin C, Swahn CG, et al. Different brain radioactivity curves in a PET study with [^{11}C]β-CIT labelled in two different positions. Nucl Med Biol 1999;26:343–50.

89. Larsen NA, Turner JM, Stevens J, et al. Crystal structure of a bacterial cocaine esterase. Nat Struct Biol 2002;9:17–21.

90. Clarke RL, Daum SJ, Gambino AJ, et al. Compounds affecting the central nervous system. 4. 3β-Phenyltropane-2-carboxylic esters and analogs. J Med Chem 1973;16:1260–7.

91. Boja JW, Carroll FI, Rahman MA, et al. New, potent cocaine analogs: ligand binding and transport studies in rat striatum. Eur J Pharmacol 1990;184: 329–32.

92. Carroll FI, Gao Y, Rahman MA, et al. Synthesis, ligand binding, QSAR, and CoMFA study of 3β-(p-substituted phenyl)tropane-2β-carboxylic acid methyl esters. J Med Chem 1991;34:2719–25.

93. Carroll FI, Lewin AH, Boja JW, et al. Cocaine receptor: biochemical characterization and structure-activity relationships of cocaine analogues at the dopamine transporter. J Med Chem 1992;35:969–81.

94. Kuhar MJ, McGirr KM, Hunter RG, et al. Studies of selected phenyltropanes at monoamine transporters. Drug Alcohol Depend 1999;56:9–15.

95. Cook CD, Carroll FI, Beardsley PM. Cocaine-like discriminative stimulus effects of novel cocaine and 3-phenyltropane analogs in the rat. Psychopharmacology 2001;159:58–63.

96. Singh S. Chemistry, design, and structure-activity relationship of cocaine antagonists. Chem Rev 2000;100:925–1024.

97. Jin C, Navarro HA, Page K, et al. Synthesis and monoamine transporter binding properties of 2β-[3'-(substituted benzyl)isoxazol-5-yl]- and 2β-[3'-methyl-4'-(substituted phenyl)isoxazol-5-yl]-3β-(substituted phenyl)tropanes. Bioorg Med Chem 2008;16:6682–8.

98. Jin C, Navarro HA, Carroll FI. Development of 3-phenyltropane analogues with high affinity for the dopamine and serotonin transporters and low affinity for the norepinephrine transporter. J Med Chem 2008;51:8048–56.

99. Boja JW, Patel A, Carroll FI, et al. [^{125}I]RTI-55: a potent ligand for dopamine transporters. Eur J Pharmacol 1991;194:133–4.

100. Meltzer PC, Liang AY, Brownell AL, et al. Substituted 3-phenyltropane analogs of cocaine: synthesis, inhibition of binding at cocaine recognition sites, and positron emission tomography imaging. J Med Chem 1993;36:855–62.

101. Wong DF, Yung B, Dannals RF, et al. In vivo imaging of baboon and human dopamine transporters by positron emission tomography using [^{11}C]WIN 35,428. Synapse 1993;15:130–42.

102. Wilson AA, DaSilva JN, Houle S. In vivo evaluation of [^{11}C]- and [^{18}F]-labelled cocaine analogues as potential dopamine transporter ligands for positron emission tomography. Nucl Med Biol 1996;23:141–6.

103. Farde L, Halldin C, Müller L, et al. PET study of [^{11}C]β-CIT binding to monoamine transporters in the monkey and human brain. Synapse 1994;16: 93–103.

104. Någren K, Halldin C, Müller L, et al. Comparison of [^{11}C]methyl triflate and [^{11}C]methyl iodide in the synthesis of PET radioligands such as [^{11}C]β-CIT and [^{11}C]β-CFT. Nucl Med Biol 1995;22:965–70.

105. Harada N, Ohba H, Fukumoto D, et al. Potential of [^{18}F]β-CFT-FE (2β-carbomethoxy-3β-(4-fluorophenyl)-8-(2- [^{18}F]fluoroethyl)nortropane) as a dopamine transporter ligand: a PET study in the conscious monkey brain. Synapse 2004;54:37–45.

106. Haaparanta M, Bergman J, Laakso A, et al. [^{18}F]CFT ([^{18}F]WIN 35,428), a radioligand to study the dopamine transporter with PET: biodistribution in rats. Synapse 1996;23:321–7.

107. Laakso A, Bergman J, Haaparanta M, et al. [^{18}F]CFT ([^{18}F]WIN 35,428), a radioligand to study the dopamine transporter with PET: characterization in human subjects. Synapse 1998;28:244–50.

108. Rinne JO, Nurmi E, Ruottinen HM, et al. [^{18}F]FDOPA and [^{18}F]CFT are both sensitive PET markers to detect presynaptic dopaminergic hypofunction in early Parkinson's disease. Synapse 2001;40:193–200.

109. Kämäräinen EL, Kyllönen T, Airaksinen A, et al. Preparation of [^{18}F]β-CFT-FP and [^{11}C]β-CFT-FP, selective radioligands for visualisation of the dopamine transporter using positron emission tomography (PET). J Labelled Comp Radiopharm 2000; 43:1235–44.

110. Koivula T, Marjamäki P, Haaparanta M, et al. Ex vivo evaluation of N-(3- [^{18}F]fluoropropyl)-2β-carbomethoxy-3β-(4-fluorophenyl)nortropane in rats. Nucl Med Biol 2008;35:177–83.

111. Owens MJ, Morgan WN, Plott SJ, et al. Neurotransmitter receptor and transporter binding profile of antidepressants and their metabolites. J Pharmacol Exp Ther 1997;283:1305–22.

112. Hiemke C, Härtter S. Pharmacokinetics of selective serotonin reuptake inhibitors. Pharmacol Ther 2000;85:11–28.

113. Neumeyer JL, Tamagnan G, Wang S, et al. N-substituted analogs of 2β-carbomethoxy-3β-(4'-iodophenyl)tropane (β-CIT) with selective affinity to dopamine or serotonin transporters in rat forebrain. J Med Chem 1996;39:543–8.

114. Neumeyer JL, Wang S, Gao Y, et al. N-ω-Fluoroalkyl analogs of (1 R)-2β-carbomethoxy-3β-(4-iodophenyl)-tropane (β-CIT): radiotracers for positron emission tomography and single photon emission computed tomography imaging of dopamine transporters. J Med Chem 1994;37:1558–61.

115. Carroll FI, Abraham P, Lewin AH, et al. Isopropyl and phenyl esters of 3β-(4-substituted phenyl)tropan-2β-carboxylic acids: potent and selective compounds for the dopamine transporter. J Med Chem 1992;35:2497–500.

116. Baldwin RM, Zea-Ponce Y, Al-Tikriti M, et al. Regional brain uptake and pharmacokinetics of [^{123}I] N-ω-fluoroalkyl-2β-carboxy-3β-(4-iodophenyl)nortropane esters in baboons. Nucl Med Biol 1995;22:211–9.

117. Kuikka JT, Bergström KA, Ahonen A, et al. Comparison of iodine-123 labelled 2β-carbomethoxy-3β-(4-iodophenyl)tropane and 2β-carbomethoxy-3β-(4-iodophenyl)- N-(3-fluoropropyl)nortropane for imaging of the dopamine transporter in the living human brain. Eur J Nucl Med 1995;22:356–60.

118. Halldin C, Farde L, Lundkvist C, et al. [^{11}C]β-CIT-FE, a radioligand for quantitation of the dopamine transporter in the living brain using positron emission tomography. Synapse 1996;22:386–90.

119. Lundkvist C, Halldin C, Ginovart N, et al. [^{18}F]β-CIT-FP is superior to [^{11}C]β-CIT-FP for quantitation of the dopamine transporter. Nucl Med Biol 1997;24:621–7.

120. Chaly T, Dhawan V, Kazumata K, et al. Radiosynthesis of [^{18}F] N-3-fluoropropyl-2-β-carbomethoxy-3-β-(4-iodophenyl) nortropane and the first human study with positron emission tomography. Nucl Med Biol 1996;23:999–1004.

121. Kazumata K, Dhawan V, Chaly T, et al. Dopamine transporter imaging with fluorine-18-FPCIT and PET. J Nucl Med 1998;39:1521–30.

122. Ma Y, Dhawan V, Mentis M, et al. Parametric mapping of [^{18}F]FPCIT binding in early stage Parkinson's disease: a PET study. Synapse 2002;45:125–33.

123. Robeson W, Dhawan V, Belakhlef A, et al. Dosimetry of the dopamine transporter radioligand ^{18}F-FPCIT in human subjects. J Nucl Med 2003;44:961–6.

124. Yaqub M, Boellaard R, van Berckel BNM, et al. Quantification of dopamine transporter binding using [^{18}F]FP-β-CIT and positron emission tomography. J Cereb Blood Flow Metab 2007;27:1397–406.

125. Lee SJ, Oh SJ, Chi DY, et al. One-step high-radiochemical-yield synthesis of [^{18}F]FP-CIT using a protic solvent system. Nucl Med Biol 2007;34:345–51.

126. Goodman MM, Keil R, Shoup TM, et al. Fluorine-18-FPCT: a PET radiotracer for imaging dopamine transporters. J Nucl Med 1997;38:119–26.

127. Goodman MM, Kilts CD, Keil R, et al. ^{18}F-labeled FECNT: a selective radioligand for PET imaging of brain dopamine transporters. Nucl Med Biol 2000;27:1–12.

128. Votaw JR, Howell LL, Martarello L, et al. Measurement of dopamine transporter occupancy for multiple injections of cocaine using a single injection of [F-18]FECNT. Synapse 2002;44:203–10.

129. Deterding TA, Votaw JR, Wang CK, et al. Biodistribution and radiation dosimetry of the dopamine transporter ligand [^{18}F]FECNT. J Nucl Med 2001;42:376–81.

130. Tipre DN, Fujita M, Chin FT, et al. Whole-body biodistribution and radiation dosimetry estimates for the PET dopamine transporter probe ^{18}F-FECNT in non-human primates. Nucl Med Commun 2004;25:737–42.

131. Voll RJ, McConathy J, Waldrep MS, et al. Semi-automated preparation of the dopamine transporter ligand [^{18}F]FECNT for human PET imaging studies. Appl Radiat Isot 2005;63:353–61.

132. Chen ZP, Wang SP, Li XM, et al. A one-step automated high-radiochemical-yield synthesis of ^{18}F-FECNT from mesylate precursor. Appl Radiat Isot 2008;66:1881–5.

133. Davis MR, Votaw JR, Bremner JD, et al. Initial human PET imaging studies with the dopamine transporter ligand ^{18}F-FECNT. J Nucl Med 2003;44:855–61.

134. Zoghbi SS, Shetty U, Ichise M, et al. PET imaging of the dopamine transporter with ^{18}F-FECNT: a polar radiometabolite confounds brain radioligand measurements. J Nucl Med 2006;47:520–7.

135. Cumming P, Yokoi F, Chen A, et al. Pharmacokinetics of radiotracers in human plasma during positron emission tomography. Synapse 1999;34:124–34.

136. Gillings NM, Bender D, Falborg L, et al. Kinetics of the metabolism of four PET radioligands in living minipigs. Nucl Med Biol 2001;28:97–104.

137. Greuter HNJM, van Ophemert PLB, Luurtsema G, et al. Optimizing an online SPE-HPLC method for

analysis of (R)- [^{11}C]1-(2-chlorophenyl)- N-methyl- N-(1-methylpropyl)-3-isoquinolinecarboxamide [(R)-[^{11}C]PK11195] and its metabolites in humans. Nucl Med Biol 2005;32:307–12.

138. Luurtsema G, Molthoff CFM, Schuit RC, et al. Evaluation of (R)- [^{11}C]verapamil as PET tracer of P-glycoprotein function in the blood-brain barrier: kinetics and metabolism in the rat. Nucl Med Biol 2005;32:87–93.

139. Shetty HU, Zoghbi SS, Liow JS, et al. identification and regional distribution in rat brain of radiometabolites of the dopamine transporter PET radioligand [^{11}C]PE2I. Eur J Nucl Med Mol Imaging 2007;34:667–78.

140. Luurtsema G, Schuit RC, Takkenkamp K, et al. Peripheral metabolism of [^{18}F]FDDNP and cerebral uptake of its labelled metabolites. Nucl Med Biol 2008;35:869–74.

141. Chaly T Jr, Matacchieri R, Dahl R, et al. Radiosynthesis of [^{18}F] N-3-fluoropropyl-2-β-carbomethoxy-3-β(4' methylphenyl) nortropane (FPCMT). Appl Radiat Isot 1999;51:299–305.

142. Chitneni SK, Garreau L, Cleynhens B, et al. Improved synthesis and metabolic stability analysis of the dopamine transporter ligand [^{18}F]FECT. Nucl Med Biol 2008;35:75–82.

143. Gu XH, Zong R, Kula NS, et al. Synthesis and biological evaluation of a series of novel N- or O-fluoroalkyl derivatives of tropane: potential positron emission tomography (PET) imaging agents for the dopamine transporter. Bioorg Med Chem Lett 2001;11:3049–53.

144. Peng X, Zhang A, Kula NS, et al. Synthesis and amine transporter affinities of novel phenyltropane derivatives as potential positron emission tomography (PET) imaging agents. Bioorg Med Chem Lett 2004;14:5635–9.

145. Wuest F, Berndt M, Strobel K, et al. Synthesis and radiopharmacological characterization of 2β-carbo-2'- [^{18}F]fluoroethoxy-3β-(4-bromo-phenyl)-tropane ([^{18}F]MCL-322) as a PET radiotracer for imaging the dopamine transporter (DAT). Bioorg Med Chem 2007;15:4511–9.

146. Mitterhauser M, Wadsak W, Mien LK, et al. Synthesis and biodistribution of [^{18}F]FE@CIT, a new potential tracer for the dopamine transporter. Synapse 2005;55:73–9.

147. Ettlinger DE, Häusler D, Wadsak W, et al. Metabolism and autoradiographic evaluation of [^{18}F]FE@CIT: a comparison with [^{123}I]β-CIT and [^{123}I]FP-CIT. Nucl Med Biol 2008;35:475–9.

148. Xing D, Chen P, Keil R, et al. Synthesis, biodistribution, and primate imaging of fluorine-18 labeled 2β-Carbo-1'-fluoro-2-propoxy-3β-(4-chlorophenyl)tropanes: ligands for the imaging of dopamine transporters by positron emission tomography. J Med Chem 2000;43:639–48.

149. Mach RH, Nader MA, Ehrenkaufer RL, et al. Fluorine-18-labeled tropane analogs for PET imaging studies of the dopamine transporter. Synapse 2000;37:109–17.

150. Chen P, Kilts CD, Camp VM, et al. Synthesis, characterization and in vivo evaluation of (N-(E)-4- [^{18}F]fluorobut-2-en-1-yl)-2β-carbomethoxy-3β-(4-substituted-phenyl)nortropanes for imaging DAT by PET. J Labelled Comp Radiopharm 1999; 42(Suppl 1):S400.

151. Goodman MM, Chen P. Fluoroalkenyl Nortropanes. 2000:World Patent Application WO2000064490. Published November 2, 2000.

152. Chalon S, Hall H, Saba W, et al. Pharmacological characterization of (E)- N-(4-Fluorobut-2-enyl)-2β-carbomethoxy-3β-(4'-tolyl)nortropane (LBT-999) as a highly promising fluorinated ligand for the dopamine transporter. J Pharmacol Exp Ther 2006;317: 147–52.

153. Dollé F, Emond P, Mavel S, et al. Synthesis, radiosynthesis and in vivo preliminary evaluation of [^{11}C]LBT-999, a selective radioligand for the visualisation of the dopamine transporter with PET. Bioorg Med Chem 2006;14:1115–25.

154. Dollé F, Hinnen F, Emond P, et al. Radiosynthesis of [^{18}F]LBT-999, a selective radioligand for the visualization of the dopamine transporter with PET. J Labelled Comp Radiopharm 2006;49: 687–98.

155. Dollé F, Helfenbein J, Hinnen F, et al. One-step radiosynthesis of [^{18}F]LBT-999: a selective radioligand for the visualization of the dopamine transporter with PET. J Labelled Comp Radiopharm 2007;50:716–23.

156. Saba W, Valette H, Schöllhorn-Peyronneau MA, et al. [^{11}C]LBT-999: a suitable radioligand for investigation of extra-striatal dopamine transporter with PET. Synapse 2007;61:17–23.

157. Stehouwer JS, Chen P, Voll RJ, et al. PET imaging of the dopamine transporter with [^{18}F]FBFNT. J Labelled Comp Radiopharm 2007;50(Suppl 1): S335.

158. Carroll FI, Kotian P, Dehghani A, et al. Cocaine and 3β-(4'-substituted phenyl)tropane-2β-carboxylic acid ester and amide analogues: new high-affinity and selective compounds for the dopamine transporter. J Med Chem 1995; 38:379–88.

159. Dworkin SI, Lambert P, Sizemore GM, et al. RTI-113 administration reduces cocaine self-administration at high occupancy of dopamine transporter. Synapse 1998;30:49–55.

160. Cook CD, Carroll FI, Beardsley PM. RTI 113, a 3-phenyltropane analog, produces long-lasting cocaine-like discriminative stimulus effects in rats and squirrel monkeys. Eur J Pharmacol 2002;442: 93–8.

161. Wilcox KM, Lindsey KP, Votaw JR, et al. Self-administration of cocaine and the cocaine analog RTI-113: relationship to dopamine transporter occupancy determined by PET neuroimaging in rhesus monkeys. Synapse 2002;43:78–85.

162. Tsukada H, Nishiyama S, Kakiuchi T, et al. Isoflurane anesthesia enhances the inhibitory effects of cocaine and GBR12909 on dopamine transporter: PET studies in combination with microdialysis in the monkey brain. Brain Res 1999;849: 85–96.

163. Miyamoto S, Leipzig JN, Lieberman JA, et al. Effects of ketamine, MK-801, and amphetamine on regional brain 2-deoxyglucose uptake in freely moving mice. Neuropsychopharmacology 2000; 22:400–12.

164. Tsukada H, Harada N, Nishiyama S, et al. Ketamine decreased striatal [^{11}c]raclopride binding with no alterations in static dopamine concentrations in the striatal extracellular fluid in the monkey brain: multiparametric PET studies combined with microdialysis analysis. Synapse 2000;37:95–103.

165. Mizugaki M, Nakagawa N, Nakamura H, et al. Influence of anesthesia on brain distribution of [^{11}C]methamphetamine in monkeys in positron emission tomography (PET) study. Brain Res 2001;911:173–5.

166. Tsukada H, Nishiyama S, Kakiuchi T, et al. Ketamine alters the availability of striatal dopamine transporter as measured by [^{11}C]β-CFT and [^{11}C]β-CIT-FE in the monkey brain. Synapse 2001;42:273–80.

167. Elfving B, Bjørnholm B, Knudsen GM. Interference of anaesthetics with radioligand binding in neuroreceptor studies. Eur J Nucl Med Mol Imaging 2003; 30:912–5.

168. Votaw JR, Byas-Smith MG, Voll R, et al. Isoflurane alters the amount of dopamine transporter expressed on the plasma membrane in humans. Anesthesiology 2004;101:1128–35.

169. Hoffman BJ, Mezey E, Brownstein MJ. Cloning of a serotonin transporter affected by antidepressants. Science 1991;254:579–80.

170. Cortés R, Soriano E, Pazos A, et al. Autoradiography of antidepressant binding sites in the human brain: localization using [3h]imipramine and [3h]paroxetine. Neuroscience 1988;27:473–96.

171. Hrdina PD, Foy B, Hepner A, et al. Antidepressant binding sites in brain: autoradiographic comparison of [^{3}H]paroxetine and [^{3}H]imipramine localization and relationship to serotonin transporter. J Pharmacol Exp Ther 1990;252:410–8.

172. Fujita M, Shimada S, Maeno H, et al. Cellular localization of serotonin transporter mRNA in the rat brain. Neurosci Lett 1993;162:59–62.

173. Austin MC, Bradley CC, Mann JJ, et al. Expression of serotonin transporter messenger RNA in the human brain. J Neurochem 1994;62:2362–7.

174. Blakely RD, De Felice LJ, Hartzell HC. Molecular physiology of norepinephrine and serotonin transporters. J Exp Biol 1994;196:263–81.

175. Gurevich EV, Joyce JN. Comparison of [^{3}H]paroxetine and [^{3}H]cyanoimipramine for quantitative measurement of serotonin transporter sites in human brain. Neuropsychopharmacology 1996; 14:309–23.

176. Stockmeier CA, Shapiro LA, Haycock JW, et al. Quantitative subregional distribution of serotonin-1A receptors and serotonin transporters in the human dorsal raphe. Brain Res 1996;727:1–12.

177. Kish SJ, Furukawa Y, Chang LJ, et al. Regional distribution of serotonin transporter protein in postmortem human brain. Is the cerebellum a SERT-free brain region? Nucl Med Biol 2005; 32:123–8.

178. Chinaglia G, Landwehrmeyer B, Probst A, et al. Serotonergic terminal transporters are differentially affected in Parkinson's disease and progressive supranuclear palsy: an autoradiographic study with [^{3}H]citalopram. Neuroscience 1993; 54:691–9.

179. Cash R, Raisman R, Ploska A, et al. High and low affinity [^{3}H]imipramine binding sites in control and parkinsonian brains. Eur J Pharmacol 1985;117: 71 80.

180. Blier P, de Montigny C. Serotonin and drug-induced therapeutic responses in major depression, obsessive-compulsive and panic disorders. Neuropsychopharmacology 1999;21:91S–8S.

181. Chaouloff F, Berton O, Mormede P. Serotonin and stress. Neuropsychopharmacology 1999;21: 28S–32S.

182. Lucki I. The spectrum of behaviors influenced by serotonin. Biol Psychiatry 1998;44:151–62.

183. Mann JJ. Role of the serotonergic system in the pathogenesis of major depression and suicidal behavior. Neuropsychopharmacology 1999;21: 99S–105S.

184. Mann JJ, Brent DA, Arango V. The neurobiology and genetics of suicide and attempted suicide: a focus on the serotonergic system. Neuropsychopharmacology 2001;24:467–77.

185. Owens MJ, Nemeroff CB. Role of serotonin in the pathophysiology of depression: focus on the serotonin transporter. Clin Chem 1994;40:288–95.

186. Owens MJ, Nemeroff CB. The serotonin transporter and depression. Depress Anxiety 1998;8(Suppl 1): 5–12.

187. Purselle DC, Nemeroff CB. Serotonin transporter: a potential substrate in the biology of suicide. Neuropsychopharmacology 2003;28:613–9.

188. Benmansour S, Cecchi M, Morilak DA, et al. Effects of chronic antidepressant treatments on serotonin transporter function, density, and mRNA level. J Neurosci 1999;19:10494–501.

189. Benmansour S, Owens WA, Cecchi M, et al. Serotonin clearance in vivo is altered to a greater extent by antidepressant-induced downregulation of the serotonin transporter than by acute blockade of this transporter. J Neurosci 2002;22:6766–72.

190. Ramsey IS, De Felice LJ. Serotonin transporter function and pharmacology are sensitive to expression level. J Biol Chem 2002;277:14475–82.

191. Kugaya A, Sanacora G, Staley JK, et al. Brain serotonin transporter availability predicts treatment response to selective serotonin reuptake inhibitors. Biol Psychiatry 2004;56:497–502.

192. Mirza NR, Nielsen EØ, Troelsen KB. Serotonin transporter density and anxiolytic-like effects of antidepressants in mice. Prog Neuropsychopharmacol Biol Psychiatry 2007;31:858–66.

193. Stokes PE. Ten years of fluoxetine. Depress Anxiety 1998;8(Suppl 1):1–4.

194. Shiue CY, Shiue GG, Cornish KG, et al. PET study of the distribution of [^{11}C]fluoxetine in a monkey brain. Nucl Med Biol 1995;22:613–6.

195. Mukherjee J, Das MK, Yang ZY, et al. Evaluation of the binding of the radiolabeled antidepressant drug, ^{18}F-fluoxetine in the rodent brain: an in vitro and in vivo study. Nucl Med Biol 1998;25:605–10.

196. Shank RP, Vaught JL, Pelley KA, et al. McN-5652: a highly potent inhibitor of serotonin uptake. J Pharmacol Exp Ther 1988;247:1032–8.

197. Suehiro M, Scheffel U, Dannals RF, et al. A PET radiotracer for studying serotonin uptake sites: carbon-11-McN-5652Z. J Nucl Med 1993;34:120–7.

198. Szabo Z, Kao PF, Scheffel U, et al. Positron emission tomography imaging of serotonin transporters in the human brain using [^{11}C](+)McN5652. Synapse 1995;20:37–43.

199. Zessin J, Eskola O, Brust P, et al. Synthesis of S-([^{18}F]fluoromethyl)-(+)-McN5652 as a potential PET radioligand for the serotonin transporter. Nucl Med Biol 2001;28:857–63.

200. Marjamäki P, Zessin J, Eskola O, et al. S- [^{18}F]fluoromethyl-(+)-McN5652, a PET tracer for the serotonin transporter: evaluation in rats. Synapse 2003;47:45–53.

201. Brust P, Hinz R, Kuwabara H, et al. In vivo measurement of the serotonin transporter with (S)-([18F]fluoromethyl)-(+)-McN5652. Neuropsychopharmacology 2003;28:2010–9.

202. Brust P, Zessin J, Kuwabara H, et al. Positron emission tomography imaging of the serotonin transporter in the pig brain using [^{11}C](+)-McN5652 and S-([^{18}F]fluoromethyl)-(+)-McN5652. Synapse 2003;47:143–51.

203. Kretzschmar M, Brust P, Zessin J, et al. Autoradiographic imaging of the serotonin transporter in the brain of rats and pigs using S-([^{18}F]fluoromethyl)-

204. Hashimoto K, Goromaru T. High-affinity [^{3}H]6-nitroquipazine binding sites in rat brain. Eur J Pharmacol 1990;180:273–81.

205. Karramkam M, Dollé F, Valette H, et al. Synthesis of a fluorine-18-labelled derivative of 6-nitroquipazine, as a radioligand for the in vivo serotonin transporter imaging with PET. Bioorg Med Chem 2002;10:2611–23.

206. Lee BS, Chu S, Lee KC, et al. Syntheses and binding affinities of 6-nitroquipazine analogues for serotonin transporter: part 3. A potential 5-HT transporter imaging agent, 3-(3- [^{18}F]fluoropropyl)-6-nitroquipazine. Bioorg Med Chem 2003;11:4949–58.

207. Mehta NB, Hollingsworth CEB, Brieaddy LE, et al. Halogen substituted diphenylsulfides. 1990: European Patent Application EP0 402 097 A1. Published December, 12, 1990.

208. Ferris RM, Brieaddy L, Mehta N, et al. Pharmacological properties of 403U76, a new chemical class of 5-hydroxytryptamine and noradrenaline reuptake inhibitor. J Pharm Pharmacol 1995;47:775–81.

209. Huang Y, Hwang DR, Narendran R, et al. Comparative evaluation in nonhuman primates of five PET radiotracers for imaging the serotonin transporters: [11C]McN5652, [11C]ADAM, [11C]DASB, [11C]DAPA, and [11C]AFM. J Cereb Blood Flow Metab 2002;22:1377–98.

210. Jarkas N, Votaw JR, Voll RJ, et al. Carbon-11 HOMADAM: a novel PET radiotracer for imaging serotonin transporters. Nucl Med Biol 2005;32:211–24.

211. Jarkas N, McConathy J, Votaw JR, et al. Synthesis and characterization of eadam: a selective radioligand for mapping the brain serotonin transporters by positron emission tomography. Nucl Med Biol 2005;32:75–86.

212. Huang Y, Narendran R, Bae S, et al. A PET imaging agent with fast kinetics: synthesis and in vivo evaluation of the serotonin transporter ligand [^{11}C]2-[2-dimethylaminomethylphenylthio]-5-fluorophenylamine ([^{11}C]AFA). Nucl Med Biol 2004;31:727–38.

213. Shiue GG, Choi SR, Fang P, et al. N, N-Dimethyl-2-(2-amino-4-^{18}F-fluorophenylthio)-benzylamine (4-^{18}F-ADAM): an improved PET radioligand for serotonin transporters. J Nucl Med 2003;44:1890–7.

214. Huang Y, Hwang DR, Bae S, et al. A new positron emission tomography imaging agent for the serotonin transporter: synthesis, pharmacological characterization, and kinetic analysis of [^{11}C]2-[2-(dimethylaminomethyl)phenylthio]-5-fluoromethylphenylamine ([^{11}C]AFM). Nucl Med Biol 2004;31:543–56.

215. Zhu Z, Guo N, Narendran R, et al. The new PET imaging agent [^{11}C]AFE is a selective serotonin transporter ligand with fast brain uptake kinetics. Nucl Med Biol 2004;31:983–94.

216. Huang Y, Bae S, Zhu Z, et al. Fluorinated diaryl sulfides as serotonin transporter ligands: synthesis, structure-activity relationship study, and in vivo evaluation of fluorine-18-labeled compounds as PET imaging agents. J Med Chem 2005;48: 2559–70.

217. Oya S, Choi SR, Hou C, et al. [18]F(2-[2-Amino-5-fluorophenyl)thio]- N, N-dimethyl-benzenmethanamine as a PET imaging agent for serotonin transporters. J Labelled Comp Radiopharm 2003; 46(Suppl 1):S164.

218. Oya S, Choi SR, Coenen H, et al. New PET imaging agent for the serotonin transporter: [18F]ACF (2-[(2-amino-4-chloro-5-fluorophenyl)thio]- N, N-dimethyl-benzenmethanamine). J Med Chem 2002;45:4716–23.

219. Parhi AK, Wang JL, Oya S, et al. 2-(2'-((Dimethylamino)methyl)-4'-(fluoroalkoxy)-phenylthio)benzenamine derivatives as serotonin transporter imaging agents. J Med Chem 2007;50:6673–84.

220. Jarkas N, Voll RJ, Williams L, et al. Synthesis and in vivo evaluation of halogenated N, N-dimethyl-2-(2'-amino-4'-hydroxymethylphenylthio)benzylamine derivatives as PET serotonin transporter ligands. J Med Chem 2008;51:271–81.

221. Oya S, Choi SR, Hou C, et al. 2-((2-((Dimethylamino)-methyl)phenyl)thio)-5-iodophenylamine (ADAM): an improved serotonin transporter ligand. Nucl Med Biol 2000;27:249–54.

222. Wilson AA, Ginovart N, Schmidt M, et al. Novel radiotracers for imaging the serotonin transporter by positron emission tomography: synthesis, radiosynthesis, and in vitro and ex vivo evaluation of 11C-labeled 2-(phenylthio)araalkylamines. J Med Chem 2000;43:3103–10.

223. Houle S, Ginovart N, Hussey D, et al. Imaging the serotonin transporter with positron emission tomography: initial human studies with ^{11}C]DAPP and ^{11}C]DASB. Eur J Nucl Med 2000;27:1719–22.

224. Ginovart N, Wilson AA, Meyer JH, et al. Positron emission tomography quantification of [11C]-DASB binding to the human serotonin transporter: modeling strategies. J Cereb Blood Flow Metab 2001;21:1342–53.

225. Frankle WG, Huang Y, Hwang DR, et al. Comparative evaluation of serotonin transporter radioligands ^{11}C-DASB and ^{11}C-McN 5652 in healthy humans. J Nucl Med 2004;45:682–94.

226. Frankle WG, Narendran R, Huang Y, et al. Serotonin transporter availability in patients with schizophrenia: a positron emission tomography imaging study with [11C]DASB. Biol Psychiatry 2005;57: 1510–6.

227. Nye JA, Votaw JR, Jarkas N, et al. Compartmental modeling of ^{11}C-HOMADAM binding to the serotonin transporter in the healthy human brain. J Nucl Med 2008;49:2018–25.

228. Huang Y, Zhu Z, Bae SA, et al. Comparison of three F-18 labeled PET ligands for the serotonin transporter: radiosynthesis and in vivo imaging studies in baboon. J Labelled Comp Radiopharm 2003; 46(Suppl 1):S57.

229. Fang P, Shiue GG, Shimazu T, et al. Synthesis and evaluation of N, N-dimethyl-2-(2-amino-5- [18]F]fluorophenylthio)benzylamine (5- [18]F]-ADAM) as a serotonin transporter imaging agent. Appl Radiat Isot 2004;61:1247–54.

230. Wang JL, Parhi AK, Oya S, et al. 2-(2'-((Dimethylamino)methyl)-4'-(3- [18]F]fluoropropoxy)-phenylthio)benzenamine for positron emission tomography imaging of serotonin transporters. Nucl Med Biol 2008;35:447–58.

231. Owens MJ, Knight DL, Nemeroff CB. Second-generation SSRIs: human monoamine transporter binding profile of escitalopram and R-fluoxetine. Biol Psychiatry 2001;50:345–50.

232. Elfving B, Wiborg O. Binding of S-citalopram and paroxetine discriminates between species. Synapse 2005;55:280–2.

233. Tejani-Butt SM. [3]H]Nisoxetine: a radioligand for quantitation of norepinephrine uptake sites by autoradiography or by homogenate binding. J Pharmacol Exp Ther 1992;260:427–36.

234. Cheetham SC, Viggers JA, Butler SA, et al. [3]H]Nisoxetine - a radioligand for noradrenaline reuptake sites: correlation with inhibition of ^{3}H]noradrenaline uptake and effects of DSP-4 lesioning and antidepressant treatments. Neuropharmacology 1996; 35:63–70.

235. Stehouwer JS, Jarkas N, Zeng F, et al. Synthesis, radiosynthesis, and biological evaluation of carbon-11 labeled 2β-carbomethoxy-3β-(3-((Z)-2-haloethenyl)phenyl)nortropanes: candidate radioligands for in vivo imaging of the serotonin transporter with positron emission tomography. J Med Chem 2006;49:6760–7.

236. Wong EHF, Sonders MS, Amara SG, et al. Reboxetine: a pharmacologically potent, selective, and specific norepinephrine reuptake inhibitor. Biol Psychiatry 2000;47:818–29.

237. Goodman MM, Chen P, Plisson C, et al. Synthesis and characterization of iodine-123 labeled 2β-carbomethoxy-3β-(4'-((Z)-2-iodoethenyl)phenyl)nortropane: a ligand for in vivo imaging of serotonin transporters by single-photon-emission tomography. J Med Chem 2003;46:925–35.

238. Plaznik A, Danysz W, Kostowski W, et al. Interaction between noradrenergic and serotonergic brain systems as evidenced by behavioral and biochemical effects of microinjections of adrenergic agonists and antagonists into the medial raphe nucleus. Pharmacol Biochem Behav 1983;19:27–32.

239. Ordway GA, Stockmeier CA, Cason GW, et al. Pharmacology and distribution of norepinephrine

transporters in the human locus coeruleus and raphe nuclei. J Neurosci 1997;17:1710–9.

240. Ressler KJ, Nemeroff CB. Role of serotonergic and noradrenergic systems in the pathophysiology of depression and anxiety disorders. Depress Anxiety 2000;12(Suppl 1):2–19.

241. Emond P, Vercouillie J, Innis R, et al. Substituted diphenyl sulfides as selective serotonin transporter ligands: synthesis and in vitro evaluation. J Med Chem 2002;45:1253–8.

242. Garg S, Thopate SR, Minton RC, et al. 3-Amino-4-(2-((4- [^{18}F]fluorobenzyl)methylamino)methylphenylsulfanyl)benzonitrile, an F-18 fluorobenzyl analogue of DASB: synthesis, in vitro binding, and in vivo biodistribution studies. Bioconjug Chem 2007;18:1612–8.

243. Mavel S, Vercouillie J, Garreau L, et al. Docking study, synthesis, and in vitro evaluation of fluoro-MADAM derivatives as SERT ligands for PET imaging. Bioorg Med Chem 2008;16:9050–5.

244. Boja J, Kuhar MJ, Kopajtic T, et al. Secondary amine analogues of 3β-(4'-substituted phenyl)tropane-2β-carboxylic acid esters and N-norcocaine exhibit enhanced affinity for serotonin and norepinephrine transporters. J Med Chem 1994;37:1220–3.

245. Blough BE, Abraham P, Lewin AH, et al. Synthesis and transporter binding properties of 3β-(4'-alkyl-, 4'-alkenyl-, and 4'-alkynylphenyl)nortropane-2β-carboxylic acid methyl esters: serotonin transporter selective analogs. J Med Chem 1996;39:4027–35.

246. Blogh BE, Abraham P, Mills AC, et al. 3β-(4-Ethyl-3-iodophenyl)nortropane-2β-carboxylic acid methyl ester as a high-affinity selective ligand for the serotonin transporter. J Med Chem 1997;40:3861–4.

247. Tamagnan G, Baldwin RM, Kula NS, et al. Synthesis and monoamine transporter affinity of 2β-carbomethoxy-3β-(2'-, 3'- or 4'-substituted) biphenyltropanes. Bioorg Med Chem Lett 2000;10:1783–5.

248. Emond P, Helfenbein J, Chalon S, et al. Synthesis of tropane and nortropane analogues with phenyl substitutions as serotonin transporter ligands. Bioorg Med Chem 2001;9:1849–55.

249. Bois F, Baldwin RM, Kula NS, et al. Synthesis and monoamine transporter affinity of 3'-analogs of 2-β-carbomethoxy-3-β-(4'-iodophenyl)tropane (β-CIT). Bioorg Med Chem Lett 2004;14:2117–20.

250. Tamagnan G, Alagille D, Fu X, et al. Synthesis and monoamine transporter affinity of new 2β-carbomethoxy-3β-[4-(substituted thiophenyl)]phenyltropanes: discovery of a selective SERT antagonist with picomolar potency. Bioorg Med Chem Lett 2005;15:1131–3.

251. Tamagnan G, Alagille D, Fu X, et al. Synthesis and monoamine transporter affinity of new 2β-carbomethoxy-3β-[aryl or heteroaryl]phenyltropanes. Bioorg Med Chem Lett 2006;16:217–20.

252. Bergström KA, Halldin C, Hall H, et al. In vitro and in vivo characterisation of Nor-β-CIT: a potential radioligand for visualisation of the serotonin transporter in the brain. Eur J Nucl Med 1997;24:596–601.

253. Helfenbein J, Sandell J, Halldin C, et al. PET examination of three potent cocaine derivatives as specific radioligands for the serotonin transporter. Nucl Med Biol 1999;26:491–9.

254. Stehouwer JS, Plisson C, Jarkas N, et al. Synthesis, radiosynthesis, and biological evaluation of carbon-11 and fluorine-18 (N-fluoroalkyl) labeled 2β-carbomethoxy-3β-(4'-(3-furyl)phenyl)-tropanes and -nortropanes: candidate radioligands for in vivo imaging of the serotonin transporter with positron emission tomography. J Med Chem 2005;48:7080–3.

255. Plisson C, Jarkas N, McConathy J, et al. Evaluation of carbon-11-labeled 2β-carbomethoxy-3β-[4'-((Z)-2-iodoethenyl)phenyl]nortropane as a potential radioligand for imaging the serotonin transporter by PET. J Med Chem 2006;49:942–6.

256. Plisson C, Stehouwer JS, Voll RJ, et al. Synthesis and in vivo evaluation of fluorine-18 and iodine-123 labeled 2β-carbo(2-fluoroethoxy)-3β-(4'-((Z)-2-iodoethenyl)phenyl)nortropane as a candidate serotonin transporter imaging agent. J Med Chem 2007;50:4553–60.

257. Stehouwer JS, Jarkas N, Zeng F, et al. Synthesis, radiosynthesis, and biological evaluation of fluorine-18-labeled 2β-carbo(fluoroalkoxy)-3β-(3'-((Z)-2-haloethenyl)phenyl)nortropanes: candidate radioligands for in vivo imaging of the serotonin transporter with positron emission tomography. J Med Chem 2008;51:7788–99.

258. Pacholczyk T, Blakely RD, Amara SG. Expression cloning of a cocaine- and antidepressant-sensitive human noradrenaline transporter. Nature 1991;350:350–4.

259. Schroeter S, Apparsundaram S, Wiley RG, et al. Immunolocalization of the cocaine- and antidepressant-sensitive 1-norepinephrine transporter. J Comp Neurol 2000;420:211–32.

260. Sara SJ. The locus coeruleus and noradrenergic modulation of cognition. Nat Rev Neurosci 2009;10:211–23.

261. Rommelfanger KS, Weinshenker D. Norepinephrine: the redheaded stepchild of Parkinson's disease. Biochem Pharmacol 2007;74:177–90.

262. Biederman J, Spencer T. Attention-deficit/hyperactivity disorder (ADHD) as a noradrenergic disorder. Biol Psychiatry 1999;46:1234–42.

263. Bymaster FP, Katner JS, Nelson DL, et al. Atomoxetine increases extracellular levels of norepinephrine and dopamine in prefrontal cortex of rat: a potential mechanism for efficacy in attention deficit/hyperactivity disorder. Neuropsychopharmacology 2002;27:699–711.

264. Southwick SM, Bremner DJ, Rasmusson A, et al. Role of norepinephrine in the pathophysiology

and treatment of posttraumatic stress disorder. Biol Psychiatry 1999;46:1192–204.

265. Ressler KJ, Nemeroff CB. Role of norepinephrine in the pathophysiology and treatment of mood disorders. Biol Psychiatry 1999;46:1219–33.

266. Van Moffaert M, Dierick M. Noradrenaline (norepinephrine) and depression: role in aetiology and therapeutic implications. CNS Drugs 1999;12:293–305.

267. Zhu MY, Klimek V, Dilley GE, et al. Elevated levels of tyrosine hydroxylase in the locus coeruleus in major depression. Biol Psychiatry 1999;46:1275–86.

268. Ahern TH, Javors MA, Eagles DA, et al. The effects of chronic norepinephrine transporter inactivation on seizure susceptibility in mice. Neuropsychopharmacology 2006;31:730–8.

269. Klimek V, Stockmeier C, Overholser J, et al. Reduced levels of norepinephrine transporters in the locus coeruleus in major depression. J Neurosci 1997;17:8451–8.

270. Logan J, Ding YS, Lin KS, et al. Modeling and analysis of PET studies with norepinephrine transporter ligands: the search for a reference region. Nucl Med Biol 2005;32:531–42.

271. Ding YS, Lin KS, Logan J. PET imaging of norepinephrine transporters. Curr Pharm Des 2006;12:3831–45.

272. Schou M, Pike VW, Halldin C. Development of radioligands for imaging of brain norepinephrine transporters in vivo with positron emission tomography. Curr Top Med Chem 2007;7:1806–16.

273. Patient selection and antidepressant therapy with reboxetine, a new selective norepinephrine reuptake inhibitor. J Clin Psychiatry 1998;59(Suppl 14).

274. Brenner E, Baldwin RM, Tamagnan G. Asymmetric synthesis of (+)-(S, S)-reboxetine via a new (S)-2-(hydroxymethyl)morpholine preparation. Org Lett 2005;7:937–9.

275. Ding YS, Lin KS, Garza V, et al. Evaluation of a new norepinephrine transporter PET ligand in baboons, both in brain and peripheral organs. Synapse 2003;50:345–52.

276. Wilson AA, Johnson DP, Mozley D, et al. Synthesis and in vivo evaluation of novel radiotracers for the in vivo imaging of the norepinephrine transporter. Nucl Med Biol 2003;30:85–92.

277. Schou M, Halldin C, Sóvágó J, et al. Specific in vivo binding to the norepinephrine transporter demonstrated with the PET radioligand, (S, S)- [11C]MeNER. Nucl Med Biol 2003;30:707–14.

278. Schou M, Halldin C, Sóvágó J, et al. PET evaluation of novel radiofluorinated reboxetine analogs as norepinephrine transporter probes in the monkey brain. Synapse 2004;53:57–67.

279. Schou M, Halldin C, Pike VW, et al. Post-mortem human brain autoradiography of the norepinephrine transporter using (S, S)- [^{18}F]FMeNER-D$_2$. Eur Neuropsychopharmacol 2005;15:517–20.

280. Seneca N, Andree B, Sjöholm N, et al. Whole-body biodistribution, radiation dosimetry estimates for the PET norepinephrine transporter probe (S, S)-[^{18}F]FMeNER-D$_2$ in non-human primates. Nucl Med Commun 2005;26:695–700.

281. Takano A, Halldin C, Varrone A, et al. Biodistribution and radiation dosimetry of the norepinephrine transporter radioligand (S, S)- [^{18}F]FMeNER-D$_2$: a human whole-body PET study. Eur J Nucl Med Mol Imaging 2008;35:630–6.

282. Seneca N, Gulyás B, Varrone A, et al. Atomoxetine occupies the norepinephrine transporter in a dose-dependent fashion: a PET study in nonhuman primate brain using (S, S)- [18F]FMeNER-D2. Psychopharmacology 2006;188:119–27.

283. Takano A, Gulyás B, Varrone A, et al. Imaging the norepinephrine transporter with positron emission tomography: initial human studies with (S, S)-[^{18}F]FMeNER-D$_2$. Eur J Nucl Med Mol Imaging 2008;35:153–7.

284. Lin KS, Ding YS, Kim SW, et al. Synthesis, enantiomeric resolution, F-18 labeling and biodistribution of reboxetine analogs: promising radioligands for imaging the norepinephrine transporter with positron emission tomography. Nucl Med Biol 2005;32:415–22.

285. Ding YS, Lin KS, Logan J, et al. Comparative evaluation of positron emission tomography radiotracers for imaging the norepinephrine transporter: (S, S) and (R, R) enantiomers of reboxetine analogs ([11C]methylreboxetine, 3-Cl-[11C]methylreboxetine and [18F]fluororeboxetine), (R)- [11C]nisoxetine, [11C]oxaprotiline and [11C]lortalamine. J Neurochem 2005;94:337–51.

286. Zeng F, Jarkas N, Stehouwer JS, et al. Synthesis, in vitro characterization, and radiolabeling of reboxetine analogs as potential PET radioligands for imaging the norepinephrine transporter. Bioorg Med Chem 2008;16:783–93.

287. Zeng F, Mun J, Jarkas N, et al. Synthesis, radiosynthesis, and biological evaluation of carbon-11 and fluorine-18 labeled reboxetine analogues: potential positron emission tomography radioligands for in vivo imaging of the norepinephrine transporter. J Med Chem 2009;52:62–73.

288. Hara K, Yanagihara N, Minami K, et al. Ketamine interacts with the noradrenaline transporter at a site partly overlapping the desipramine binding site. Naunyn Schmiedebergs Arch Pharmacol 1998;358:328–33.

289. Blough BE, Holmquist CR, Abraham P, et al. 3α-(4-Substituted phenyl)nortropane-2β-carboxylic acid methyl esters show selective binding at the norepinephrine transporter. Bioorg Med Chem Lett 2000;10:2445–7.

290. Hoepping A, Johnson KM, George C, et al. Novel conformationally constrained tropane analogues by 6-endo-trig radical cyclization and stille coupling: switch

of activity toward the serotonin and/or norepinephrine transporter. J Med Chem 2000;43:2064–71.

291. Tamiz AP, Smith MP, Kozikowski AP. Design, synthesis and biological evaluation of 7-azatricyclodecanes: analogues of cocaine. Bioorg Med Chem Lett 2000;10:297–300.

292. Zhou J, Zhang A, Kläss T, et al. Biaryl analogues of conformationally constrained tricyclic tropanes as potent and selective norepinephrine reuptake inhibitors: synthesis and evaluation of their uptake inhibition at monoamine transporter sites. J Med Chem 2003;46:1997–2007.

293. Carroll FI, Tyagi S, Blough BE, et al. Synthesis and monoamine transporter binding properties of 3α-(substituted phenyl)nortropane-2β-carboxylic acid methyl esters: norepinephrine transporter selective compounds. J Med Chem 2005;48:3852–7.

294. Zhou J, Kläß T, Johnson KM, et al. Discovery of novel conformationally constrained tropane-based biaryl and arylacetylene ligands as potent and selective norepinephrine transporter inhibitors and potential antidepressants. Bioorg Med Chem Lett 2005;15:2461–5.

295. Zeng F, Jarkas N, Owens MJ, et al. Synthesis and monoamine transporter affinity of front bridged tricyclic 3β-(4'-halo or 4'-methyl)phenyltropanes bearing methylene or carbomethoxymethylene on the bridge to the 2β-position. Bioorg Med Chem Lett 2006;16:4661–3.

296. Eildal JNN, Andersen J, Kristensen AS, et al. From the selective serotonin transporter inhibitor citalopram to the selective norepinephrine transporter inhibitor talopram: synthesis and structure-activity relationship studies. J Med Chem 2008;51:3045–8.

297. McConathy J, Owens MJ, Kilts CD, et al. Synthesis and biological evaluation of [¹¹C]talopram and [¹¹C]talsupram: candidate PET ligands for the norepinephrine transporter. Nucl Med Biol 2004; 31:705–18.

Index

Note: Page numbers of article titles are in **boldface** type.

A

[^{18}F]A-84,543 analogs, for nicotinic acetylcholine receptors, 93
[^{11}C]-Acetate
　for myocardial carbohydrate metabolism, 77
　for myocardial oxygen consumption, 73
　for myocardial perfusion, 70
Acetylcholine receptors, nicotinic, radioligands for, **89–100**
Alzheimer's disease, nicotinic acetylcholine receptors in, 92
[^{13}N]-Ammonia, for myocardial perfusion, 70, 72–73
Angiogenesis, **17–38**
　biology of, 18
　functional imaging of, 19–20
　PET imaging of, 20–30
　　fibronectin, 29
　　functional, 21
　　integrins, 21–25
　　matrix metalloproteinases, 28–29
　　sensitivity and specificity of, 20
　　vascular endothelial growth factors and receptors, 25–28
　　versus CT, 20
　　versus MR imaging, 19–20
　　versus SPECT, 20
　structural imaging of, 18–19
　therapies based on, 17–18
Angiopoietins, 29–30
Arginine-Glycine-Aspartic acid (RGD)-containing components, for angiogenesis, 22–25
Atherosclerosis
　inflammation evaluation in, 79–80
　matrix metalloproteinases in, 29
Attention-deficit–hyperactivity disorder, monoamine transporters in. *See* Monoamine transporters.
Autonomic nervous system, cardiac, radiotracers for, 80–82
[^{18}F]AZAN (2-(6-[^{18}F]Fluoro-2,3′-bipypridin-5′-yl)-7-methyl-7-aza-bicyclo[2.2.1]heptane), for nicotinic acetylcholine receptors, 96–97

B

[^{64}Cu]BAT compounds, for neuroendocrine tumors, 54
Benzamide analogs, conformationally flexible, for proliferative status measurement, 9–11
Bevacizumab, for angiogenesis, 25–26
Bitistatin-DOTA conjugate, copper-labeled, for neuroendocrine tumors, 55–56

[^{18}F]-BMS747158-02 (pyridaben analog), for myocardial perfusion, 70–71
Brain, nicotinic acetylcholine receptor radioligands for, **89–100**
BrdU (5-bromodeoxyuridine), for proliferative status measurement, 2–4
5-Bromodeoxyuridine (BrdU), for proliferative status measurement, 2–4
[^{18}F]Bromo-2′-fluoro-2′-deoxyuridine (FBAU), for proliferative status measurement, 4

C

Carbohydrate metabolism, myocardial, radiotracers for, 74–76
[^{11}C]-Carbon monoxide, for angiogenesis, 21
[^{15}O]-Carbon monoxide, for angiogenesis, 21
Cardiomyopathy
　innervation evaluation in, 81
　nonischemic dilated, metabolism assessment in, 77–78
Cardiovascular system, radiotracers for, **69–87**
　list of, 69–70
　of innervation, 80–82
　of metabolism, 73–80
　of myocardial perfusion, 69–73
CB-TE2A (somatostatin analog), for neuroendocrine tumors, 54
CD276, in angiogenesis, 29–30
Cerebral nicotinic acetylcholine receptor radioligands, **89–100**
Cetuximab, copper-labeled, 56–57
[^{11}C]-C-GB67 (prazoxin derivative), for cardiac innervation evaluation, 81
[^{11}C]-CGP12177, for cardiac innervation evaluation, 80–01
[^{11}C]-CGP12388, for cardiac innervation evaluation, 81
CGS 25,966 (fluorinated matrix metalloproteinase inhibitor), for angiogenesis, 29
CGS 27,023A (fluorinated matrix metalloproteinase inhibitor), for angiogenesis, 29
(S,E)-2-Chloro-5-((1-[11C]methylpyrrolidin-2-yl)methoxy)-3-(2-(pyridin-4-yl)vinyl)pyridine ([11C]Me-PVC), for nicotinic acetycholine receptors, 90, 93
Cigarette smoking, nicotinic acetylcholine receptor occupancy in, 92
Cocaine, dopamine transporter binding to, 103
Colorectal cancer, copper radiopharmaceuticals for, 56

PET Clin 4 (2009) 129–133
doi:10.1016/S1556-8598(09)00098-4
1556-8598/09/$ – see front matter © 2009 Elsevier Inc. All rights reserved.

Moving?

Make sure your subscription moves with you!

To notify us of your new address, find your **Clinics Account Number** (located on your mailing label above your name), and contact customer service at:

Email: journalscustomerservice-usa@elsevier.com

800-654-2452 (subscribers in the U.S. & Canada)
314-447-8871 (subscribers outside of the U.S. & Canada)

Fax number: 314-447-8029

Elsevier Health Sciences Division
Subscription Customer Service
3251 Riverport Lane
Maryland Heights, MO 63043

*To ensure uninterrupted delivery of your subscription, please notify us at least 4 weeks in advance of move.

Printed and bound by CPI Group (UK) Ltd, Croydon, CR0 4YY

03/10/2024

01040362-0001